T0396685

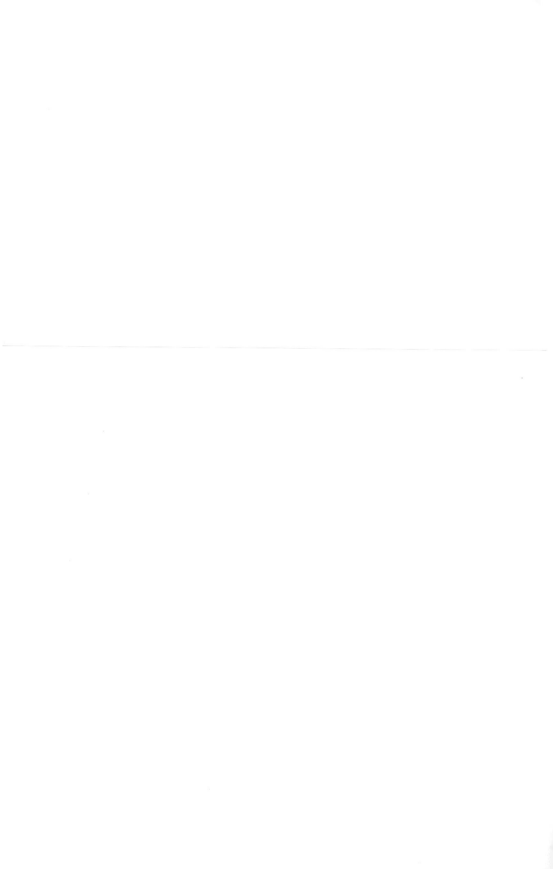

Liposomes in Analytical Methodologies

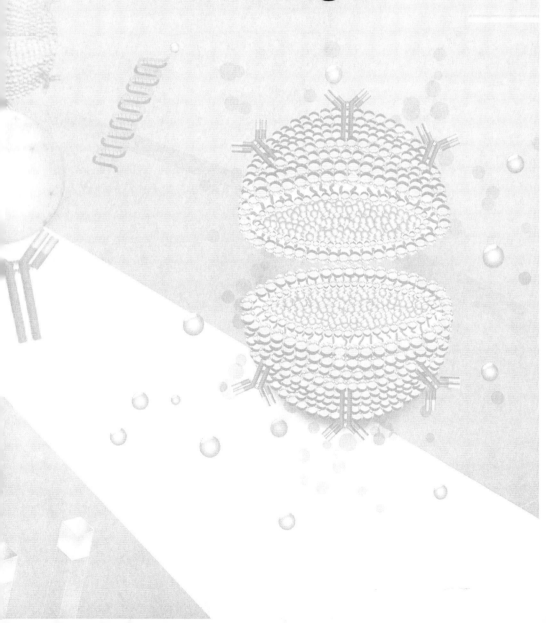

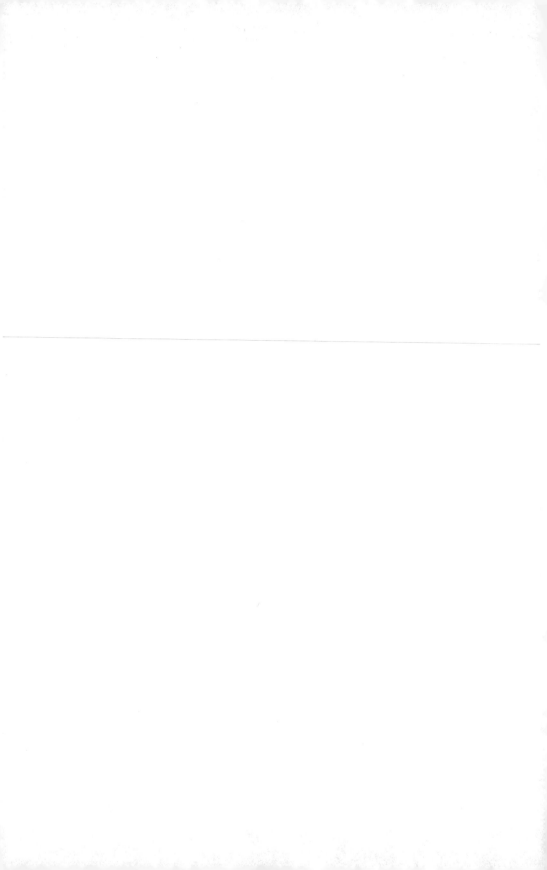

Liposomes
in Analytical
Methodologies

edited by
Katie A. Edwards

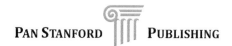

PAN STANFORD PUBLISHING

Published by

Pan Stanford Publishing Pte. Ltd.
Penthouse Level, Suntec Tower 3
8 Temasek Boulevard
Singapore 038988

Email: editorial@panstanford.com
Web: www.panstanford.com

British Library Cataloguing-in-Publication Data
A catalogue record for this book is available from the British Library.

Liposomes in Analytical Methodologies

Copyright © 2016 Pan Stanford Publishing Pte. Ltd.

ISBN 978-981-4669-26-9 (Hardcover)
ISBN 978-981-4669-27-6 (eBook)

Printed in the USA

Contents

Preface

Liposomes have widely been investigated and employed in the drug delivery realm to afford protection of sensitive encapsulants, prolonged release, and targeting to selected tissues. While this is by far the most notable area, liposomes are also widely used in cosmetic formulations, food processing, and as models of cell membranes. These well-researched areas have been covered in numerous scientific publications and texts. However, liposomes have been investigated since the 1970s for diagnostic applications and as a unique modification to traditional analytical techniques. The aim of this book is to bring together the works of researchers working in the area of analytical method development using liposomes. The text is intended to both garner interest to those new to the field as well as provide detail to researchers seeking to expand their analytical repertoire. Topics covered include liposome usage in biosensors, pharmacological studies, PCR, array-based platforms, capillary electrophoresis, and imaging. Chapter 1 provides an introduction to liposome-based analyses and the work covered throughout the book, while the remaining chapters provide focused discussion in their respective areas. While many of the key areas of research are covered in depth, it is of course not possible to capture all of the historical and modern developments in the field in this level of detail. It is hoped that the extensive reference lists provided within will facilitate further inquiry.

I am grateful for the immersion into liposome research many years ago in the laboratory of Dr. Richard Durst and the opportunities provided by Dr. Antje Baeumner. Thank you both for the inspiration and friendship over the years. This book would not have been possible without the authors to this book and their thorough contributions. I am also indebted to Pan Stanford Publishing, namely Sarabjeet Garcha, Arvind Kanswal, and Stanford Chong. Thank you for your patience and interest in this project.

Katie Edwards

Chapter 1

Analytical Utility of Liposomes: From Past to Present

Katie A. Edwards

Department of Biological and Environmental Engineering,
Cornell University, 140 Riley-Robb Hall, Ithaca, New York 14853, USA

kae24@cornell.edu

The formation of closed structures by aqueous suspensions of phospholipids and impermeability of the resulting structures to encapsulated ions was first reported by Bangham, Standish, and Watkins in 1965.[1] Later termed liposomes in 1968,[2] the formation of these synthetic structures that comprise lipid bilayers encompassing aqueous spaces was a significant finding that paved the way for numerous applications, including their usage as model cell membranes, drug-delivery agents, and components of cosmetic formulations. The importance of these applications has been well reviewed in many sources[3,4] and hence will be touched on briefly within this text. The focus of this book is instead on a well-researched but perhaps less well-publicized area of liposome research, which is that of the utility of liposomes as analytical tools. As will be described within, soon after their discovery, liposomes began to find their place in analytical chemistry and biochemistry beginning in the 1970s.[5] Many of the properties

Liposomes in Analytical Methodologies
Edited by Katie A. Edwards
Copyright © 2016 Pan Stanford Publishing Pte. Ltd.
ISBN 978-981-4669-26-9 (Hardcover), 978-981-4669-27-6 (eBook)
www.panstanford.com

that made them well suited for the above applications, such as the internal space to encapsulate a large payload of hydrophilic molecules and its inherent protection from exterior stresses, could be exploited in unique analytical methodologies, offering advantages over existing technologies and approaches not possible with other systems. For example, the amphiphilic nature of the bilayer could be used to incorporate hydrophobic biorecognition elements such as membrane receptors, which would be otherwise challenging, if not impossible, to retain activity in aqueous systems. This introductory chapter is intended to provide a primer for readers entering the field or a refresher for those with existing background to understand some of the fundamentals and utility of liposomes for analytical purposes. It is by no means an exhaustive review of all publications in their respective fields, but a sampling of some of the more well-researched approaches. The great work of many liposome pioneers in their respective areas is introduced within but is captured in detail in the chapters to follow.

1.1   Introduction to Liposomes

In their most simple form, liposomes are often described as a spherical lipid bilayer surrounding an aqueous core. The lipid bilayer of liposomes is composed of double chain, amphiphilic lipids with their nonpolar, hydrophobic tails aligned with each other and their polar, hydrophilic headgroups oriented toward the exterior aqueous solution or directed toward the inner aqueous core (Fig. 1.1).

Planar lipid bilayers are formed with a similar architecture, though form linear structures, and are often confined to surfaces rather than to discrete solution-phase structures.[6] Liposomes with a single lipid bilayer are termed unilamellar vesicles, and their classification according to size is generally such that small unilamellar vesicles typically have sizes between 20 and 100 nm; those with diameters between 100 nm and 1 µm are generally termed large unilamellar vesicles; and liposomes above 1 µm are termed giant unilamellar vesicles.[7,8] Unilamellar liposomes comprise a single bilayer encapsulating an aqueous core, and multilamellar liposomes comprise multiple concentric bilayers with encapsulation possible both within the core and between adjacent bilayers (Fig. 1.2).

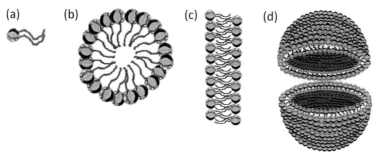

Figure 1.1 (a) Lipid structure with hydrophilic headgroup represented by a grey sphere and hydrophobic tails, (b) micelle formed from single-chain amphiphiles, (c) lipid bilayer, and (d) the liposome structure yielded from lipids forming a bilayer with their hydrophilic headgroups oriented toward the inner cavity and external solution while their hydrophobic tails are oriented away from these aqueous environments.

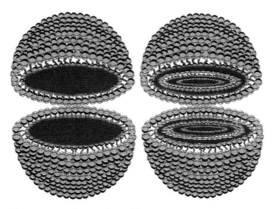

Figure 1.2 Structure of a unilamellar vesicle with encapsulation (blue) within the aqueous core (left) versus a multilamellar vesicle with encapsulation between bilayers (right).

Such liposomes are often termed multilamellar vesicles (MLVs). These bilayered species are in contrast to micelles, which are lipid monolayers formed from single-chain lipids, such as fatty acids and detergents, with their hydrophobic tails directed away from the aqueous environment while their polar headgroups are directed toward it (Fig. 1.1). Lipids having a headgroup and a hydrocarbon area that are similar and cylindrical in shape tend to form bilayer structures, whereas those that are cone shaped due to a larger headgroup than the hydrocarbon tail region tend to assemble into micelles.[9] The double hydrocarbon chains of lipids that form liposomes are typically too bulky for micelle formation, hence such lipids typically do not form micelles.[10] Reverse micelles are effectively the opposite configuration where polar headgroups are oriented inward, while nonpolar tails are directed toward an exterior nonaqueous environment. The structures formed may be predicted by the packing parameter, which takes into account the area of the lipid headgroup and the volume and length of the hydrocarbon tail.[11] All such species form through self-assembly orienting the hydrophobic portions and hydrophilic portions of their amphipathic components in accordance with their lowest energy states. The hydrocarbon tails are held both by van der Waals and hydrophobic forces, while electrostatic and hydrogen bonding interactions take place between the polar headgroups and water on each side of the bilayer.

The liposomal lipid bilayer is typically composed of a mixture of phospholipids, either synthetic or naturally derived, and cholesterol. Phospholipids are amphiphilic molecules consisting of two long fatty acid tails forming a hydrophobic portion, which are linked via esters through glycerol to a phosphate group and hydrophilic headgroup. Derivatives of the zwitterionic phosphatidylcholine (PC) are commonly employed for liposome preparation, and natural PCs are widespread constituents of plant and mammalian tissues. Many liposome preparations, especially in the early years, utilized egg PC, which is a naturally derived mixture of both unsaturated and saturated PCs with predominantly 16–18 carbon tails.[12] The heterogeneity and potential for peroxidation of unsaturated egg PC led researchers to seek more stable, reproducible, and easily characterized alternatives.[13,14] Over the years, synthetic phospholipids have had increased commercial production, offering on-demand availability, consistency, and purity in preparation. The structure of the 16 carbon symmetric 1,2-dipalmitoyl-sn-glycero-3-phosphocholinedipalmitoyl (DPPC) is shown in Fig. 1.3. Other common derivatives include shorter and longer chains, such as lauryl, myristoyl, and stearoyl, with 12 (DLPC), 14 (DMPC), and 18 (DSPC) carbon chains, respectively. The hydrocarbon chains of such lipids intercalate into the hydrophobic portion of the bilayer, while the polar headgroups extend into the aqueous environments on either side of the bilayer.

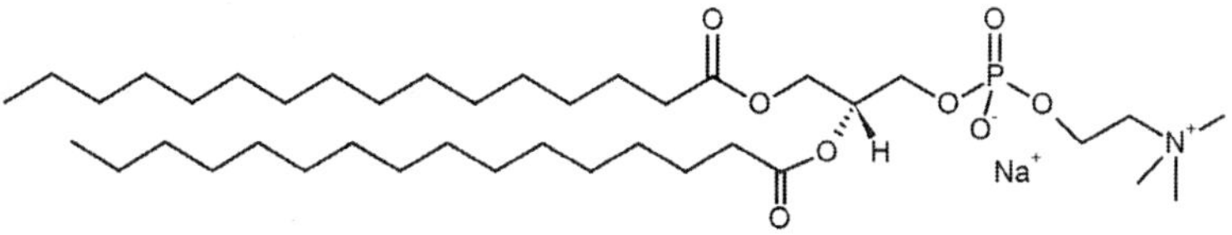

Figure 1.3 Structure of 1,2-dipalmitoyl-*sn*-glycero-3-phosphocholine (DPPC).

Liposomes often incorporate negatively charged phospholipids such as dipalmitoylphosphatidylglycerol (DPPG) or dipalmitoylphosphatidyl-serine (DPPS) or positively charged lipids such as 1,2-dioleoyl-3-trimethylammonium-propane (DOTAP) (Fig. 1.4) to prevent aggregation as well as to confer desired electrostatic properties.[15,16] Such lipids have been suggested to improve the encapsulation efficiency of multilamellar vesicles due to increased electrostatic repulsion between the bilayers.[17]

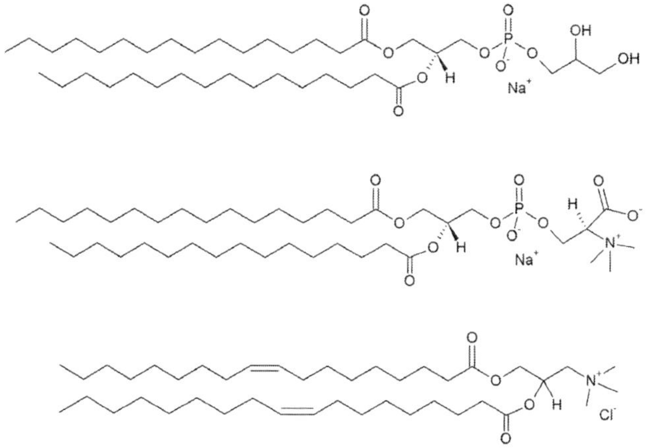

Figure 1.4 Structure of 1,2-dipalmitoyl-*sn*-glycero-3-phospho-(1′-rac-glycerol) (DPPG) (top), 1,2-dipalmitoyl-*sn*-glycero-3-phospho-L-serine (DPPS) (middle), sodium salts, and 1,2-dioleoyl-3-trimethylammonium-propane, chloride salt (DOTAP) (bottom).

Cholesterol, the structure of which is shown in Fig. 1.5, in a simple sense, imparts reduced permeability to charged and water-soluble molecules by effectively filling in gaps or defects in the lipid bilayer. The steroid moiety of cholesterol is believed to lie parallel to the hydrophobic tails of the phospholipids within the bilayer, while its 3β-hydroxyl function is directed toward the aqueous medium on both sides of the bilayer.[18] The hydroxyl function does impart a degree of amphipathy on the otherwise hydrophobic molecule; however, it does not extend into the polar headgroup region of the bilayer[18] and instead is believed to lie in close proximity to the ester carbonyl of the phospholipids.[19] The hydroxyl groups of cholesterol have also been used to allow for covalent modifications of preformed liposomes,[20] while the hydrophobic structure allows for the direct incorporation of cholesterol-modified molecules during liposome preparation. Examples of the latter include preparation of DNA reporter probe or aptamer-modified liposomes through the incorporation of cholesteryl-modified DNA sequences during liposome prepara-tion.[21,22]

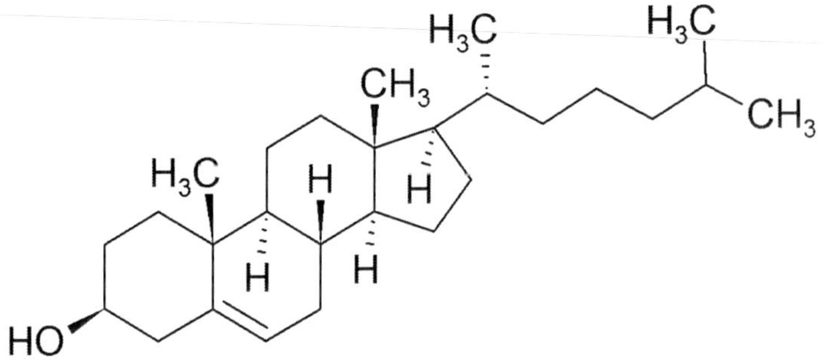

Figure 1.5   Structure of cholesterol.

The hydrophobic nature of the bilayer allows for the availability and presentation of molecules otherwise challenging for aqueous environments, such as cholesterol. For example, one of the difficulties in early assays for cholesterol 7 alpha-hydrolase (cytochrome P450 7A1) activity, an enzyme responsible for the breakdown of cholesterol in vivo and whose deficiency has been linked to gallstone formation, was the poor aqueous solubility of its cholesterol substrate. Assays attempted to overcome this through solubilization of the substrate in surfactants; however, this had deleterious effects on enzyme activity.[23,24] Instead, utilizing liposome-embedded cholesterol as a substrate, an enzymatic assay was successfully developed without the loss of enzyme activity concomitant with surfactant-based substrate solubilization.[24] A similar strategy to assess phospholipase activity was developed commercially as a fluorescence assay using a lipophilic substrate embedded in DOPC/DOPG liposomes (EnzChek® Phospholipase A2 Assay Kit, Life Technologies).[25]

Lipids have a characteristic transition temperature (T_c), which represents the temperature at which they transform from a solid, or "gel" phase, to a liquid or fluid phase. The temperature at which this transition occurs is dependent on the lipid chain length, degree of unsaturation, presence of chain side groups, as well as the structure of the hydrophilic headgroup. An increase of 14–17°C results for every two methylene units in saturated hydrocarbon chains. For example, the T_c values of DMPC, DPPC, and DSPC are 23, 41, and 55°C, respectively.[26,27] Substituting the phosphatidylcholine headgroup in DPPC for a phosphatidylethanol-amine group in DPPE results in an increase in the T_c to 60°C, whereas substitution for phosphatidyl glycerol in DPPG yields no change from 41°C.[28] By contrast, this transition temperature decreases with the degree of unsaturation or side groups in the hydrocarbon chain.[27] Collectively, hydration of lipid mixtures above the transition temperature of the composite lipids is necessary to afford a fluid state, which greatly facilitates manipulations required during preparation. Numerous methods for liposome preparation exist, including most commonly reverse phase evaporation, freeze-thaw, dehydration/rehydration, thin-film hydration, sonication, and detergent dialysis. The choice of method depends on the desired properties of the liposomes and the nature of the material to be encapsulated. Excellent reviews of preparation methodologies are available in several review articles.[9,27,29-31]

Lipids with specific functional groups are commonly employed to impart the ability to covalently link the lipid bilayer to biorecognition elements such as antibodies or DNA probes or to surfaces for the purpose of immobilization. For example, 1,2-dipalmitoyl-*sn*-glycero-3-phosphoethanolamine (DPPE), 1,2-dipalmitoyl-*sn*-glycero-3-phospho-ethanolamine-*N*-(glutaryl), and 1,2-dipalmitoyl-*sn*-glycero-3-phospho-thioethanol impart amine, carboxylic acid, and sulfydryl functionalities as lipid headgroups, respectively (Fig. 1.6). Among many crosslinking options, such functional groups may be linked to sulfhydryls using sulfosuccinimidyl-4-(*N*-malei midomethyl)cyclohexane-1-carboxylate (sulfo-SMCC),[32] amines using 1-ethyl-3-(3-dimethylaminopropyl) carbodiimide (EDC),[33] and maleimide-derivatized biomolecules or support surfaces, respectively.[34] Conjugation to polyethylene glycol (PEG)-based lipids with functional groups at the distal ends of the PEG chains has been shown to improve accessibility and recognition of relatively bulky liposome structures.[35] An excellent overview of covalent modifications of liposomes is provided in Chapter 2 by Dr. Hsiao-Wei Wen and colleagues.

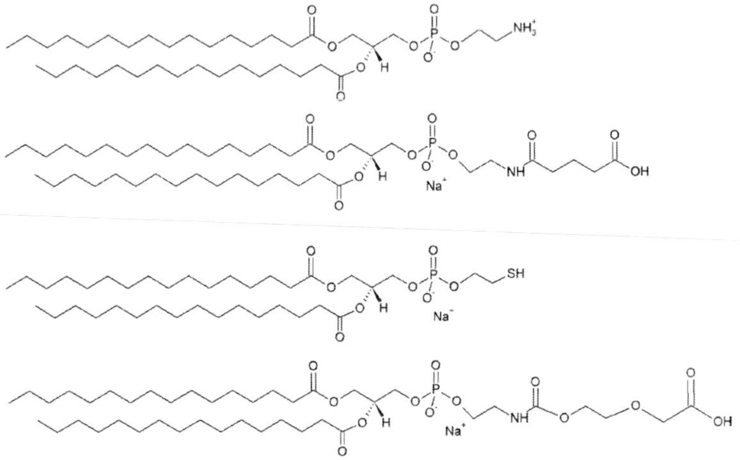

Figure 1.6 Structure of 1,2-dipalmitoyl-*sn*-glycero-3-phosphoethano-lamine (DPPE) (top), 1,2-dipalmitoyl-*sn*-glycero-3-phosphoethanolamine-*N*-(glutaryl) (second), 1,2-dipalmitoyl-*sn*-glycero-3-phosphothioethanol sodium salts (third), and 1,2-distearoyl-*sn*-glycero-3-phosphoethanolamine-*N*-[carboxy (polyethylene glycol)-2000] (ammonium salt) (*n* = 45, DSPE-PEG(2000) carboxylic acid) (bottom).

Covalent modification to bilayer lipids may be carried out after the liposomes have formed in aqueous solution. Water-soluble crosslinking reagents allow biologically relevant molecules to be linked to the liposome surface without unduly harsh conditions. The approach for coupling depends on the availability of useable functional groups on the biorecognition element as well as maintaining binding properties after conjugation. Appropriate coupling conditions must be chosen to minimize the impact of conjugation on the viability of intact liposomes. Conditions employed during coupling can yield to loss of bilayer integrity and loss of encapsulated materials, aggregation of liposomes, and covalent crosslinking of vesicles if the stoichiometry of reagents is not carefully maintained. Alternatively, covalent modification of desired molecules may be made initially with lipids to allow for their incorporation within the lipid bilayer when added during liposome preparation. This approach is well suited for small molecules that can tolerate the organic solvents required to solubilize the lipids.[36,37] The lipid tails of such conjugates partition within the bilayer, while the covalently linked small molecule remains at the headgroup surface, with distance from the bilayer depending on the inclusion and length of hydrophilic spacers. Additionally, one must also consider whether the conjugate, especially in the case of sensitive biomolecules such as enzymes or antibodies, can tolerate the conditions for liposome preparation if added prior to liposome formation. These conditions can include organic solvents, sonication, detergents, and elevated temperatures.

Not limited to synthetic small-molecule conjugates, naturally occurring molecules that possess hydrophobic moieties may be incorporated during preparation to afford recognition sites.[38] For example, gangliosides are glycosphingolipids that are predominantly found in brain and neuronal cell membranes and, among other functions, serve as receptors for viruses and bacterial toxins. These molecules are composed of a carbohydrate-linked lipid with the sialic acid portion extending into the aqueous environment and their hydrophobic tails partitioning within the lipid tails of the bilayer upon liposome incorporation (Fig. 1.7).

GM1

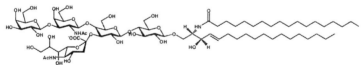

Figure 1.7   Structure of GM1 ganglioside.[39] Reprinted from Ref. [39], Copyright 2012, with permission from Elsevier. http://dx.doi. org/10.1016/j.bbamem.2012.07.010.

Aside from cholesterol, zwitterionic, charged, and functional group modified lipids, specialized lipids may be included in the preparations to confer desired properties. Liposomes may be prepared with diacetylenic lipids, which may subsequently be polymerized using UV light.[40,41] Such compositions yield colored liposomes that are both environmentally responsive in terms of their spectra and more resistant to leakage of contents following stresses such as solvents or surfactants.[42] Other options include pH-sensitive lipids such as *N*-(4-carboxybenzyl)-*N*,*N*-dimethyl-2,3-bis(oleoyloxy)propan-1-aminium (DOBAQ), which exhibits pH-dependent ionization,[43] or lysolipids, such as 1-palmitoyl-2-hydroxy-*sn*-glycero-3-phosphocholine, which are single alkyl chain lipids that enhance the kinetics of liposome permeability and lower their transition temperatures.[44] Other investigators have used unsaturated lipids such as dioleoylphosphatidylethanolamine (DOPE) to impart a degree of instability to their formulation in conjunction with antibody labeling, making their liposomes sensitive to localized changes in bilayer architecture and subsequent disruption upon target binding.[45] The understanding of various lipids and their impact on liposomes structure is a subject worthy of many volumes in and of itself and the reader is referred thorough reviews for more detailed descriptions.[27,46–48]

1.2 Liposomes in Drug Delivery

In the drug-delivery realm, liposomes have offered advantages such as reducing toxicity to peak levels of free drug, prolonged exposure through delayed release or reduced clearance, enhanced chemical stability of encapsulants, and improved accumulation within target tissues and tumors.[49,50] These benefits stem from the unique architecture of both the interior cavity as well as the lipid bilayer. The interior cavity may be used to encapsulate high concentrations of therapeutic formulations, while their exteriors may be conjugated to or incorporated with poorly soluble therapeutic agents or labeled with antibodies or other biorecognition elements to facilitate targeting.[49] The aqueous compartments in the interior cavity of unilamellar liposomes or between the lipid bilayers of multilamellar liposomes provide, relatively speaking, a considerable volume for encapsulation. This space can be used to encapsulate a large payload of hydrophilic therapeutic molecules as well as restrict their degradation and distribution to unintended tissues. The lipid bilayer is of the order of 4 nm thick, leaving a theoretical internal volume of 4×10^{-13} µL per 100 nm unilamellar liposome assuming a spherical structure.

This may not seem to be a considerable volume at first glance, but if encapsulations of small molecules are carried out at high concentrations, the theoretical number of encapsulated molecules approaches 25,000 per liposome even at a modest 100 mM starting concentration. All things being equal, additionally, encapsulation per liposome increases with increasing liposome size. The molecules confined within the liposome can circulate with delayed release and degradation, and when used in conjunction with specific targeting, the amount of a therapeutic that can be delivered per specific binding event can be greatly improved. Active targeting has been accomplished through tissue-specific molecules such as antibodies,[51] glycolipids,[52,53] proteins,[54] aptamers,[55] or small molecules[56,57] immobilized on liposome surfaces to allow for recognition by cell-specific receptors. Such biorecognition entities may be directly tagged with therapeutic molecules; however, the stoichiometry of drug to antibody that is possible while retaining the efficacy of both is relatively small. As an example, an estimated 28,000 molecules of daunomycin, an anti-neoplastic agent, entrapped per 100 nm liposome can yield an antibody to drug ratio of ∼1:1000 versus ∼1:1 for directly conjugated drug molecules.[58-60] Of course, various factors such as steric access, multivalency, and electrostatic repulsion play a role that separates observed performance from this possible ideal; however, the enhanced amount of drug that can be delivered via liposomes remains considerable.

The relatively large size of liposomes not only offers the benefit of a large delivery payload, it is also advantageous from a targeting standpoint. Targeting of liposomes to desired tissues stems from specific biorecognition events and via size discrimination. The comparatively large size of liposomes versus free drug molecules restricts their accumulation in healthy tissues, which have continuous endothelial barriers, but yields accumulation in cancerous tissues due to the increased permeability of tumor endothelia.[61-63] This is known as the enhanced permeability and retention (EPR) effect and has proven to be beneficial for passive targeting of tumor cells by liposomes as well as other macromolecular or nanoparticle species.[64] Similarly, for doxorubicin, a cancer chemotherapeutic with known cardiac toxicity, liposomal formulations are advantageous as they restrict passage of this drug on a size basis from tight capillary junctions in cardiac tissue.[65] Despite the benefits of increased encapsulation and selective targeting, there are, however, limitations imposed on the maximum liposome size as well. The maximum size is hindered due to the rapid clearance of larger particles by the reticuloendothelial system (RES) and thus resulting short circulation times.[66,67] Clearance is dependent on many parameters, including lipid composition and charge, but size remains a significant factor.[61]

Despite these benefits, early investigations into the use of liposomes as drug-delivery vehicles yielded lackluster performance due to poor stability, inefficient encapsulation of drug molecules, and rapid clearance by phagocytosis.[68,69] However, further study into bilayer composition and liposome structure led to more efficient species with greater utility.[68] As a result, in 1995, a PEGylated formulation encapsulating the chemotherapeutic agent doxorubicin (Doxil®) yielded the first liposome-based drug approved for human use.[70] PEG chains on the liposomal exterior provide a hydrophilic steric barrier yielding benefits, including minimizing nonspecific protein adsorption, and effectively increasing circulation time through reducing recognition by the RES system as well as minimizing the impact of lipid formulation on clearance.[71,72] Incorporation of gangliosides has served much the same purpose.[73,74] Liposomes encapsulating chemotherapeutic agents such as doxorubicin, daunorubicin, and cytarabine have been used commercially to treat Kaposi's sarcoma,[75,76] ovarian cancer,[77,78] and neoplastic meningitis.[79] Other liposome-based drugs include encapsulated amphotericin B (Ambisome®) for the treatment of severe fungal and parasitic infections[80,81]; bupivacaine (Exparel®) or morphine (DepoDur®) for pain management[82,83]; and vincristine (Marqibo®) for the treatment of refractory acute lymphoblastic leukemia.[84,85] Aside from intravenous routes, liposomes have been used for dermal, transdermal, inhalational, and occular drug administration,[86–88] with commercial products, including liposome-encapsulated amikacin (Arkiface®), a nebulized antibiotic for the treatment of resistant lung infections, and verteporfin (Visudyne®), an ocular treatment for macular degeneration.[89] The enzyme bacteriophage T4 endonuclease 5 (T4N5) has been shown to be effective in repairing DNA damage resulting from the genetic disease xeroderma pigmentosum, which causes hypersensitivity to UV light. Delivery of this sensitive enzyme through the stratum corneum could be improved via liposomal encapsulation when applied as a topical lotion.[90-94] Advances in targeting via brain-specific molecules such as anti-transferrin receptor antibodies and rabies virus glycoprotein peptides have been made taking advantage of liposomes to allow passage of encapsulated drugs through the blood–brain barrier.[58,60,95-98] Liposomes have also been used as delivery agents for gene therapy with benefits, including relatively minimal adverse effects versus viral delivery methods while still maintaining good gene transfer efficiency.[99-103] The usage of liposomes as adjuvants and carriers in the development of vaccines has been widely investigated, with FDA-approved formulations available against viruses such as hepatitis A (Epaxel®)[104] and influenza (Inflexal®).[105] A variety of other medical applications are currently in advanced clinical trials.[106] Novel advances, including triggered release using pH,[107,108] temperature,[109-111] and magnetic field[112] sensitive liposomes have come under increasing study to improve distribution to target tissues and reduce nonspecific toxicity. Readers are directed to several excellent review articles for further background and recent developments on therapeutics relying on liposomes for delivery and performance.[11,60,101,113,114]

Aside from drug-delivery applications, liposomes have been employed in many other areas, including animal care, cosmetics, and food science.[115-118] For example, they have been investigated to enhance cryopreservation of spermatozoa,[119-121] and those encapsulating follicle-stimulating hormone have been used to facilitate embryo transfer in cattle.[122] Similar to their use as topical drug-delivery agents, liposomes are widely used in cosmetics, facilitating transport of both hydrophilic and hydrophobic molecules such as vitamins and moisture-restoring lipids to the stratum corneum.[69,123] They are also utilized in the food industry, offering improved flavor and nutrient delivery as well as enhanced antimicrobial activity[116] and stability of light- or oxygen-sensitive components.[124] For example, liposomes encapsulating enzymes or substrates have been used to accelerate the cheese-ripening process[125] and those encapsulating antioxidants have shown enhanced bioavailability.[126]

1.3   Liposomes in Analytical Applications

Beyond the more widely known utility of liposomes for drug delivery, liposomes have also been employed for analytical purposes spanning over several decades for many diverse applications. Their utility in an analytical sense stems from many of the same features that are advantageous for drug delivery (Fig. 1.8). As opposed to utilizing bilayer-tagged recognition molecules to allow targeting toward selected tissues, this recognition capacity using, for example, antibodies, DNA probes, and aptamers, instead can be directed toward binding analytes of interest.[22,127,128] Rather than a therapeutic payload, the large internal volume of liposomes instead allows for encapsulation of high concentrations of measurable species such as visible dyes, fluorescent dyes, electrochemical markers, chemluminescent markers, and electrogenerated chemiluminescent species.[127,129-132] Instead of protecting sensitive therapeutics from degradation and prolonging in vivo circulation time, the cloistered internal space may be used to enhance the stability of sensitive biomolecules such as DNA or enzymes

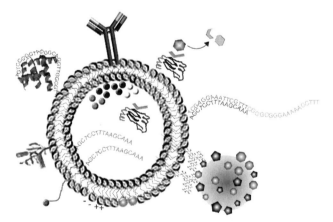

Figure 1.8   Features of liposomes for analytical applications: The bilayer may be tagged with biorecognition elements such as antibodies, enzymes, DNA probes, gangliosides, small molecules, and periplasmic binding proteins or lipophilic signaling species; interactions may occur with charged headgroups or with lipid tails; the interior may encapsulate hydrophilic molecules capable of providing signaling or for further amplification; the liposomes themselves afford applications based on mass or refractive index changes.

used for signal amplification as well as serve as selective microreactors.[133,134] In lieu of utilizing the amphiphilic nature and charge of the lipid bilayer to promote drug incorporation, unique modes of separation have resulted when liposomes are employed as a pseudo-stationary phase in chromatographic and electrophoretic separations.[135-137] Rather than relying on the lipid bilayer to facilitate passive delivery across cell membranes, it may be used to further understanding and characterization of drug interactions. Instead of relying on the relatively large size to afford passive targeting, "passive" signaling using properties inherent to the liposomes themselves, such as relatively large refractive indices and mass, allows them to be employed in surface plasmon resonance (SPR) and piezoelectric-based detection schemes.[138-140] The following text will introduce readers to some of these applications, but making no claim to be comprehensive, readers are also encouraged to seek review articles spanning several decades.[8,141-146]

1.3.1 Intact Liposomes in Signal Transduction

Liposomes employed for signaling purposes may be utilized both as intact and lysed species. Among the earliest examples of the analytical utility of intact liposomes are agglutination assays, which are traditionally carried out with antibody- or antigen-conjugated latex beads. If present, the multivalent target analyte or antibody, respectively, can be bound to multiple beads causing them to form clumps, which can be visualized. This assay format, originally described in 1956 for the assay of rheumatoid factor,[147] has since been expanded to numerous other analytes of clinical interest. In 1980, the principle behind this format was extended to liposome agglutination. These early investigations focused on determining antibody specificity by monitoring increases in turbidity as a function of binding to liposomal lipid bilayer-incorporated glycosphingolipids and subsequent agglutination.[148] Here, liposomes prepared with asialo GM2 gangliosides were incubated in the presence of anti-asialo GM2 antibodies. An increase in the turbidity of the sample, monitored at 340 nm, was observed with GM2 liposomes but not with control liposomes devoid of GM2. The extent was dependent on the type of antibodies (IgG or IgM) as well as the GM2 coverage on the liposomes. This approach was subsequently applied to the study of lectin binding by sugar-modified liposomes[149]; polysaccharides by lectin-conjugated liposomes[150]; and assay of C-reactive protein and tuberculosis antigens via liposomes conjugated to anti-CRP antibodies[151] and anti-glycolipid antibodies,[152] respectively, among others. Assay formats have extended beyond monitoring turbidity differences to piezoelectric sensors[153] and point-of-care card formats relying on visible detection.[152,154] The principle behind the liposome agglutination assay format is shown in Fig. 1.9a. Figure 1.9b illustrates the use of blue-dye-encapsulating liposomes with bilayer containing cardiolipin, which agglutinate in the presence of syphilis antibodies.[155]

(a)

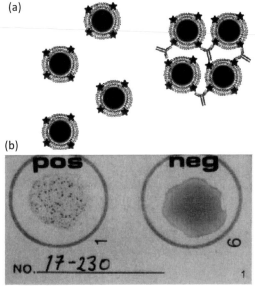

(b)

Figure 1.9 (a) Liposome agglutination assay principle: (left) no agglutination in the absence of sample antibodies; (right) liposomes form networks with multivalent antibodies. (b) Liposomes composed of cardiolipin, lecithin, and cholesterol encapsulating the blue dye erioglaucine in the presence of human sera positive and negative for syphilis. Agglutination, evidenced by visible complex formation, in the positive sample was due to interactions between anti-syphilis antibodies and liposomal cardiolipin.[155] Reprinted from Ref. [155], Copyright 1986, with permission from Elsevier. http://www.sciencedirect.com/science/article/pii/002217598690075X.

In agglutination assays, liposomes with bilayer-embedded or encapsulating dye may be used to generate a visible signal upon interaction with multivalent antibodies or antigens.[152,155] In the mid-1980s, sulforhodamine B-encapsulating liposomes, patented for use in various analytical applications by Becton Dickinson and Company, were instead employed to provide signal enhancement in solid-phase immunoassays.[156,157] Such technology was introduced commercially in the form of the BD Qtest®, a flow-through immunoassay with visible readout for Group A *Streptococcus* and the ColorPAC™ lateral-flow sandwich immunoassay for *Clostridium difficile* toxin A.[158,159–162] Both assays utilized antibody-conjugated dye-encapsulating liposomes to yield a highly visible magenta symbol or line in the presence of their respective antigens upon binding in spatially defined regions. Such visible-dye-encapsulating liposomes were employed in lieu of industry standard colloidal gold and dyed latex beads to yield visible lines or patterns similar to those observed in home-pregnancy tests.[163] Numerous other qualitative and semi-quantitative lateral-flow and similar assay applications for analytes of national security, environmental monitoring, point-of-care, and food safety interests using liposomes subsequently emerged.[164–168]

One common format is the sandwich lateral-flow immunoassay where an antibody against the analyte of interest is immobilized in a line on a nitrocellulose membrane (Fig. 1.10). In the presence of the analyte, a sandwich complex forms between the immobilized capture antibody, the analyte in the sample, and a second detection antibody directed to a different epitope on the analyte. The latter is conjugated to a detectable species, which results in a visible line in the presence of the analyte. In the absence of analyte, no sandwich complex forms, and thus no signal results. The sandwich assay format requires that the analyte has either different epitopes or multiple copies of the same epitope in order for two biorecognition elements, such as antibodies or DNA probes, to bind. This, by necessity, requires that the analyte is a relatively large molecule.

For small-molecule analytes, competitive assay formats, which require only one biorecognition element, are more appropriate. In such formats, for example, a fixed concentration of labeled antigen and antigen potentially present in the sample compete for a limited amount of antibody. In the absence of analyte, the maximum amount of labeled antigen can bind to the antibody, whereas less labeled antigen can bind as the analyte concentration decreases. Hence, the signal proportionally decreases with increasing analyte concentration. This indirect relationship can be somewhat counterintuitive for interpretation by the end user. In 1995, Roberts and Durst devised a method to yield a proportional signal for small-molecule analytes by engineering size discrimination into traditional lateral-flow technology while utilizing liposome agglutination.[166] In the liposome immunoaggregation (LIA) assay, antigen-tagged visible-dye-encapsulating liposomes formed a network of complexes in the presence of their respective antibodies. This prevented their migration via capillary action up a limited porosity nitrocellulose membrane (Fig. 1.11a). The degree of aggregation was reduced when antigens were also present in the sample, as they would compete with liposomes for antibody binding. Liposomes that were not involved in the complexes could migrate and be captured at a zone specific to an additional tag on the liposomes (Fig. 1.11b).[166]

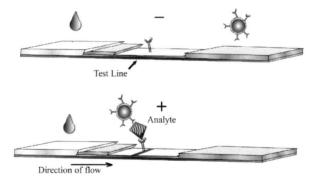

Figure 1.10 Example use of intact liposomes to provide signaling capabilities. Liposomes encapsulating high concentrations of visible dyes may be used to provide an optical signal. As an example, a sandwich lateral-flow assay, similar to a home-pregnancy test, yields a yes/no or semi-quantitative result proportional to analyte concentration. Shown here, liposomes encapsulating the magenta dye sulforhodamine B and tagged with a monoclonal antibody bind to one epitope on the analyte, which is captured by another monoclonal antibody immobilized on the membrane, which is directed toward a different epitope. In the absence of analyte, no signal results in the location of the immobilized antibody. In the presence of analyte, a sandwich complex forms yielding a visible result.

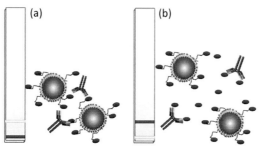

Figure 1.11   Liposome immunoaggregation assay.[166] (a) In the absence of analyte, analyte-conjugated liposomes form large complexes with antibody, which are unable to migrate up the lateral-flow assay membrane. (b) In the presence of analyte, the analyte-specific antibody interacts with the analyte, leaving the liposomes to and be captured. This novel competitive assay format offers an increasing signal intensity with increasing analyte concentration. Drawn from text described in Ref. [166].

This novel competitive assay format allowed for a signal directly proportional to the analyte concentration resulting from the encapsulation of high concentrations of visible dyes and downstream capture of the uncomplexed liposomes. This and adaptation of liposome-based immunological assays to those suited for nucleic acid detection were only a few of the many liposome-based technologies developed in the laboratories of Dr. Richard Durst. Numerous investigators have since developed point-of-use sensors based on these early innovative technologies, increasing the breadth of utility and advancing methodologies, many of which will be described by Dr. Hsiao-Wei Wen and colleagues in Chapter 2.

Aside from consumer-friendly "home-pregnancy style" assays, intact liposomes have been used in innovative manners in other well-known laboratory-based formats. One example is that of blotting techniques, which rely on visualization of binding events on a solid phase to determine the presence of specific nucleic acids and proteins from often complex mixtures in a qualitative and quantitative manner. For example, in a traditional Western blot, proteins are first separated based on size using gel electrophoresis, then the separated proteins are transferred to a membrane, which is later probed by antigen-specific antibodies and functionalized enzymes capable of binding to the antibodies. The subsequent addition of an appropriate substrate yields a visible or luminescent signal proportional to the analyte concentration at its location on the membrane. Rather than using enzymes for signaling, liposomes have been shown to provide a viable and advantageous alternative. Intact liposomes conjugated to antibodies and encapsulating enzymes have been employed in Western blotting using an external precipitating substrate (Fig. 1.12).[169,170] In this application, the bilayer was permeable to the soluble form of the substrate, but not the encapsulated enzymes nor precipitated product of the enzymatic conversion. Such liposomes reduced diffusion since the product of the enzymatic conversion was retained within the confines of the bilayer and improved the sensitivity by two orders of magnitude over antibodies directly conjugated to liposomes due to greater enzyme to antibody ratios.[170]

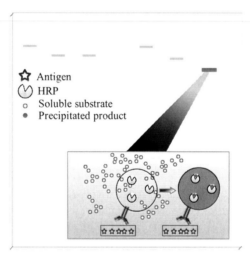

Figure 1.12 Liposome immunoblotting assay.[170] Protein antigens previously separated by SDS-PAGE and transferred to a PVDF membrane were probed with antibody-tagged, horseradish peroxidase (HRP)-encapsulating liposomes. A substrate soluble to the lipid bilayer precipitated within the liposomes upon enzymatic conversion, yielding improved sensitivity over antibody–enzyme conjugates alone. Drawn from text described in Ref. [170].

In another example, liposomes encapsulating a fluorescent dye were used as a signaling reagent in a dot blot method to quantify apurinic/apyrimidinic sites in genomic DNA.[171] Here, an avidin-coated slide served to bind DNA via electrostatic interactions between positively charged amine groups of the protein and the negative backbone of the DNA. An aldehyde reactive probe, which reacts with apurinic or apyrimidinic sites in DNA and functionalizes them with biotin, was used to identify sites of DNA damage. Streptavidin, followed by biotinylated sulforhodamine B-encapsulating liposomes, were utilized to form a fluorescent complex in proportion to the concentration of abasic sites in the DNA (Fig. 1.13). In contrast to direct fluorescence labeling or enzymatic amplification, this approach yielded greater sensitivity and avoided the time dependence of signal amplification, respectively.

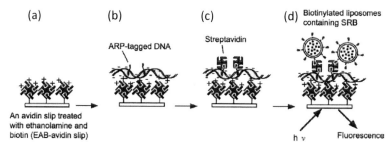

Figure 1.13   Liposome-based detection of apurinic/apyrimidinic sites in DNA.[171] Avidin was immobilized onto a glass slide serving to capture DNA by electrostatic interactions. Streptavidin formed a bridge between the biotin group introduced by the aldehyde reactive probe to the DNA and biotinylated liposomes encapsulating 1.5 mM sulforhodamine B (SRB). The apurinic/apyrimidinic sites in the DNA were quantified via fluorescence of the dye within the liposomes. Reprinted from Ref. [171], Copyright 2004, with permission from Elsevier. http://www.sciencedirect.com/science/article/pii/S0003269704005512.

In the aforementioned method, the concentration of encapsulated fluorescent dye was sufficient to attain the desired level of detection. However, fluorescent dyes, such as calcein, carboxyfluorescein, fluorescein, and sulforhodamine B,[172-175] undergo self-quenching when encapsulated within liposomes at high concentrations. In systems relying on intact liposomes for fluorescence detection, the concentration of the fluorescent dye must be carefully optimized to achieve maximal fluorescence, while avoiding the self-quenching and loss of signal that occurs at higher concentrations.

In another laboratory-based platform, liposomes encapsulating non-quenched concentrations of fluorescent dyes have been utilized in flow cytometry.[176] To maximize fluorescence intensity, liposomes were prepared encapsulating carboxyfluorescein and sulforhodamine at concentrations of 10 mM and 1 mM, respectively. Dye concentrations above this were found to yield self-quenching of fluorescence. In a subsequent comparison of protein A conjugated to carboxyfluorescein-encapsulating liposomes versus that conjugated to fluorescein isothiocyanate (FITC) for cell staining, a 15-fold greater signal was observed with the former when CF was encapsulated at a 10 mM concentration for flow cytometry analyses.

In lieu of relying on visualization or measurement of encapsulated marker molecules, other sensing approaches utilizing intact liposomes have resulted from the ability to tailor the lipid bilayer composition. For example, the lipid bilayer may be tagged with fluorescent dyes either by post-formation conjugation or incorporation of fluorescent lipids during liposome preparation.[177,178] Fluorescent lipids contribute significantly to the measurable signal even when dyes are also encapsulated within the interior volume.[179,180] Both approaches to generation of fluorescent liposomes have been successfully employed in a variety of assay formats, relying on fluorescent species either encapsulated,[181,182] attached to the lipid bilayer,[178,181] or both.[180,183] For example, intact fluorescent liposomes both encapsulating and with bilayer-tagged dyes have been utilized in microarray formats. Such arrays derive their addressing capabilities through oligonucleotide sequence,[181] protein–lipid specificity recognition,[180] or other means in a spatially distinct manner (Fig. 1.14).

One example, which will be reviewed by Dr. Chien-Sheng Chen and colleagues in Chapter 3, is a proteome microarray where liposomes incorporating both fluorescent lipids and specific phosphatidylinositides were used to study interactions between these lipids and immobilized yeast proteins. Since liposomes encapsulating self-quenching concentrations of fluorescent dye require lysis to detect any appreciable fluorescence signal, they are not appropriate for detection in high-density microarray platforms. To broaden the application of fluorescent liposomes in proteome microarrays, Lu et al.[150] constructed non-quenched fluorescent (NQF) liposomes by optimizing the sulforhodamine B concentration inside the liposomal vesicles as well as the lissamine rhodamine B-dipalmitoyl phosphatidylethanol present in the liposomal bilayers. The NQF liposome was able to amplify the fluorescent signal without a lysis step and thus could be directly applied to real-time assays or high-density microarrays. Through the combination of NQF liposome and proteome microarrays, the high-throughput identification of new lipid-binding proteins was realized.

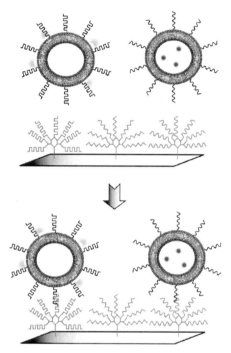

Figure 1.14 Sequence-specific recognition of immobilized DNA in an array format afforded by liposomes conjugated with DNA probes and either bilayer-tagged or encapsulating fluorescent dyes.[181] Adapted from Ref. [181], Copyright 2006, with permission from American Chemical Society. http://pubs. acs.org/doi/abs/10.1021/bc050273p.

Aside from the utilization of visible or fluorescent dyes, the bulky liposome structure and lipid bilayer itself provide other detection opportunities unique to liposomes. Due to their inherent size and impact on refractive index, liposomes have been used to enhance the signal in SPR applications (Fig. 1.15).[138] In a sandwich immunoassay for interferon-γ using SPR, liposomes were used to enhance the signal of the detector antibody, yielding an approximately 40,000-fold improvement in sensitivity.

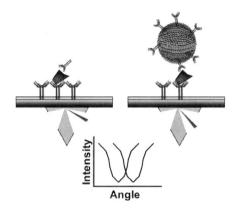

Figure 1.15   Surface plasmon resonance using liposomal amplification in a sandwich immunoassay.

Time-resolved luminescence has been accomplished using a technique named Liposome Resonance Energy Transfer (Fig. 1.16).[184–186] Hydrophobic europium chelates, such as Eu^{3+} complexed with 4,4,4-trifluoro-1-(2-napthalenyl)-1,3-butanedione (NTA) and trioctylphosphine oxide (TPO), embedded in the liposomal bilayer served as donors, while fluorescently labeled molecules binding to the liposome surface served as acceptors.[186]

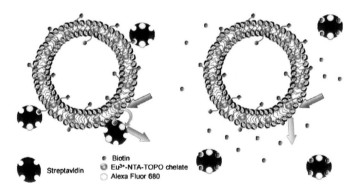

Streptavidin

● Biotin
◎ Eu^{3+}-NTA-TOPO chelate
○ Alexa Fluor 680

Figure 1.16   Liposome resonance energy transfer. Biotin in the sample competes with biotin-tagged, europium chelate-labeled liposomes for streptavidin-tagged AlexaFluor 680. Energy transfer occurs between donor and acceptor, resulting in a decrease in the signal at the acceptor wavelength when free biotin is present. Adapted from Ref. [186], Copyright 2009, with permission from Elsevier. http://www.sciencedirect.com/science/article/pii/S0003269708006556.

In this competitive assay format, aside from the europium chelate in the bilayer, the liposomes were also functionalized with biotin. Biotin as an analyte competed with the biotinylated liposomes for the available streptavidin, which was labeled with the fluorescent dye Alexa Fluor 680. The fluorescence of the acceptor molecules decreased as the free biotin concentration increased. Another novel advance that offers great sensing potential relies on the inclusion of lipophilic electrochemically active species in the lipid bilayer to impart redox capabilities to liposomes.[187]

As noted above, array formats are typically intended for the multiplex analysis of hundreds to thousands of analytes in a single assay, usually identified through probing defined locations on the immobilization surface. Some of the challenges with such conventional formats include spatial limitations on the number of resolvable species and expense associated with appropriate deposition equipment. This was addressed in a recent study where DNA-probe modified liposomes with sequence-specific lipid compositions were used as a barcode forming the detection portion in a sandwich hybridization assay (Fig. 1.17).[188] In this approach, the chemical composition of the lipids was identified by time-of-flight secondary ion mass spectrometry and correlated

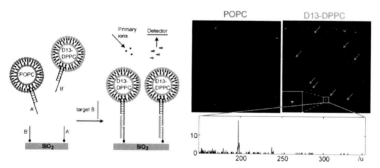

Figure 1.17 Liposomes with different lipid compositions serving as chemical barcodes form sandwich hybridization complexes with target DNA in a sequence-specific manner. Lipids from the liposomes participating in the complexes are subsequently analyzed by time-of-flight secondary ion mass spectrometry.[188] Reprinted from Ref. [188], Copyright 2010, with permission from American Chemical Society. http://pubs.acs.org/doi/abs/10.1021/nl904208y.

to the amount of target sequences partaking in the sandwich complex. The vast diversity possible in lipid compositions used for liposome preparation suggests this approach affords yet unrealized opportunities for multiplexed detection.

Lastly, a rapidly developing area of research is the use of polymerizable liposomes to afford signaling capabilities. For example, polydiacetylenic lipids polymerized by UV light yield conjugated diacetylene backbones,[189] which when incorporated into lipid bilayers can undergo conformational changes in response to various stimuli, including pH, mechanical stress, and molecular recognition (Fig. 1.18).[190,191] These conformational changes yield a colorimetric response, which can be visualized or monitored via spectrophotometry, which is enhanced when such lipid bilayers are formed as liposomes offering the opportunity for higher polymer density.[192]

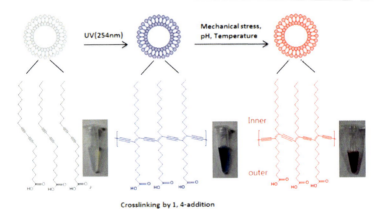

Figure 1.18 Chemical structure of polydiacetylene and its chromatic properties following UV polymerization and mechanical stress, pH, and temperature changes.[191] Chemical structures were drawn with ChemDraw, Perkin Elmer, Inc. Reprinted from Ref. [191] (http://www.mdpi.com/1424-8220/12/7/9530) under the Creative Commons Attribution License.

The sensing opportunities for such materials were embarked upon in the early 1990s[193] leading to liposomes employed as colorimetric sensors to detect influenza virus, *Escherichia coli*, and identification of bacterial lipopolysaccharides.[192,194–196] Such sensors rely on the visible transition from blue to red upon binding events, though PDA-liposome research has extended into monitoring fluorescence changes as well.[197] Numerous diverse technologies using PDA liposomes, including array-based platforms for selective potassium and mercury detection,[198,199] which were developed in the laboratory of Dr. Jinsang Kim, will be detailed in Chapter 4.

1.3.2 Lysed Liposomes in Signal Transduction

Rather than measurement of the intact species, other assays instead have relied on the quantification of entrapped marker molecules, such as fluorophores, electroactive species, or DNA probes released upon liposome lysis.[127,200,201] When employed in such a manner, liposomes may be readily substituted for enzymes in traditional formats. For example, following the final washing step in heterogeneous assays such as enzyme-linked immuno-sorbent assays (ELISAs), liposomes encapsulating fluorescent or electrochemical markers may simply be lysed instantaneously with surfactant, solvent, or other means to release their measurable contents.[202] An example of this using a nucleic acid sandwich hybridization format is shown in Fig. 1.19.

The first reported assay utilizing this strategy employed liposomes encapsulating sulforhodamine B, a water-soluble, highly visible, and highly fluorescent dye, with their bilayers tagged with a digoxigenin–lipid conjugate.[127] These liposomes competed with sample digoxigenin for limited available anti-digoxigenin antibody coated onto polypropylene tubes. The liposomes remaining bound to the antibodies were then lysed with surfactant and visible signal read at 565 nm. This early finding formed the basis for a variety of later platforms relying on measurement of released materials, including high-throughput microtiter plate-based assays,[203-207] flow-injection analysis systems,[208-210] intricate point-of-care assays,[211] and microfluidic platforms.[212,213]

For fluorescence measurements, release of dyes encapsulated at high concentrations upon lysis into the external medium overcomes self-quenching effects and results in an increase in the fluorescence intensity. Example dyes for such purposes have included sulforhodamine B, fluorescein, carboxyfluorescein, and calcein,[214-216] generally due to their high water solubility, quantum yields, and affordability. Comparing the incremental values of fluorescence intensity versus that from complete surfactant-induced lysis makes for a facile measure of liposome integrity.

Liposomes stored below their transition temperature generally exhibit improved retention of encapsulants, which is beneficial for long-term usage. Our lab has demonstrated excellent stability of liposomes encapsulating sulforhodamine B dye under both refrigerated (4°C) and ambient (21°C) conditions for over 400 days, while storage of these same liposomes at 41°C and 52°C led to pronounced loss of encapsulant and, therefore, function.[204]

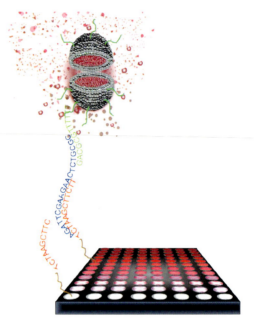

Figure 1.19 Example use of lysed liposomes to provide signaling capabilities. Liposomes encapsulating high concentrations of fluorescent dyes may be used to provide a quantitative fluorescence signal. As an example, a sandwich hybridization assay in a microtiter plate format, similar in operation to the antibody and enzyme-based counterpart ELISA, yields quantitative result proportional to analyte concentration. Shown here, liposomes encapsulating fluorescent dye and tagged with a DNA reporter probe (green) bind to one portion of the target nucleic acid sequence (blue), which is captured by an immobilized DNA capture probe (red) directed toward a different portion of the target sequence. After washing away unbound materials, the liposomes participating in the sandwich complex are lysed, releasing their fluorescent dye and yielding a quantitative signal proportional to the concentration of the target species.

Using these liposomes, a sandwich immunoassay for myoglobin in human serum samples was developed and fully optimized for detection with streptavidin-conjugated horseradish peroxidase (HRP), alkaline phosphatase, or liposomes encapsulating sulforhodamine B.[204] Even with the most sensitive fluorescent substrates commercially available for both enzymes, such liposomes were found to provide an approximately 1.4 times lower limit of detection over both HRP and alkaline phosphatase. More significant than a lower limit of detection, however, was the markedly greater sensitivity than enzyme-based detection, which improved the limit of quantification and concentration discrimination possible between small analyte concentration increments. For example, the maximum signal to noise attainable with sulforhodamine B-encapsulating liposomes reached 736:1 versus 158 and 120:1 for HRP and alkaline phosphatase, respectively (Fig. 1.20).

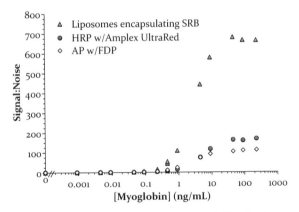

Figure 1.20 Sandwich immunoassay for myoglobin in human serum samples using streptavidin-conjugated HRP with Amplex UltraRed, Alkaline phosphatase with fluorescein diphosphate, or sulforhodamine B-encapsulating liposomes for signal amplification of the biotinylated anti-myoglobin reporter antibody.[204] Signal-to-noise ratios for fluorescence detection were calculated by dividing the response at each myoglobin concentration by that in the absence of myoglobin. With kind permission from Springer Science+Business Media, reprinted from Ref [204], Copyright 2013. http://link.springer.com/ article/10.1007%2Fs00216-013-6807-3.

One advantage of lysed liposome strategies over enzymatic amplification is the instantaneous signal, as compared to the time-dependent enzymatic conversion of substrate to measurable product. This has proven to be advantageous in flow-based systems, such as flow-injection analysis and microfluidic sensors where implementation of appropriate substrate–enzyme ratios in a transient regime and reliance on time-dependent enzymatic conversion is not practical.[210,212,217] Not only the signal obtained through instantaneous lysis reduces the time to result, but also the use of liposomes lessens reliance on additional potentially expensive and complicated substrate preparations necessary for enzymatic amplification.[204] Reliance on the measurement of contents released from liposomes has provided considerable signal enhancement over such markers alone when they are used directly as a single label. For example, antibody-conjugated liposomes encapsulating HRP yielded an approximately 27 times lower limit of detection than HRP-antibody conjugates in a sandwich immunoassay.[32] Liposomes encapsulating fluorescein were reported to provide a 1000-fold increase in sensitivity over a fluorophore-labeled antibody in a sandwich hybridization-based flow-injection analysis system.[218] Where such direct comparisons have been made, the liposome-based systems have allowed for significant enhancement over single labels. The potential for liposome amplification is, however, often not fully realized as liposomes impart steric and multivalency effects, which block or occupy, respectively, some binding sites available otherwise to smaller, less reactive labels.

1.3.2.1 Assays relying on complement-mediated lysis

While solvent- or surfactant-mediated lysis is most commonly used to afford release of liposomal contents, lysis can also be more selectively accomplished, which opens up opportunities for homogeneous assay formats. Among analytical labels, liposomes have the unique ability to activate the complement system, which is composed of roughly 30 serum proteins and serves as an initial defense mechanism by the host against infection.[219] These proteins bind in an ordered fashion to antibodies directed against cell surface antigens and cause lysis of the cellular structure. In the case of liposomes, if an antibody binds to an antigen accessible on their surface in the presence of serum, a cascade of complement protein binding events ensue leading to liposome lysis and release of contents (Fig. 1.21).[220,221]

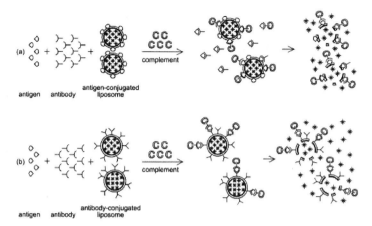

Figure 1.21 Antibody–antigen interactions promote liposome lysis in the presence of complement.[141] (Top) A competitive format where the presence of the antigen in the sample reduces interactions between antigen-conjugated liposomes and free antibody and (bottom) a sandwich format where antigen in the sample forms a complex between free antibody and antibody-conjugated liposomes. In both cases, complement induces liposome lysis in proportion to the antigen–antibody complexes formed on the liposome surface. Reprinted from Ref. [141], Copyright 1997, with permission from Elsevier Science, B.V. http://www.sciencedirect.com/science/article/pii/S0022175997000410.

This formed the basis for many early assays initiating in the 1970s, with key benefits including the homogeneous format and concomitant lack of need for separation or washing steps.[5,222] The spin membrane immunoassay (SMIA) utilized liposome-entrapped spin labels, which were released by complement upon antibody binding to the lipid bilayer.[221,223] The released spin labels containing unpaired electrons yielded enhanced signals upon dilution into the bulk medium, which could then be quantified by electron spin resonance (ESR) spectroscopy, and offered handling and disposal advantages over widely used radioimmunoassays.[221] Aside from the novel formats made possible by the use of the complement system, liposomes offered a high concentration of spin labels available for release per binding event. This yielded improved sensitivity over the precursor spin immunoassay (SIA) format, which utilized spin labels directly conjugated to binding entities.[5,224,225]

Later advances utilized the same hapten-complement system approach as in the SMIA but relied on entrapment of enzymes rather than spin labels. The advantages of enzyme entrapment included avoidance of quenching of spin labels by biological fluids as well as expensive equipment required for ESR signal measurement.[222] In one example of this format, theophylline-tagged liposomes, prepared from lipids conjugated to this small molecule and entrapping the enzyme HRP, were used in a competitive assay format for theophylline, a bronchodilator drug with a narrow therapeutic index.[222] These liposomes were mixed with a known concentration of anti-theophylline antibodies, a complement source, and samples potentially containing theophylline. In the presence of the analyte, competition of the sample theophylline with the theophylline-tagged liposomes for the available anti-theophylline antibodies resulted in reduced complement-induced lysis. In the absence of the analyte, complement-induced lysis was maximal. The amount of enzyme released from the liposomes was thus inversely proportional to the analyte concentration. The released enzyme was then used to catalyze substrate conversion, effectively relying on the depletion of oxygen in the surrounding media, which could be monitored using amperometric detection.

In a commercially available kit (Autokit CH50, available from Wako Diagnostics), enzyme-encapsulating liposomes are used to assess complement activity in human serum.[226] This assay relies on dinitrophenol (DNP)-tagged liposomes encapsulating glucose-6-phosphate dehydrogenase, which are added to anti-DNP antibodies, an appropriate enzyme substrate, and human serum samples. Complement present in the serum sample is activated by the binding of anti-DNP to the liposomes, which results in their subsequent lysis. Released enzyme becomes available to act on the external substrate yielding a spectrophotometric response proportional to the complement activity. This can be used for the diagnosis of disease states, including systemic lupus erythematosus and rheumatoid arthritis.

Other entrapped species used with complement-mediated assay designs included electroactive species,[227] fluorescent dyes,[215,216,228-230] and enzyme substrates.[231] Taking advantage of the quenching of fluorescent dyes when encapsulated at high concentrations, the Liposome Immune Lysis Assay (LILA) again relied on the same concepts of complement-induced lysis, but fluorescent signal was instead generated upon lysis through dilution of the previously encapsulated dye into the surrounding media.[229] This format was successfully used to measure a range of analytes, including antibodies,[229] inflammatory proteins,[232] plant toxins,[216] and mycotoxins[233] as well as to determine the concentrations of gangliosides on cell surfaces.[234]

1.3.2.2 Assays utilizing lysis via cytolytic agents

Reliance on animal-derived serum for use toward liposome lysis via complement was relatively expensive due to the high concentrations of complement needed to allow lysis to proceed with reasonable kinetics.[235] Additionally, certain lipid formulations were prone to nonspecific lysis induced by complement in the absence of antibody–antigen binding.[236] As such, alternatives were sought, including lysis by enzymes such as phospholipase C[237,238] or pore-forming peptides, such as melittin, the primary component of honey bee venom.[239] Assays have been devised using analyte–melittin conjugates, which induce liposome lysis, but may be inhibited by the addition of analyte-specific antibody. The antibody inhibits melittin-induced liposome lysis by binding to the conjugate, hence more, free antibody equates to reduced lysis. Competitive effects between sample analyte and these conjugates for the available antibody can yield a concentration-dependent response and has formed the basis for numerous assays.[235,240]

In one example of this format, liposomes encapsulating alkaline phosphatase were mixed with anti-digoxin antibodies, samples potentially containing digoxin, and a melittin conjugate prepared from an analogue of digoxin (Fig. 1.22).[235] The melittin–digoxin conjugate and sample digoxin competed for the available antibodies. The resulting degree of liposome lysis was directly proportional to the concentration of digoxin as its increasing concentrations allowed for more, free melittin conjugate. The enzyme released could then participate in colorimetric substrate conversion, the rate of which was monitored over time and correlated to the analyte concentration.

In a similar approach, a competitive assay for the aminoglycoside antibiotic gentamycin was developed using a conjugate of the analyte with phospholipase C.[237] A fixed concentration of anti-gentamycin antibodies was available, which could inhibit the activity of the enzyme conjugate toward lysis of the fluorescent-dye-encapsulating liposomes. Similar to the assay for digoxin, in the presence of the analyte, more free conjugate was available to lyse the liposomes and an increase in the fluorescence intensity resulted. One advantage to these approaches over prior complement-mediated assays was that they were more universal as a single batch of liposomes could be used for many analytes since the liposomes themselves did not require functionalization with a specific analyte.

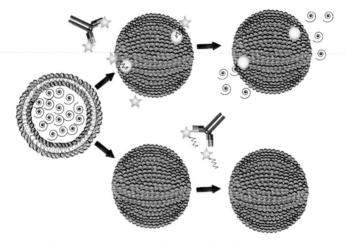

Figure 1.22   Liposomes encapsulating alkaline phosphatase were added to antigen–melittin conjugates in the presence of antigen-specific antibodies. In the presence of sample analyte (top), a competition with the melittin conjugates exists for the available antibody and more free conjugates are available to lyse the liposomes and generate signal from released enzyme in the presence of substrate. (Bottom) In the absence of analyte, the antigen–mellitin conjugates are bound by antibodies and liposome lysis is inhibited.[235] Drawn from text described in Ref. [235].

Beyond the quantification of a specific analyte, this approach can be applied for the qualitative and quantitative analysis of inhibitors of lytic events. In a novel approach, a high-throughput screening assay for compounds that can inhibit hepatitis C virus was developed. Researchers took advantage of the pore-forming properties of the viral protein p7, which forms multimeric channel structures following insertion into lipid membranes.[241] As p7 is necessary for virus activity, compounds that can inhibit this protein are targets for pharmaceutical development. In this novel assay format, compounds that potentially could inhibit p7 activity were combined with p7, followed by liposomes encapsulating self-quenching concentrations of fluorescein in 384-well microtiter plates. p7 formed pores in the liposomal lipid bilayers, which yielded the release of encapsulated dye and marked increase in fluorescence intensity due to overcoming the self-quenching effects. Mixtures without inhibiting compounds yielding maximal pore formation and mixtures without p7 yielding no pore formation served as positive and negative controls, respectively. Inhibitors of p7 yielded reduced liposome lysis as determined by either kinetic or end-point measurements. Specificity of inhibitors toward p7 was demonstrated against mellitin. Some challenges in the development of this assay included isolation of an active form of the p7 protein, which retained its activity without yielding nonspecific liposome lysis. This was accomplished by developing a detergent-free isolation procedure for the protein as well as determining appropriate buffer conditions that minimized nonspecific aggregate formation. Second, the lipid composition was found to be critical for retaining p7 activity and concomitant assay performance, with the requirement for a high percentage of negatively charged lipids (PA) in conjunction with lipids typical to natural cell membranes.

Rather than making use of cytolytic species as reagents in quantitative assays, such species may also be targeted in assay formats made uniquely possible with liposomes. For example, liposomes encapsulating 2,6-dichlorophenolindophenol, an electrochemical mediator, were used in a lysis-based assay intended to differentiate pathogenic from nonpathogenic strains of bacteria (Fig. 1.23).[242] In this assay, hemolytic and non-hemolytic strains of *Listeria monocytogenes* and *Escherichia coli* were incubated with liposomes, the former of which was capable of inducing lysis. The mediator released from the liposomes was then detected amperometrically.

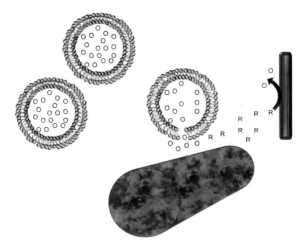

Figure 1.23 Amperometric signal generation by hemolytic bacteria: (1) Liposome containing entrapped mediator (oxidized, O). (2) Action of bacterial enzymes releases mediator, which is reduced by the cell. (3) Reduced mediator (•) is reoxidized at detector to generate signal.[242] Adapted from Ref. [242], Copyright 1995, with kind permission from Springer Science and Business Media. http://link.springer.com/article/10.1007%2FBF00160823.

Similarly, in a heterogeneous assay format, liposomes encapsulating potassium ferrohexacyanide were immobilized onto an electrode and used to assess the presence of streptolysin, a staphylococcal pore-forming toxin.[243] When present, the toxin increased the permeability of the bilayer resulting in leakage of the encapsulated marker. A linear relationship between the concentration of pore-forming toxin and current was obtained via amperometry. In another variant, liposomes encapsulating fluorescent dyes have been employed to detect pore-forming hemolysins, such as those excreted from the foodborne pathogen *L. monocytogenes*.[244] While these assays were not specific to the identities of the lytic species, such liposome-based biosensors provide an effective measure of agents responsible for cell lysis.

Other sensing modalities have made use of embedding ion-selective channels into the lipid bilayer. For example, gramicidin, a naturally occurring antimicrobial peptide, can form transmembrane channels in lipid bilayers from its dimeric structure, which are selectively permeable to monovalent cations.[245,246] Taking advantage of this selectivity in one sensor, the addition of gramicidin yielded the formation of channels through the liposomal lipid bilayer, which were permeable to hydrogen ions (Fig. 1.24).[247] pH-sensitive dyes encapsulated within liposomes under acidic conditions yielded an increase in fluorescence intensity with efflux of protons. The utility of this sensor design lied within the distortion of the channels that occurred upon analyte–antigen recognition on the liposome surface. As the native channels were shorter than the bilayer thickness, localized changes of the bilayer structure due to binding events resulted in greater fractions of open channels.[248] The resulting kinetics of hydrogen ion passage was altered in an analyte-concentration-dependent manner and the resulting fluorescence increase could be utilized in a homogeneous format.

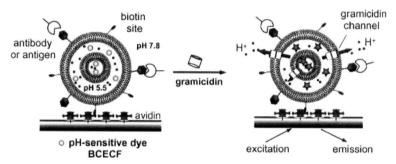

Figure 1.24 Liposomes tagged with biotin encapsulating a pH-sensitive dye at lower pH were immobilized onto an avidin surface in an external solution of higher pH. Antibody–antigen recognition events at the liposome surface yielded gramicidin channels, release of protons, and a measurable fluorescence signal from the pH-sensitive dye. Reprinted from Ref. [247], Copyright 2007, with permission from Elsevier. http://www.sciencedirect.com/science/article/pii/S0003269707004629.

Using a similar principle, pH-sensitive dye-encapsulating liposomes functionalized with antibodies against the growth hormone somatostatin and growth hormone releasing factor were employed in an array format utilizing gramicidin to afford pore formation.[182] In this format, liposomes were functionalized with target-specific antibody fragments and reversibly immobilized via cleavable disulfide linkages onto a glass slide. The liposomes were then incubated with their respective target molecules, followed by gramicidin. In the presence of the antigens, distortion of the bilayer upon recognition affected the monomer–dimer kinetics of gramicidin and yielded an increase in fluorescence intensity in spatially distinct regions in the array.

1.3.2.3 Modern advances

Among the many technologies developed in the laboratory of Dr. Antje Baeumner, advances in the combination of liposomes with microfluidics are of significant note. Novel microfluidic designs allowing for sequential introduction of reagents needed for multi-step sandwich immunoassays and hybridization assays have been developed with the requirement for limited user intervention. Many of these technologies take advantage of the existing and cutting-edge approaches for biosensing such as the use of dendrimeric surfaces, magnetic nanoparticles, and electrospun nanofibers to promote interactions through increased surface area and functional sites. Work toward total microanalysis systems for RNA detection from pathogenic organisms, such as *Cryptosporidium parvum*,[249] Dengue virus,[250] and feline calicivirus,[251] including provisions for multianalyte detection in parallel[252] will be detailed in Chapter 5. In this chapter, an overview of the progress in liposome formation in microfluidic devices is also available.

Numerous developments focusing on liposome-based electrochemical detection have materialized in the laboratory of Dr. Ja-An Annie Ho. Electrochemical measurements offer low-cost instrumentation, rapid and sensitive response, and ease of miniaturization.[253] Liposomes encapsulating electrochemically active species, such as hexaammineruthenium(III) chloride,[253] potassium ferricyanide,[211,254] and ferrocene,[255] have been utilized in various embodiments in conjunction with advances in the field of electrochemical biosensing. For example, liposomes encapsulating potassium ferrocyanide and functionalized with GM1 were used in a sandwich assay with an immobilized capture antibody. The unique feature of this assay was that the antibody was coupled to PEDOT, a conducting polymer, coated onto Nafion-supported carbon nanotubes. This, in accompaniment with the high concentrations of electrochemically active encapsulant, contributed to the efficiency of the assay leading to a limit of detection of

1 fg/mL (100 µL volume) via square-wave stripping voltammetry.[254] In another embodiment utilizing biotin-tagged potassium ferrocyanide encapsulating liposomes, a competitive assay for the small-molecule biotin (vitamin B7) was developed utilizing gold nanoparticles coated with a polyelectrolyte as a working electrode. The increased surface area, efficient electron transfer, and measurable species made available by the lysed liposomes resulted in an impressive detection limit of 9.1 pg biotin in a 4.5 µL volume.[211] These technologies and other advances will be detailed by Dr. Ho and colleagues in Chapter 6.

However, the utility of lysed liposomes does not necessarily conclude with end-point measurement of released materials. By taking advantage of encapsulation of dsDNA reporters, secondary signal amplification strategies can be devised. The technique of liposome-PCR was invented and developed in the laboratories of Dr. Jeffery Mason and Dr. Timothy O'Leary. In this exquisite approach, liposomes encapsulating dsDNA reporters and tagged with GM1 or GT1b gangliosides were first employed as the detection portion of a sandwich assay for cholera toxin and botulinum toxin, respectively, using an immobilized antibody for analyte capture.[201] Rather than directly detecting the bound liposomes or encapsulants within, the DNA released by surfactant-induced lysis served as reporters subsequently quantified by real-time PCR. This approach achieved remarkable sensitivity yielding detection limits of 0.02 fg/mL for both toxins. This was not only a marked improvement over conventional approaches such as ELISAs,[256] but also over modern advances, including immuno-PCR[257] and other liposome-based assays.[164,177,258,259] For example, this approach yielded a substantially better limit of detection than that achieved using a similarly designed antibody-GM1 sandwich liposome-based assay, which instead relied on the measurement of released fluorescent dye following liposome lysis.[258] Measurement of sulforhodamine B allowed for the detection of 340 pg/mL of cholera toxin, which was sufficient for the cell culture application under investigation, but paled in comparison to sensitivity possible with the liposome-PCR amplification approach. This unique and versatile assay design will be detailed in Chapter 7 and may very well set the bar for sensitive, yet practical, future methods.

Novel developments in the fields of drug delivery and liposome characterization offer exciting potential in the analytical realm. As noted previously, liposomes responsive to magnetic fields, pH, and temperature have been shown to selectively release their contents under the appropriate conditions in vivo. Yet these stresses have seen little usage in analytical platforms to date. One recent development centered around the use of pH-sensitive liposomes and a lipid bilayer-embedded hydrophobically modified glucose oxidase. These liposomes were used in an assay for glucose, in which the enzymatic conversion of glucose to gluconic acid resulted in a decrease in pH and concomitant release of encapsulated calcein, which was measured by fluorescence (Fig. 1.25).[260]

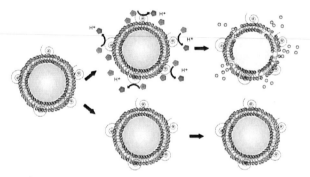

Figure 1.25 pH-sensitive liposomes with bilayer-embedded glucose oxidase and encapsulating calcein experience a decrease in pH with enzymatic conversion of glucose to gluconic acid. In the presence of sample glucose, the decrease in pH results in the release of encapsulated calcein and an increase in fluorescence intensity (top), whereas in the absence of glucose, liposomes retain their encapsulated dye at self-quenching concentrations (bottom).[260] Drawn from text described in Ref. [260].

In another recent advance, the analytical utility of thermally responsive liposomes was demonstrated when such liposomes were used as detection species in a sandwich immunoassay for carcinoembryonic antigen.[32] These liposomes, which included a thermally sensitive lysolipid in their bilayers, were shown to release encapsulated enzyme upon elevation of temperature in the surrounding medium. The released enzyme could subsequently be used for amperometric signal generation proportional to the amount of analyte present. The benefits of this approach included not only signal amplification due to numerous enzyme molecules within the liposomes available per analyte recognition event, but also specific to the lysis method, the retention of enzyme activity and avoidance of potential interferences with detection versus chemical means such as surfactants or solvents.

From the perspective of manipulation, liposomes with iron oxide nanoparticles embedded within the lipid bilayer and encapsulating fluorescent dye have recently been developed as analytical reagents. Their potential, as demonstrated in microfluidics and microtiter plate platforms, will be described in Chapter 8, affording the high sensitivity concomitant with liposome-based amplification, yet providing directional control and overcoming mass transfer limitations to binding events in heterogeneous assay formats otherwise associated with these sub-micron sized particles (Fig. 1.26). Existing and potential magnetic liposome applications for analysis are discussed as well.

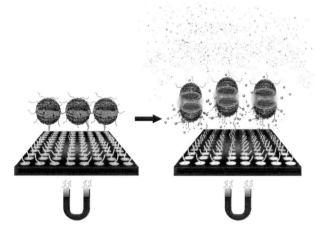

Figure 1.26 DNA-functionalized liposomes with bilayer-embedded iron oxide and encapsulating sulforhodamine B. In the sandwich hybridization assay depicted here, the liposomes can be drawn to the underlying target hybridized to the surface immobilized capture probe via a magnet. This serves to help overcome mass transport limitations of these bulky particles with molecules bound at a surface. Reprinted from *Anal Chem*, 2014, 86(13), pp. 6610–6616, Copyright 2014, with permission from the American Chemical Society. http://pubs.acs.org/doi/abs/10.1021/ac501219u.

1.3.3 Liposomes as Cellular Mimics

Given the similarity of the liposomal lipid bilayer to that of natural cell membranes, the structure of liposomes lends them to utility as cell mimics to study various interactions. Liposomes have been prepared as model membranes to replicate properties of specific cell types through modifying lipid composition,[261] varying surface charge,[262,263] and through the incorporation of membrane-bound receptors.[264,265] Such liposomes have been used to study a variety of biologically relevant interactions, including those between proteins and lipids[266]; membrane–protein interactions[267]; virus attachment[268,269]; drug–membrane interactions[270]; and permeation characteristics.[2] Some of these studies rely on specific receptor–ligand interactions, whereas others utilize the amphiphilic nature of the lipid bilayer itself. As an example of the former, the lipid bilayer of liposomes provides a suitable environment for reconstitution of gangliosides. As discussed in Section 1.1, gangliosides are composed of a carbohydrate-linked lipid, with the sialic acid portion extending into the aqueous environment and their hydrophobic tails partitioning within the lipid tails of the bilayer. These molecules are natural components of many cell types, predominantly neuronal cells, and serve as receptors for viruses and bacterial toxins. Specific examples include ganglioside GD1a, GT1b, and GM1 for Sendai virus,[261,271] tetanus toxin,[272,273] and cholera toxin,[274] respectively. Such molecules reconstituted within the lipid bilayer of liposomes have been used to present antigens for vaccine development,[275] to study organ distribution of drugs,[276] and to study disease correlated with anti-ganglioside activity.[277]

1.3.3.1 Membrane interactions

From an analytical perspective, one of the areas where liposome-based assays have made the broadest impact is in the assessment of chemical/drug–membrane interactions. The traditional predictor of lipophilic properties and membrane interactions has been the octanol–water partition coefficient, which assesses the extent of partitioning of a solute between octanol, an organic solvent with a nonpolar tail and polar hydroxyl headgroup, and an immiscible aqueous phase. Partitioning has historically been carried out by manual agitation, then assessment of the resulting amount of solute residing within each phase then correlated to pharmacokinetics, nonspecific toxicity, and bioavailability of therapeutics, industrial chemicals, and environmental pollutants.[278] Liposome-based methods were subsequently developed, which relied instead on partitioning of solutes into formed vesicles, rather than an organic solvent. Advantages include closer similarity to natural cell membranes as both electrostatic interactions and amphiphilic properties can be accounted for; the ability to change lipid composition to better mimic certain cell types, and consequently, better prediction of biological effects.[279-281]

Early liposome-based methods relied on labor-intensive equilibrium dialysis or ultracentrifugation to separate bound and free solutes,[282] whereas subsequent approaches utilized immobilized liposomes in solid-phase microextraction (SPME),[283] chromatography,[284-288] and capillary electrophoresis (CE),[285,289,290] which allowed for reduced assay times and lower solute concentrations.[290] In an example of the latter technique, liposomes were incorporated as a pseudo-stationary phase in capillary electrophoresis, a combination known as liposome electrokinetic chromatography (LEKC).[290] Solutes could partition into the liposome phase to varying degrees depending on their structures, which subsequently affected their migration times, and the retention factors were found to be directly proportional to the liposome–water partition coefficient. This approach could yield results in minutes, versus hours or days required of equilibrium-based methods, and has been applied to the study of pesticides,[291] antibiotics,[292] and anesthetics.[293] In another approach, using the aforementioned PDA liposomes, a method that relied on the extent of color change upon drug–membrane interaction was developed to determine the affinity constant of various drugs, including cardiac β-blockers and anesthetics, to lipid membranes.[270] The method showed strong correlation with results from standard octanol–water partitioning for neutral nonpolar compounds. It has been suggested that liposome-based approaches are more selective than the standard octanol–water system, with the former better able to account for electrostatic interactions as well as having closer resemblance to cell membranes due to the ordered structure of the bilayer.[281,294,295]

Several conventional and emerging liposome/lipid bilayer-based methodologies are available to study interactions and partitioning,[296-298] many of which are based on changes in refractive index/SPR.[273,299–301] For example, by immobilizing liposomes with different lipid compositions, the affinity and kinetics of the anti-fungal agent amphotericin B could be evaluated using SPR.[302] Similarly, the interactions between liposomes with varying lipid compositions and immobilized recombinant human erythropoietin were characterized using Bio-Layer Interferometry.[303] Immobilized liposomes form the basis for commercially available SPR assays (Biacore S51) to aid in absorption, distribution, metabolism, and excretion (ADME) studies.[304] In one method centered on the permeation characteristics of solutes, immobilized liposomes were incubated with mellitin, followed by sucrose. The pores formed by mellitin allowed sucrose to permeate into the liposomes, which could be monitored by local changes in refractive index.[300] In another method, unmodified liposomes or those with an embedded transmembrane pore were first equilibrated with high concentrations of uncharged solutes, followed by rapid exchange to a buffer devoid of such solutes.[301] The subsequent efflux of solutes from within the liposome either by passive means or via the membrane pore could be monitored over time using the change in refractive index by SPR. Other liposome-based methodologies measure partitioning as a function of pH via titrations[294] or flow cytometry.[305] Novel work toward this end includes the usage of a fluorescein–lipid conjugate, which, when embedded in the bilayer, serves as a pH-sensitive probe of interactions with analytes due to both adsorption and penetration.[296,306] This and other novel work of Dr. Marek Langner and colleagues will be reviewed in Chapter 9.

Orienting biologically active molecules in liposomal lipid bilayers has allowed for the development of immobilization surfaces, which retain the requisite recognition and binding capacity.[307] Noted previously was the ability to incorporate hydrophobic biorecognition elements such as gangliosides[38] and cholesterol-modified synthetic DNA sequences,[21,22] which otherwise require complicated post-formation conjugation chemistries or simply are energetically unfavorable. However, this strategy is not limited to these common biorecognition elements. Taking advantage of the ability to incorporate hydrophobic biorecognition elements, lipid bilayer-incorporated mycolic acids (MAs), extracted from cell wall lipids of *Mycobacterium tuberculosis*, were used to provide recognition capabilities in a waveguide-based assay for tuberculosis diagnosis.[308] MAs are fatty acids composed of two asymmetric hydrocarbon chains: one long β-hydroxy chain and one shorter α-alkyl chain. Patients with TB have a high prevalence of antibodies against MAs, though in conditions such as HIV, immunosuppression can limit antibody development to these and other relevant antigens.[309,310] Given the high mortality rate of coinfection and difficulty in detecting TB by standard methods, an assay targeting MAs is of clinical importance. However, standard ELISAs were reportedly unable to provide the requisite specificity and sensitivity against MAs.[309] Direct immobilization of such molecules led to poor physiological presentation and significant cross-reactivity with anti-cholesterol antibodies present in human serum.[311] Overcoming these difficulties, in this assay, liposomes with MA-incorporated in their lipid bilayers were immobilized and the binding of anti-MA antibodies from patient sera was observed in real time by the resulting change in refractive index. Further advances led to an SPR-based assay known as the MAs antibody real-time inhibition test, which utilized immobilized liposomes presenting MAs in competition with the same for anti-MA antibodies in serum.[308,311] Other lipid-based surfaces utilizing liposomes for SPR measurements have been formulated.[273,312] For example, immobilization of liposomes with gangliosides incorporated within the lipid bilayer allowed for the study of bacterial toxin binding affinity and kinetics. The benefits of this approach included those inherent to SPR, which are real-time, label-free measurements, while taking advantage of the lipid bilayer to present glycolipid receptors in an analogous manner to that found in natural cell membranes.[273]

In an innovative advance, a three-dimensional matrix utilizing liposomes for SPR studies was devised.[313,314] Liposomes were immobilized to the surface via complementary base pairing between bilayer-embedded cholesterol-modified DNA probes and biotinylated DNA linked to the surface by neutravidin. This approach helped to maintain the liposome structure versus direct immobilization. Subsequent liposome layers were assembled using cholesterol-modified sequences complementary to those on the previous liposome layer. The amphiphilic nature of the lipid bilayer allowed for the reconstitution of transmembrane proteins in an environment similar to natural cell membranes, thus retaining their function.[315] Utilizing a multilayer approach and the ability to reconstitute high densities of such proteins, some of the sensitivity limitations inherent to SPR-based techniques could be overcome. This method required taking into account the exponential decay in signal measured with distance from the surface. This technology has been commercialized in a kit (memLAYER) by Layerlab AB for use with the Bio-Rad ProteOn™ XPR36 system, an SPR-based instrument that can monitor 36 interactions in parallel.

1.3.3.2 Lipid-signaling applications

The hydrophobic nature and cell mimicry of liposomes also make them of great practicality for studying lipid-based signaling, which, when malfunctioning in living systems, has been implicated in tumorigenesis, metabolic diseases, and inflammatory processes.[316] Lipids such as diacylglycerol (DAG), phosphatidic acid (PA), and phosphatidylinositol phosphates (PIP$_n$s) are important in cell-signaling pathways and serve to bind soluble receptors in vivo such as members of the protein kinase C (PKC) family.[267] Liposomes offer the ability to solubilize and present these hydrophobic structures in a manner consistent with that of the conformation and composition of natural cell membranes. Toward this end, a solution-phase liposome aggregation assay was developed, which relied on the increase in turbidity associated with lipid interactions.[317] In a method intended for high-throughput analysis of protein-membrane binding, intact liposomes prepared with DAG and PS in their lipid composition were immobilized in wells of microtiter plates via a biotin-streptavidin linkage.[267] PKCα, which is known to interact with DAG and PS, was added and that bound was subsequently detected via antibodies against PKCα with enzymatic-based chemiluminescence detection.

In another high-throughput approach, liposomes were used to present lipid-based substrates for the assessment of lipid kinase activity in a homogeneous format.[318] Liposomes composed of negatively charged phospholipids were prepared incorporating the substrate PI(5)P (D-*myo*-phosphatidylinositol-5-phosphate) in their bilayers. The charge of the lipid composition ensured appropriate association by phosphatdylinositol kinases (PIPK) and the liposome presentation of the substrate was used to ensure appropriate enzyme activity. The PIPK under investigation was introduced in the presence of the liposomes, ATP, and potentially inhibiting compounds. The PIPK phosphorylates liposomal PI(5)P at the expense of phosphate groups from the supplied ATP thus yielding ADP. Subsequent to the enzymatic reaction, commercially available assays such as the Kinase-Glo® assay served to quantify the amount of ATP remaining via chemiluminescence or the Transcreener® FP assay, which quantified the amount of ADP produced via a displacement assay based on fluorescence polarization. This liposome-based method showed great promise due to the ability to present in the lipid bilayer otherwise intractable substrates as well as the facile combination of liposome with commercially available and widely accepted high-throughput methodologies for measuring kinase activity.

1.3.4 Liposomes in Separations

The unique hydrophilic and hydrophobic nature of liposomes provides for separation mechanisms when used as supports in chromatographic or electrophoretic techniques. For example, in the technique of immobilized liposome chromatography (ILC) developed in the late 1980s, liposomes were associated with gel beads used as a stationary phase either through hydrophobic interactions or entrapment within.[319] Liposomes could be covalently immobilized within gel beads or via avidin-biotin linkages to better tolerate challenging elution conditions.[286,320] Increased retention times of passing solutes indicated either interactions with or partitioning into the liposomal phase versus the passing mobile phase. The first publication thereof showed that immobilized liposomes with an embedded glucose transport protein from red blood cells were capable of separation of D-glucose from L-glucose as the former was retained longer by the liposomes due to its stereospecific facilitated diffusion.[319,321] This method was subsequently employed to study competitive membrane interactions, such as D-glucose with its transport inhibitor cytochalasin B for the immobilized RBC transport protein.[322] In this analysis, retention of the transport inhibitor was decreased in the presence of glucose, the concentration dependence of which allowed for the determination of equilibrium dissociation constants.

Aside from "affinity" or specific transport retention chromatographic effects, ILC was utilized for unique modes relying on ion-exchange and hydrophobic interaction chromatography taking advantage of the charged and lipophilic nature of liposomal lipid bilayers, repectively.[323] The retention of drugs of varying hydrophobicities on immobilized liposomes has demonstrated excellent correlation with octanol–water coefficients and has been shown to serve as a strong predictor of drug permeability of epithelial cells.[288,324] Quantification of association constants into liposomes has been accomplished by calculating the amount of free solutes following chromatographic separation.[287]

Immobilized artificial membrane (IAM) chromatography was developed to serve much the same purpose, utilizing phospholipids covalently conjugated to silica supports.[325,326] Example IAM supports include phosphatidylcholines bound through amide linkages to aminopropylsilica particles, which residual amine groups remain either unmodified or capped to yield neutral amides.[327] IAM analyses have shown a strong correlation to the octanol–water coefficient for local anaesthetics.[328] However, given the amphiphilic nature of phospholipids, with solutes containing polar moieties, correlations to K_{ow} were less concrete, hence the mechanisms beyond interactions related to hydrophobicity needed to be taken into account.[329] This required mathematically understanding the differences between the lipophilic octanol–water parameter versus the retention coefficient obtained for IAM with purely aqueous mobile phases to account for ionic and specific structural interactions. This ultimately led to a strong correlation to partition coefficients related to drug permeability through human skin and a good model for what could be anticipated with in vivo barriers. One advantage of the IAM technique is that the lipid-based supports are commercially available, from vendors such as Regis Technologies,[327] though it remained limited in its correlation to membrane processes as this approach utilized effectively modeled a lipid monolayer rather than the complexities associated with a bilayer.[290]

Both ILC and IAM have been widely investigated as a predictor of biological interactions, including affinity parameters and determination of association and dissociation rate constants,[330] though few investigations have taken advantage of the unique resolving potential, especially of ILC. However, used in conjunction with mass spectrometry, ILC was used to identify and predict the permeability of a mixture of compounds present in a Chinese herbal medicine.[331] By varying the lipid content of the immobilized liposomes and composition and pH of the mobile phase, a better understanding of the bioactivity was attained for complex mixture of two traditional Chinese medicines commonly used in a combined prescription.[332] Recent advances have included an immobilized liposome column in two-dimensional separations in conjunction with reverse phase chromatography[333,334]; an affinity column allowing for competition between environmental bisphenol A (BPA) and BPA-phospholipase A2 conjugates, preceding a column with immobilized fluorophore-encapsulating liposomes, which relies on fluorescence detection[335]; and ILC methodology developed to study unique interactions with nucleic acids and phospholipids.[336] ILC and IAM are discussed in Chapters 9 and 10. Readers are directed to several excellent review articles for further discussion on these techniques as well.[319,337]

As introduced in the preceding section, liposomes have also been employed as pseudo-stationary phases in electrophoretic applications.[136] In that example, liposomes were employed to study drug–membrane partitioning. However, the utility of liposomes and lipid-based materials in capillary electorphoresis expands beyond such applications, for example, affording unique phases for separations. Separations of basic proteins driven by electrostatic interactions[338]; affinity-based separations of known activators versus inhibitors through liposome incorporation of membrane–protein transporters[339]; and enantiomeric separations allowing for separation of L-tryptophan and D-tryptophan have been accomplished using liposome-based CE.[340] The work in the laboratory of Dr. Susanne Wiedmer, which includes applications of LEKC as well as the development of numerous unique liposome-based coatings for CE, will be presented in Chapter 10. Her thorough work on ensuring stable coatings during preparation and usage has been influential in overcoming stability issues while improving performance and application potential.[340-342]

1.3.5 Liposomes in Imaging

Introduced previously in Section 1.3.1 were various applications using liposomes as intact species. These applications required that the vesicles retained their structure during the course of the analyses.

In microscopy applications, GM1 ganglioside embedded fluorescent liposomes have been utilized to provide visualization and signal proportional to cholera toxin binding events on human epithelial cells.[179] These liposomes were specifically formulated to afford recognition of the toxin through sandwich complex formation with the ganglioside on both the cells and the liposomes, yet avoid fusion of these species. The dual-labeled approach allowed for visualization of intact liposomes via microscopy, subsequent to sensitive binding measurements made through lysis and fluorescence measurements of released dye. A specific example was the visualization of cholera toxin binding events on epithelial cells in a culture model. In this assay, the fluorescent tag of the GM1-tagged lipid bilayer provided visualization of intact vesicles in microscopy (Fig. 1.27), followed by surfactant-induced release of encapsulated fluorescent contents for sensitive quantitative assessments in a plate reader (Fig. 1.28).[179]

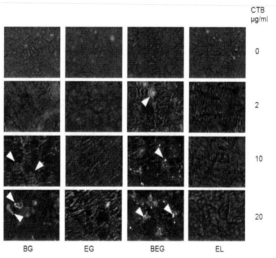

Figure 1.27 Fluorescence/Brightfield images of Caco-2 epithelial layers incubated with cholera toxin B and probed with GM1 ganglioside modified liposomes. Liposomes with GM1 ganglioside and (a) bilayer tagged with lissamine rhodamine PE, (b) encapsulating 150 mM SRB, (c) both bilayer tagged and encapsulating, and (d) encapsulating SRB, but not labeled with GM1 were used to probe Caco-2 cells incubated with 0, 2, 10, and 20 µg/ml CTB. Arrows indicate bound liposomes. Magnification is 40×. Reprinted from Ref. [179], Copyright 2008, with permission from Elsevier. http://www.sciencedirect.com/science/article/pii/S0003269708003278.

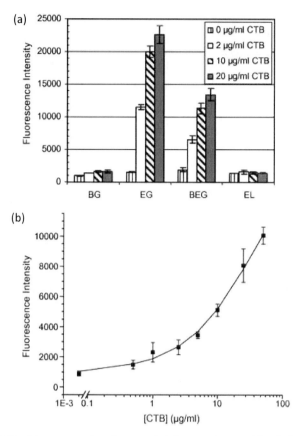

Figure 1.28 Liposomes forming sandwich complexes with cholera toxin B and Caco-2 epithelial cells were subsequently lysed to provide quantitative measurements in a fluorescence plate reader. (a) Those both encapsulating and bilayer tagged with fluorophores yielded optimal response and (b) yielded a proportional response over a range of toxin concentrations. Reprinted from Ref. [179], Copyright 2008, with permission from Elsevier. http://www.sciencedirect.com/science/article/pii/S0003269708003278.

In another application, PEGylated liposomes functionalized with anti-CD81 antibodies with fluorescently labeled lipids in their bilayers and encapsulating fluorescent dyes were employed to visualize HEK293 cells in a microfluidic device.[343] In these applications, the lipid composition was formulated to avoid nonspecific interactions of the liposomes with the cells. However, for many other studies, it is of greater benefit for the liposomes to fuse with the cells. For example, in vivo imaging applications, liposomes encapsulating paramagnetic gadolinium species,[344] iodine,[345] or bilayer-incorporated spin labels,[346] or amphiphilic gadolinium species[347] have been developed for use as medical imaging agents for MRI and CT. In such applications, the bilayer is often conjugated to antibodies to allow selective binding, subsequent to the delivery of contents by fusion to the tissue type under investigation. Benefits over the same agents administered as unencapsulated materials include improved targeting, uptake, contrast, and extended visualization time as well as reduced doses.[347-350] Utilizing fluorescent molecules, a similar approach may be taken for visualization of cell culture samples for microscopy applications. However, one of the challenges for using liposomes for such purposes includes poor fusion of the lipid bilayer with cells. Through work in the lab of Dr. Agnes Csiszár and colleagues, novel aromatic lipids in conjunction with appropriately charged lipid formulations have been developed with the result of high fusion efficiency and exceptionally vivid imaging of cells.[351] This and further work allowing visualization of membrane traffic processes while maintaining cellular function will be discussed in Chapter 11.[351,352]

1.3.6   Future Prospects

With a solid foundation from early investigations, the field of liposome-based analytics continues to evolve in exciting ways. Novel biorecognition elements have been used with liposome-based analyses. For example, liposomes conjugated to the maltose periplasmic binding protein have been shown to provide exceptional specificity toward the disaccharide maltose.[205] Furthering this line of inquiry to other periplasmic binding proteins can expand the analytical toolbox to other analytes, such as amino acids, inorganic ions, and vitamins, otherwise difficult for antibody-based strategies. Advances in the drug-delivery realm may provide new strategies for analytics—for example, liposomes conjugated to antimicrobial peptides used to deliver antimicrobial drugs to bacteria[353] may well serve as biorecognition elements in liposome-based analyses. Other approaches rely purely on chemically mediated recognition. Hegh et al. recently demonstrated that by embedding a lipophilic alkyl-amidine prosurfactant in the lipid bilayer, liposomes could be induced to release contents upon a decrease in pH, notably here, by the conversion of CO_2 to carbonic acid.[354] In this work, the addition of CO_2 yielded conversion of the prosurfactant to surfactant form, causing a change in the structure of its headgroup, destabilization of the bilayer, and release of encapsulated fluorescein.

Advances in synthetic organic chemistry may also give rise to more efficient functionalizations previously deemed prohibitive with standard chemistries; for example, "Click chemistry" approaches have been used to conjugate liposomes to sugars,[355,356] aptamers,[357] and peptides.[358] Other intriguing areas include novel means for control over liposome content release. Recent work has demonstrated lipids capable of undergoing conformational "flips," termed "flipids," in response to stimuli such as pH changes or metal complexation[359]; amino acid substitutions yielding proteins capable of serving as light-triggered gated large pores[360]; liposomes that release contents in response to a magnetic field[361,362]; and gold-coated liposomes, which can be triggered to release their contents upon stimulation with specific wavelengths of light.[363] While not currently in practice for analytical purposes, such liposomes have great potential especially in microfluidic platforms[364] where miniaturization and compartmentalization of functionalities are comparatively facile. Bridging the pharmaceutical divide, new platforms for drug testing, such as the phospholipid vesicle-based permeation assay used to assess skin or intestinal drug permeability, may reduce reliance on animal testing and provide cost-effective predictors of efficacy.[365,366] With exceptional researchers (including, but of course not limited to, the authors within) actively investigating new avenues, the outlook for novel liposome-based diagnostics and analytical platforms remains bright.

References

1. Bangham AD, Standish MM, Watkins JC. Diffusion of univalent ions across the lamellae of swollen phospholipids. *J Mol Biol.* 1965; 13(1): 238–252.

2. Sessa G, Weissmann G. Phospholipid spherules (liposomes) as a model for biological membranes. *J Lipid Res.* 1968; 9(3): 310–318.

3. Ottiger C, Wunderli-Allenspach H. Immobilized artificial membrane (IAM)-HPLC for partition studies of neutral and ionized acids and bases in comparison with the liposomal partition system. *Pharm Res.* 1999; 16(5): 643–650.

4. Razin S. Reconstruction of biological membranes. *Biochim Biophys Acta.* 1972; 265(2): 241–296.

5. Wei R, Alving CR, Richards RL, Copeland ES. Liposome spin immunoassay: A new sensitive method for detecting lipid substances in aqueous media. *J Immunol Methods.* 1975; 9(2): 165–170.

6. Andreoli TE. Planar lipid bilayer membranes. *Methods Enzymol.* 1974; 32: 513–539.

7. Lasic DD. The mechanism of vesicle formation. *Biochem J.* 1988; 256(1): 1–11.

8. Jesorka A, Orwar O. Liposomes: Technologies and analytical applications. *Annu Rev Anal Chem (Palo Alto Calif).* 2008; 1: 801–832.

9. Ulrich AS. Biophysical aspects of using liposomes as delivery vehicles. *Biosci Rep.* 2002; 22(2): 129–150.

10. Fiandaca M, Bankiewicz K. Micelles and liposomes: Lipid nanovehicles for intracerebral drug delivery. In: Kateb B, Heiss J, eds. *The Textbook of Nanoneuroscience and Nanoneurosurgery.* Boca Raton, FL: CRC Press; 2014: 51–64.

11. Balazs DA, Godbey WT. Liposomes for use in gene delivery. *J Drug Deliv.* 2011; 2011.

12. Tajima S, Sato R. Topological studies of the membrane-binding segment of cytochrome b5 embedded in phosphatidylcholine vesicles. *J Biochem.* 1980; 87(1): 123–134.

13. Arifin DR, Palmer AF. Determination of size distribution and encapsulation efficiency of liposome-encapsulated hemoglobin blood substitutes using asymmetric flow field-flow fractionation coupled with multi-angle static light scattering. *Biotechnol Prog.* 2003; 19(6): 1798–1811.

14. Huang YY, Chung TW, Wu CI. Effect of saturated/unsaturated phosphatidylcholine ratio on the stability of liposome-encapsulated hemoglobin. *Int J Pharm.* 1998; 172(1–2): 161–167.

15. Schneider T, Sachse A, Rößling G, Brandl M. Generation of contrast-carrying liposomes of defined size with a new continuous high pressure extrusion method. *Int J Pharm.* 1995; 117(1): 1–12.

16. Lesieur S, Grabielle-Madelmont C, Paternostre MT, Ollivon M. Size analysis and stability study of lipid vesicles by high-performance gel

exclusion chromatography, turbidity, and dynamic light scattering. *Anal Biochem*. 1991; 192(2): 334–343.

17. Benita S, Poly PA, Puisieux F, Delattre J. Radiopaque liposomes: Effect of formulation conditions on encapsulation efficiency. *J Pharm Sci*. 1984; 73(12): 1751–1755.

18. Yeagle PL. Cholesterol and the cell membrane. *Biochim Biophys Acta*. 1985; 822(3–4): 267–287.

19. Franks NP. Structural analysis of hydrated egg lecithin and cholesterol bilayers. I. X-ray diffraction. *J Mol Biol*. 1976; 100(3): 345–358.

20. Carroll TR, Davison A, Jones AG. Functional cholesteryl binding agents: Synthesis, characterization, and evaluation of antibody binding to modified phospholipid vesicles. *J Med Chem*. 1986; 29(10): 1821–1826.

21. Edwards KA, Baeumner AJ. Optimization of DNA-tagged dye-encapsulating liposomes for lateral-flow assays based on sandwich hybridization. *Anal Bioanal Chem*. 2006; 386(5): 1335–1343.

22. Edwards KA, Wang Y, Baeumner AJ. Aptamer sandwich assays: Human alpha-thrombin detection using liposome enhancement. *Anal Bioanal Chem*. 2010; 398(6): 2645–2654.

23. Miner-Williams W. Surfactant inhibition of cholesterol oxidase. *Clin Chim Acta*. 1980; 101(1): 77–84.

24. Junker LH, Story JA. An improved assay for cholesterol 7 alpha-hydroxylase activity using phospholipid liposome solubilized substrate. *Lipids*. 1985; 20(10): 712–718.

25. EnzChek® Phospholipase A2 Assay Kit. 2009; https://tools.lifetechnologies.com/content/sfs/manuals/mp10217.pdf. Accessed Feb. 28, 2015.

26. Ladbrooke BD, Chapman D. Thermal analysis of lipids, proteins and biological membranes. A review and summary of some recent studies. *Chem Phys Lipids*. 1969; 3(4): 304–356.

27. Szoka F, Jr., Papahadjopoulos D. Comparative properties and methods of preparation of lipid vesicles (liposomes). *Annu Rev Biophys Bioeng*. 1980; 9: 467–508.

28. Jacobson K, Papahadjopoulos D. Phase transitions and phase separations in phospholipid membranes induced by changes in temperature, pH, and concentration of bivalent cations. *Biochemistry*. 1975; 14(1): 152–161.

29. Bangham AD, Hill MW, Miller NGA. Preparation and use of liposomes as models of biological membranes. *Methods Membr Biol*. 1974; 1: 1–68.

30. Barenholz Y, Lasic DD. An overview of liposome scaled-up production and quality control. In: Barenholz Y, Lasic DD, eds. *Handbook of Nonmedical Applications of Liposomes*. Vol 3: CRC Press; 1996: 368.

31. Walde P, Ichikawa S. Enzymes inside lipid vesicles: Preparation, reactivity and applications. *Biomol Eng*. 2001; 18(4): 143–177.

32. Genc R, Murphy D, Fragoso A, Ortiz M, O'Sullivan CK. Signal-enhancing thermosensitive liposomes for highly sensitive immunosensor development. *Anal Chem*. 2011; 83(2): 563–570.

33. Kung VT, Redemann CT. Synthesis of carboxyacyl derivatives of phosphatidylethanolamine and use as an efficient method for conjugation of protein to liposomes. *Biochim Biophys Acta*. 1986; 862(2): 435–439.

34. Allen TM, Brandeis E, Hansen CB, Kao GY, Zalipsky S. A new strategy for attachment of antibodies to sterically stabilized liposomes resulting in efficient targeting to cancer cells. *Biochim Biophys Acta*. 1995; 1237(2): 99–108.

35. Maruyama K, Takizawa T, Yuda T, Kennel SJ, Huang L, Iwatsuru M. Targetability of novel immunoliposomes modified with amphipathic poly(ethylene glycol)s conjugated at their distal terminals to monoclonal antibodies. *Biochim Biophys Acta*. 1995; 1234(1): 74–80.

36. Ho RJ, Huang L. Interactions of antigen-sensitized liposomes with immobilized antibody: A homogeneous solid-phase immunoliposome assay. *J Immunol*. 1985; 134(6): 4035–4040.

37. Edwards KA, Baeumner AJ. Synthesis of a liposome incorporated 1-carboxyalkylxanthine-phospholipid conjugate and its recognition by an RNA aptamer. *Talanta*. 2007; 71(1): 365–372.

38. Redwood WR, Polefka TG. Lectin-receptor interactions in liposomes. II. Interaction of wheat germ agglutinin with phosphatidylcholine liposomes containing incorporated monosialoganglioside. *Biochim Biophys Acta*. 1976; 455(3): 631–643.

39. Rondelli V, Fragneto G, Motta S, et al. Ganglioside GM1 forces the redistribution of cholesterol in a biomimetic membrane. *Biochim Biophys Acta*. 2012; 1818(11): 2860–2867.

40. O'Brien DF, Klingbiel RT, Specht DP, Tyminski PN. Preparation and characterization of polymerized liposomes. *Ann. N. Y. Acad Sci*. 1985; 446: 282–295.

41. Johnston DS, Sanghera S, Pons M, Chapman D. Phospholipid polymers: Synthesis and spectral characteristics. *Biochim Biophys Acta*. 1980; 602(1): 57–69.

42. Hupfer B, Ringsdorf H, Schupp H. Liposomes from polymerizable phospholipids. *Chem Phys Lipids.* 1983; 33(4): 355–374.

43. Walsh CL, Nguyen J, Szoka FC. Synthesis and characterization of novel zwitterionic lipids with pH-responsive biophysical properties. *Chem Commun (Camb).* 2012; 48(45): 5575–5577.

44. Needham D, Anyarambhatla G, Kong G, Dewhirst MW. A new temperature-sensitive liposome for use with mild hyperthermia: Characterization and testing in a human tumor xenograft model. *Cancer Res.* 2000; 60(5): 1197–1201.

45. Ho RJ, Rouse BT, Huang L. Target-sensitive immunoliposomes: Preparation and characterization. *Biochemistry.* 1986; 25(19): 5500–5506.

46. Nagle JF, Tristram-Nagle S. Structure of lipid bilayers. *Biochim Biophys Acta.* 2000; 1469(3): 159–195.

47. Gregoriadis G. The carrier potential of liposomes in biology and medicine (first of two parts). *N Engl J Med.* 1976; 295(13): 704–710.

48. Gregoriadis G. The carrier potential of liposomes in biology and medicine (second of two parts). *N Engl J Med.* 1976; 295(14): 765–770.

49. Willis MC, Collins BD, Zhang T, et al. Liposome-anchored vascular endothelial growth factor aptamers. *Bioconjug Chem.* 1998; 9(5): 573–582.

50. Park JW, Benz CC, Martin FJ. Future directions of liposome- and immunoliposome-based cancer therapeutics. *Semin Oncol.* 2004; 31(6 Suppl 13): 196–205.

51. Papahadjopoulos D, Heath T, Bragman K, Matthay K. New methodology for liposome targeting to specific cells. *Ann N Y Acad Sci.* 1985; 446: 341–348.

52. Soriano P, Dijkstra J, Legrand A, et al. Targeted and nontargeted liposomes for in vivo transfer to rat liver cells of a plasmid containing the preproinsulin I gene. *Proc Natl Acad Sci U S A.* 1983; 80(23): 7128–7131.

53. Spanjer HH, Scherphof GL. Targeting of lactosylceramide-containing liposomes to hepatocytes in vivo. *Biochim Biophys Acta.* 1983; 734(1): 40–47.

54. Duzgunes N, Pretzer E, Simoes S, et al. Liposome-mediated delivery of antiviral agents to human immunodeficiency virus-infected cells. *Mol Membr Biol.* 1999; 16(1): 111–118.

55. Mann AP, Bhavane RC, Somasunderam A, et al. Thioaptamer conjugated liposomes for tumor vasculature targeting. *Oncotarget.* 2011; 2(4): 298–304.

56. Umezawa F, Eto Y. Liposome targeting to mouse brain: Mannose as a recognition marker. *Biochem Biophys Res Commun.* 1988; 153(3): 1038–1044.

57. Lee RJ, Low PS. Delivery of liposomes into cultured KB cells via folate receptor-mediated endocytosis. *J Biol Chem.* 1994; 269(5): 3198–3204.

58. Huwyler J, Wu D, Pardridge WM. Brain drug delivery of small molecules using immunoliposomes. *Proc Natl Acad Sci U S A.* 1996; 93(24): 14164–14169.

59. Pardridge WM. Vector-mediated drug delivery to the brain. *Adv Drug Deliv Rev.* 1999; 36(2–3): 299–321.

60. Schnyder A, Huwyler J. Drug transport to brain with targeted liposomes. *NeuroRx.* 2005; 2(1): 99–107.

61. Drummond DC, Meyer O, Hong K, Kirpotin DB, Papahadjopoulos D. Optimizing liposomes for delivery of chemotherapeutic agents to solid tumors. *Pharmacol Rev.* 1999; 51(4): 691–743.

62. Dvorak HF, Nagy JA, Dvorak AM. Structure of solid tumors and their vasculature: Implications for therapy with monoclonal antibodies. *Cancer Cells.* 1991; 3(3): 77–85.

63. Dudley AC. Tumor endothelial cells. *Cold Spring Harb Perspect Med.* 2012; 2(3): a006536.

64. Maeda H, Bharate GY, Daruwalla J. Polymeric drugs for efficient tumor-targeted drug delivery based on EPR-effect. *Eur J Pharm Biopharm.* 2009; 71(3): 409–419.

65. Abraham SA, Waterhouse DN, Mayer LD, Cullis PR, Madden TD, Bally MB. The liposomal formulation of doxorubicin. *Methods Enzymol.* 2005; 391: 71–97.

66. Abra RM, Hunt CA. Liposome disposition in vivo. III. Dose and vesicle-size effects. *Biochim Biophys Acta.* 1981; 666(3): 493–503.

67. Senior JH. Fate and behavior of liposomes in vivo: A review of controlling factors. *Crit Rev Ther Drug Carrier Syst.* 1987; 3(2): 123–193.

68. Lasic DD, Papahadjopoulos D. Liposomes revisited. *Science.* 1995; 267(5202): 1275–1276.

69. Lasic DD. Novel applications of liposomes. *Trends Biotechnol.* 1998; 16(7): 307–321.

70. Barenholz Y. Doxil(R)—the first FDA-approved nano-drug: Lessons learned. *J Control Release*. 2012; 160(2): 117–134.

71. Woodle MC, Lasic DD. Sterically stabilized liposomes. *Biochim Biophys Acta*. 1992; 1113(2): 171–199.

72. Working PK, Newman MS, Huang SK, Mayhew E, Vaage J, Lasic DD. Pharmacokinetics, biodistribution, and therapeutic efficacy of doxorubicin encapsulated in Stealth® liposomes. *J Liposome Res*. 1994; 4(1): 667–687.

73. Allen TM, Chonn A. Large unilamellar liposomes with low uptake into the reticuloendothelial system. *FEBS Lett*. 1987; 223(1): 42–46.

74. Fresta M, Wehrli E, Puglisi G. Enhanced therapeutic effect of cytidine-5'-diphosphate choline when associated with GM1 containing small liposomes as demonstrated in a rat ischemia model. *Pharm Res*. 1995; 12(11): 1769–1774.

75. Gilden D. KS: A new drug and, maybe, a new bug. *GMHC Treat Issues*. 1995; 9(1): 11–12.

76. FDA approves DaunoXome as first-line therapy for Kaposi's sarcoma. Food and Drug Administration. *J Int Assoc Physicians AIDS Care*. 1996; 2(5): 50–51.

77. Muggia FM. Liposomal encapsulated anthracyclines: New therapeutic horizons. *Curr Oncol Rep*. 2001; 3(2): 156–162.

78. Tejada-Berges T, Granai CO, Gordinier M, Gajewski W. Caelyx/Doxil for the treatment of metastatic ovarian and breast cancer. *Expert Rev Anticancer Ther*. 2002; 2(2): 143–150.

79. Murry DJ, Blaney SM. Clinical pharmacology of encapsulated sustained-release cytarabine. *Ann Pharmacother*. 2000; 34(10): 1173–1178.

80. Meyerhoff A. U.S. Food and Drug Administration approval of AmBisome (liposomal amphotericin B) for treatment of visceral leishmaniasis. *Clin Infect Dis*. 1999; 28(1): 42–48; discussion 49–51.

81. Baker R. Early approval for two lipid-based drugs. *Beta*. 1995: 4.

82. Vogel JD. Liposome bupivacaine (EXPAREL®) for extended pain relief in patients undergoing ileostomy reversal at a single institution with a fast-track discharge protocol: An IMPROVE Phase IV health economics trial. *J Pain Res*. 2013; 6: 605–610.

83. Angst MS, Drover DR. Pharmacology of drugs formulated with DepoFoam: A sustained release drug delivery system for parenteral administration using multivesicular liposome technology. *Clin Pharmacokinet*. 2006; 45(12): 1153–1176.

84. Hagemeister F, Rodriguez MA, Deitcher SR, et al. Long term results of a phase 2 study of vincristine sulfate liposome injection (Marqibo(®) substituted for non-liposomal vincristine in cyclophosphamide, doxorubicin, vincristine, prednisone with or without rituximab for patients with untreated aggressive non-Hodgkin lymphomas. *Br J Haematol.* 2013; 162(5): 631–638.

85. Harrison TS, Lyseng-Williamson KA. Vincristine sulfate liposome injection: A guide to its use in refractory or relapsed acute lymphoblastic leukemia. *BioDrugs.* 2013; 27(1): 69–74.

86. Schaeffer HE, Krohn DL. Liposomes in topical drug delivery. *Invest Ophthalmol Vis Sci.* 1982; 22(2): 220–227.

87. Kirjavainen M, Urtti A, Jaaskelainen I, et al. Interaction of liposomes with human skin in vitro: The influence of lipid composition and structure. *Biochim Biophys Acta.* 1996; 1304(3): 179–189.

88. Pierre MB, Dos Santos Miranda Costa I. Liposomal systems as drug delivery vehicles for dermal and transdermal applications. *Arch Dermatol Res.* 2011; 303(9): 607–621.

89. Aquaron R, Forzano O, Murati JL, Fayet G, Aquaron C, Ridings B. Simple, reliable and fast spectrofluorometric method for determination of plasma Verteporfin (Visudyne) levels during photodynamic therapy for choroidal neovascularization. *Cell Mol Biol* (*Noisy-le-grand*). 2002; 48(8): 925–930.

90. Yarosh D, Bucana C, Cox P, Alas L, Kibitel J, Kripke M. Localization of liposomes containing a DNA repair enzyme in murine skin. *J Invest Dermatol.* 1994; 103(4): 461–468.

91. Yarosh D, Klein J, O'Connor A, Hawk J, Rafal E, Wolf P. Effect of topically applied T4 endonuclease V in liposomes on skin cancer in xeroderma pigmentosum: A randomised study. Xeroderma Pigmentosum Study Group. *Lancet.* 2001; 357(9260): 926–929.

92. Sarasin A. Progress and prospects of xeroderma pigmentosum therapy. *Adv Exp Med Biol.* 2008; 637: 144–151.

93. Cafardi JA, Elmets CA. T4 endonuclease V: Review and application to dermatology. *Expert Opin Biol Ther.* 2008; 8(6): 829–838.

94. Ceccoli J, Rosales N, Tsimis J, Yarosh DB. Encapsulation of the UV-DNA repair enzyme T4 endonuclease V in liposomes and delivery to human cells. *J Invest Dermatol.* 1989; 93(2): 190–194.

95. Visser CC, Stevanovic S, Voorwinden LH, et al. Targeting liposomes with protein drugs to the blood-brain barrier in vitro. *Eur J Pharm Sci.* 2005; 25(2–3): 299–305.

96. Pardridge WM. Drug targeting to the brain. *Pharm Res.* 2007; 24(9): 1733–1744.

97. Tao Y, Han J, Dou H. Brain-targeting gene delivery using a rabies virus glycoprotein peptide modulated hollow liposome: Bio-behavioral study. *J Mater Chem.* 2012; 22(23): 11808–11815.

98. Salvati E, Re F, Sesana S, et al. Liposomes functionalized to overcome the blood-brain barrier and to target amyloid-beta peptide: The chemical design affects the permeability across an in vitro model. *Int J Nanomedicine.* 2013; 8: 1749–1758.

99. Felgner PL, Gadek TR, Holm M, et al. Lipofection: A highly efficient, lipid-mediated DNA-transfection procedure. *Proc Natl Acad Sci U S A.* 1987; 84(21): 7413–7417.

100. Caplen NJ, Gao X, Hayes P, et al. Gene therapy for cystic fibrosis in humans by liposome-mediated DNA transfer: The production of resources and the regulatory process. *Gene Ther.* 1994; 1(2): 139–147.

101. Lasic DD, Templeton NS. Liposomes in gene therapy. *Adv Drug Deliv Rev.* 1996; 20(2–3): 221–266.

102. Whitemore M, Li S, Huang L. Liposome vectors for in vivo gene delivery. *Curr Protoc Hum Genet.* 2001; Chapter 12: Unit 12 18.

103. Lee JH, Lee MJ. Liposome-mediated cancer gene therapy: Clinical trials and their lessons to stem cell therapy. *Bull Korean Chem Soc.* 2012; 33(2): 433–442.

104. Gluck R, Walti E. Biophysical validation of Epaxal Berna, a hepatitis A vaccine adjuvanted with immunopotentiating reconstituted influenza virosomes (IRIV). *Dev Biol (Basel).* 2000; 103: 189–197.

105. Gluck R. Intranasal immunization against influenza. *J Aerosol Med.* 2002; 15(2): 221–228.

106. Chang HI, Yeh MK. Clinical development of liposome-based drugs: Formulation, characterization, and therapeutic efficacy. *Int J Nanomedicine.* 7: 49–60.

107. Oberg C, Welsh N. Nonspecific delivery of substances into pancreatic islet cells by pH-sensitive liposomes in vitro. *Diabete Metab.* 1990; 16(1): 48–54.

108. Connor J, Norley N, Huang L. Biodistribution of pH-sensitive immunoliposomes. *Biochim Biophys Acta.* 1986; 884(3): 474–481.

109. Sullivan SM, Huang L. Enhanced delivery to target cells by heat-sensitive immunoliposomes. *Proc Natl Acad Sci U S A.* 1986; 83(16): 6117–6121.

110. Bassett JB, Anderson RU, Tacker JR. Use of temperature-sensitive liposomes in the selective delivery of methotrexate and cis-platinum analogues to murine bladder tumor. *J Urol.* 1986; 135(3): 612–615.

111. Sullivan SM, Huang L. Preparation and characterization of heat-sensitive immunoliposomes. *Biochim Biophys Acta.* 1985; 812(1): 116–126.

112. Liburdy RP, Tenforde TS, Magin RL. Magnetic field-induced drug permeability in liposome vesicles. *Radiat Res.* 1986; 108(1): 102–111.

113. Allen TM, Cullis PR. Liposomal drug delivery systems: From concept to clinical applications. *Adv Drug Deliv Rev.* 2012; 65(1): 36–48.

114. Langner M, Kral TE. Liposome-based drug delivery systems. *Pol J Pharmacol.* 1999; 51(3): 211–222.

115. Sadozai H, Saeidi D. Recent developments in liposome-based veterinary therapeutics. *ISRN Vet Sci.* 2013; 2013: 167521.

116. Taylor TM, Davidson PM, Bruce BD, Weiss J. Liposomal nanocapsules in food science and agriculture. *Crit Rev Food Sci Nutr.* 2005; 45(7–8): 587–605.

117. Gibbs BF, Kermasha S, Alli I, Mulligan CN. Encapsulation in the food industry: A review. *Int J Food Sci Nutr.* 1999; 50(3): 213–224.

118. Betz G, Aeppli A, Menshutina N, Leuenberger H. In vivo comparison of various liposome formulations for cosmetic application. *Int J Pharm.* 2005; 296(1–2): 44–54.

119. Wilhelm KM, Graham JK, Squires EL. Effects of phosphatidylserine and cholesterol liposomes on the viability, motility, and acrosomal integrity of stallion spermatozoa prior to and after cryopreservation. *Cryobiology.* 1996; 33(3): 320–329.

120. Padilla AW, Tobback C, Foote RH. Penetration of frozen-thawed, zona-free hamster oocytes by fresh and slow-cooled stallion spermatozoa. *J Reprod Fertil Suppl.* 1991; 44: 207–212.

121. Graham JK, Foote RH. Dilauroylphosphatidylcholine liposome effects on the acrosome reaction and in vitro penetration of zona-free hamster eggs by bull sperm: I. A fertility assay for fresh semen. *Gamete Res.* 1987; 16(2): 133–145.

122. Dees C, Stringfellow D, Schultz RD. Incorporation of a follicle stimulating hormone used for embryo transfer in cattle into multilamellar liposomes. *Theriogenology.* 1984; 21(4): 661–675.

123. Weiner N, Lieb L, Niemiec S, Ramachandran C, Hu Z, Egbaria K. Liposomes: A novel topical delivery system for pharmaceutical and cosmetic applications. *J Drug Target.* 1994; 2(5): 405–410.

124. Lu Q, Li DC, Jiang JG. Preparation of a tea polyphenol nanoliposome system and its physicochemical properties. *J Agric Food Chem.* 2011; 59(24): 13004–13011.

125. el Soda M, Pannell L, Olson N. Microencapsulated enzyme systems for the acceleration of cheese ripening. *J Microencapsul.* 1989; 6(3): 319–326.

126. Takahashi M, Uechi S, Takara K, Asikin Y, Wada K. Evaluation of an oral carrier system in rats: Bioavailability and antioxidant properties of liposome-encapsulated curcumin. *J Agric Food Chem.* 2009; 57(19): 9141–9146.

127. O'Connell JP, Campbell RL, Fleming BM, Mercolino TJ, Johnson MD, McLaurin DA. A highly sensitive immunoassay system involving antibody-coated tubes and liposome-entrapped dye. *Clin Chem.* 1985; 31(9): 1424–1426.

128. Rule GS, Montagna RA, Durst RA. Characteristics of DNA-tagged liposomes allowing their use in capillary-migration, sandwich-hybridization assays. *Anal Biochem.* 1997; 244(2): 260–269.

129. Tsukagoshi K, Okumura Y, Akasaka H, Nakajima R. Electrophoretic behavior of dyestuff-containing liposome in a capillary with original on-line chemiluminescence detection. *Anal Sci.* 1996; 12: 869–874.

130. Kannuck RM, Bellama JM, Durst RA. Measurement of liposome-released ferrocyanide by a dual-function polymer modified electrode. *Anal Chem.* 1988; 60(2): 142–147.

131. Yoon CH, Cho JH, Oh HI, et al. Development of a membrane strip immunosensor utilizing ruthenium as an electro-chemiluminescent signal generator. *Biosens Bioelectron.* 2003; 19(4): 289–296.

132. Zhan W, Bard AJ. Electrogenerated chemiluminescence. 83. Immunoassay of human C-reactive protein by using Ru(bpy)32+-encapsulated liposomes as labels. *Anal Chem.* 2006; 79(2): 459–463.

133. Nasseau M, Boublik Y, Meier W, Winterhalter M, Fournier D. Substrate-permeable encapsulation of enzymes maintains effective activity, stabilizes against denaturation, and protects against proteolytic degradation. *Biotechnol Bioeng.* 2001; 75(5): 615–618.

134. Walde P, Marzetta B. Bilayer permeability-based substrate selectivity of an enzyme in liposomes. *Biotechnol Bioeng.* 1998; 57(2): 216–219.

135. Roberts MA, Locascio-Brown L, Maccrehan WA, Durst RA. Liposome behavior in capillary electrophoresis. *Anal Chem.* 1996; 68(19): 3434–3440.

136. Zhang Y, Zhang R, Hjerten S, Lundahl P. Liposome capillary electrophoresis for analysis of interactions between lipid bilayers and solutes. *Electrophoresis.* 1995; 16(8): 1519–1523.

137. Hautala JT, Linden MV, Wiedmer SK, et al. Simple coating of capillaries with anionic liposomes in capillary electrophoresis. *J Chromatogr A.* 2003; 1004(1–2): 81–90.

138. Wink T, van Zuilen SJ, Bult A, van Bennekom WP. Liposome-mediated enhancement of the sensitivity in immunoassays of proteins and peptides in surface plasmon resonance spectrometry. *Anal Chem.* 1998; 70(5): 827–832.

139. Hyun S-J, Kim H-S, Kim Y-J, Jung II-I. Mechanical detection of liposomes using piezoresistive cantilever. *Sensor Actuat B-Chem.* 2006; 117(2): 415–419.

140. Chen H, Jiang JH, Li YF, Deng T, Shen GL, Yu RQ. A novel piezoelectric immunoagglutination assay technique with antibody-modified liposome. *Biosens Bioelectron.* 2007; 22(6): 993–999.

141. Rongen HA, Bult A, van Bennekom WP. Liposomes and immunoassays. *J Immunol Methods.* 1997; 204(2): 105–133.

142. Lasic DD, Barenholz Y. *Handbook of Nonmedical Applications of Liposomes.* Vol IV: CRC Press; 1996.

143. Gómez-Hens A, Manuel Fernández-Romero J. The role of liposomes in analytical processes. *TrAC Trends in Analytical Chemistry.* 2005; 24(1): 9–19.

144. Edwards KA, Baeumner AJ. Liposomes in analyses. *Talanta.* 2006; 68(5): 1421–1431.

145. Liu Q, Boyd BJ. Liposomes in biosensors. *The Analyst.* 2013; 138(2): 391–409.

146. Singh A, Schoeniger J, Carbonell R. Liposomes as Signal-Enhancement Agents in immunodiagnostic applications. In: Yang V, Ngo T, eds. *Biosensors and Their Applications*: Springer US; 2000: 131–145.

147. Singer JM, Plotz CM. The latex fixation test. *Am J Med.* 21(6): 888–892.

148. Uemura K-I, Yuzawa-Watanabe M, Kitazawa N, Taketomi T. Liposome agglutination and liposomal membrane immune-damage assays for the characterization of antibodies to glycosphingolipids. *J Biochem.* 1980; 87(6): 1641–1648.

149. Yoshioka H, Ohmura T, Hasegawa M, Hirota S, Makino M, Kamiya M. Synthesis of galactose derivatives that render lectin-induced agglutinating ability to liposomes. *J Pharm Sci.* 1993; 82(3): 273–275.

150. Torchilin VP, Levchenko TS, Lukyanov AN, et al. p-Nitrophenylcarbonyl-PEG-PE-liposomes: Fast and simple attachment of specific ligands, including monoclonal antibodies, to distal ends of PEG chains via p-nitrophenylcarbonyl groups. *Biochim Biophys Acta, Biomembr.* 2001; 1511(2): 397–411.

151. Ueno T, Tanaka S, Umeda M. Liposome turbidimetric assay (LTA). *Adv Drug Deliv Rev.* 1997; 24(2–3): 293–299.

152. Tiwari RP, Garg SK, Bharmal RN, Kartikeyan S, Bisen PS. Rapid liposomal agglutination card test for the detection of antigens in patients with active tuberculosis. *Int J Tuberc Lung Dis.* 2007; 11(10): 1143–1151.

153. Chen H, Jiang J-H, Li Y-F, Deng T, Shen G-L, Yu R-Q. A novel piezoelectric immunoagglutination assay technique with antibody-modified liposome. *Biosensors Bioelectron.* 2007; 22(6): 993–999.

154. Tiwari RP, Tiwari D, Garg SK, Chandra R, Bisen PS. Glycolipids of *Mycobacterium tuberculosis* strain H37Rv are potential serological markers for diagnosis of active tuberculosis. *Clin Diagn Lab Immunol.* 2005; 12(3): 465–473.

155. Kung VT, Vollmer YP, Martin FJ. Large liposome agglutination technique for the serological detection of syphilis. *J Immunol Methods.* 1986; 90(2): 189–196.

156. O'Connell JP, Piran, Uri., Wagner, Daniel B., Inventor; Becton Dickinson and Company (Franklin Lakes, NJ) assignee. Sac or liposome containing dye (sulforhodamine) for immunoassay US patent 4,695,554. March 27, 1985, 1987.

157. Campbell RL, Wagner, Daniel B., O'Connell, James P., Inventor; Becton Dickinson and Company (Franklin Lakes, NJ) assignee. Solid phase assay with visual readout. US patent 4,703,017. February 14, 1984, 1987.

158. COLOR PAC™ TOXIN A LABORATORY PROCEDURE http://www.bd.com/ds/technicalCenter/clsi/clsi-COLORPAC.pdf. Accessed August 13, 2013.

159. Gerber MA, Randolph MF, DeMeo KK. Liposome immunoassay for rapid identification of group A streptococci directly from throat swabs. *J Clin Microbiol.* 1990; 28(6): 1463–1464.

160. Ozinskas AJ. Probe design and chemical sensing. In: Lakowicz JR, ed. *Topics in Fluorescence Spectroscopy.* Vol 4. New York: Plenum Press; 1994: 449–496.

161. BD ColorPAC™ Toxin A Test. 2005; http://www.bd.com/ds/technicalCenter/promotionalFlyers/ss-colorpac.pdf. Accessed August 15, 2013.

162. Vanpoucke H, De Baere T, Claeys G, Vaneechoutte M, Verschraegen G. Evaluation of six commercial assays for the rapid detection of Clostridium difficile toxin and/or antigen in stool specimens. *Clin Microbiol Infect.* 2001; 7(2): 55–64.

163. Martorell D, Siebert ST, Durst RA. Liposome dehydration on nitrocellulose and its application in a biotin immunoassay. *Anal Biochem.* 1999; 271(2): 177–185.

164. Ahn-Yoon S, DeCory TR, Durst RA. Ganglioside-liposome immunoassay for the detection of botulinum toxin. *Anal Bioanal Chem.* 2004; 378(1): 68–75.

165. Wen HW, Borejsza-Wysocki W, DeCory TR, Durst RA. Development of a competitive liposome-based lateral flow assay for the rapid detection of the allergenic peanut protein Ara h1. *Anal Bioanal Chem.* 2005; 382(5): 1217–1226.

166. Roberts MA, Durst RA. Investigation of liposome-based immunomigration sensors for the detection of polychlorinated biphenyls. *Anal Chem.* 1995; 67(3): 482–491.

167. Ho JA, Zeng SC, Tseng WH, Lin YJ, Chen CH. Liposome–based immunostrip for the rapid detection of Salmonella. *Anal Bioanal Chem.* 2008; 391(2): 479–485.

168. Ho JA, Hsu HW. Procedures for preparing *Escherichia coli* O157: H7 immunoliposome and its application in liposome immunoassay. *Anal Chem.* 2003; 75(16): 4330–4334.

169. Kumada Y, Maehara M, Katoh S. Characteristics of microblotting assay using immunoliposomes. *J Biosci Bioeng.* 2004; 98(2): 129–131.

170. Kumada Y, Maehara M, Tomioka K, Katoh S. Liposome immunoblotting assay using a substrate-forming precipitate inside immunoliposomes. *Biotechnol Bioeng.* 2002; 80(4): 414–418.

171. Yanagisawa H, Hirano A, Sugawara M. A dot-blot method for quantification of apurinic/apyrimidinic sites in DNA using an avidin plate and liposomes encapsulating a fluorescence dye. *Anal Biochem.* 2004; 332(2): 358–367.

172. Legros F, Schietecat P, Leroy CP, Van Vooren JP. An automated micromethod for detection of lytic antimycobacterial antibodies by immune lysis of liposomes sensitized to tuberculin. *J Immunoassay.* 1989; 10(4): 359–372.

173. Tsao YS, Huang L. Sendai virus induced leakage of liposomes containing gangliosides. *Biochemistry.* 1985; 24(5): 1092–1098.

174. Van Renswoude J, Hoekstra D. Cell-induced leakage of liposome contents. *Biochemistry.* 1981; 20(3): 540–546.

175. Chen RF, Knutson JR. Mechanism of fluorescence concentration quenching of carboxyfluorescein in liposomes: Energy transfer to nonfluorescent dimers. *Anal Biochem.* 1988; 172(1): 61–77.

176. Truneh A, Machy P, Horan PK. Antibody-bearing liposomes as multicolor immunofluorescence markers for flow cytometry and imaging. *J Immunol Methods.* 1987; 100(1–2): 59–71.

177. Singh AK, Harrison SH, Schoeniger JS. Gangliosides as receptors for biological toxins: Development of sensitive fluoroimmunoassays using ganglioside-bearing liposomes. *Anal Chem.* 2000; 72(24): 6019–6024.

178. Singh AK, Kilpatrick PK, Carbonell RG. Application of antibody and fluorophore-derivatized liposomes to heterogeneous immunoassays for d-dimer. *Biotechnol Prog.* 1996; 12(2): 272–280.

179. Edwards KA, Duan F, Baeumner AJ, March JC. Fluorescently labeled liposomes for monitoring cholera toxin binding to epithelial cells. *Anal Biochem.* 2008; 380(1): 59–67.

180. Lu KY, Tao SC, Yang TC, et al. Profiling lipid-protein interactions using nonquenched fluorescent liposomal nanovesicles and proteome microarrays. *Mol Cell Proteomics.* 2012; 11(11): 1177–1190.

181. Chaize B, Nguyen M, Ruysschaert T, et al. Microstructured liposome array. *Bioconjug Chem.* 2006; 17(1): 245–247.

182. Shoji A, Sugimoto E, Orita S, et al. A reusable liposome array and its application to assay of growth-hormone-related peptides. *Anal Bioanal Chem.* 2010; 397(3): 1377–1381.

183. Bally M, Bailey K, Sugihara K, Grieshaber D, Voros J, Stadler B. Liposome and lipid bilayer arrays towards biosensing applications. *Small.* 2010; 6(22): 2481–2497.

184. Laukkanen ML, Orellana A, Keinanen K. Use of genetically engineered lipid-tagged antibody to generate functional europium chelate-loaded liposomes. Application in fluoroimmunoassay. *J Immunol Methods.* 1995; 185(1): 95–102.

185. Orellana A, Laukkanen ML, Keinanen K. Europium chelate-loaded liposomes: A tool for the study of binding and integrity of liposomes. *Biochim Biophys Acta.* 1996; 1284(1): 29–34.

186. Pihlasalo S, Hara M, Hanninen P, Slotte JP, Peltonen J, Harma H. Liposome-based homogeneous luminescence resonance energy transfer. *Anal Biochem.* 2009; 384(2): 231–237.

187. Lee HY, Jung HS, Fujikawa K, et al. New antibody immobilization method via functional liposome layer for specific protein assays. *Biosens Bioelectron.* 2005; 21(5): 833–838.

188. Gunnarsson A, Sjovall P, Hook F. Liposome-based chemical barcodes for single molecule DNA detection using imaging mass spectrometry. *Nano Lett.* 2010; 10(2): 732–737.

189. Pons M, Johnston DS, Chapman D. The optical activity and circular dichroic spectra of diacetylenic phospholipid polymers. *Biochim Biophys Acta.* 1982; 693(2): 461–465.

190. Charych DH, Nagy JO, Spevak W, Bednarski MD. Direct colorimetric detection of a receptor-ligand interaction by a polymerized bilayer assembly. *Science.* 1993; 261(5121): 585–588.

191. Kim Y-R, Jung S, Yoo Y-E, Kim SM, Jeon T-J. Synthetic biomimetic membranes and their sensor applications. *Sensors.* 2012; 12(7): 9530–9550.

192. Charych D, Cheng Q, Reichert A, et al. A "litmus test" for molecular recognition using artificial membranes. *Chem Biol.* 1996; 3(2): 113–120.

193. Reppy MA, Pindzola BA. Biosensing with polydiacetylene materials: Structures, optical properties and applications. *Chem Commun (Camb).* 2007(42): 4317–4338.

194. Reichert A, Nagy JO, Spevak W, Charych D. Polydiacetylene liposomes functionalized with sialic acid bind and colorimetrically detect influenza virus. *J Am Chem Soc.* 1995; 115: 1146–1147.

195. Su YL, Li JR, Jiang L, Cao J. Biosensor signal amplification of vesicles functionalized with glycolipid for colorimetric detection of *Escherichia coli. J Colloid Interface Sci.* 2005; 284(1): 114–119.

196. Rangin M, Basu A. Lipopolysaccharide identification with functiona-lized polydiacetylene liposome sensors. *J Am Chem Soc.* 2004; 126(16): 5038–5039.

197. Ji E, Ahn DJ, Kim J. The fluorescent polydiacetylene liposome. *Bull Korean Chem Soc.* 2003; 24(5): 667–670.

198. Lee J, Kim HJ, Kim J. Polydiacetylene liposome arrays for selective potassium detection. *J Am Chem Soc.* 2008; 130(15): 5010–5011.

199. Lee J, Jun H, Kim J. Polydiacetylene–liposome microarrays for selective and sensitive mercury(II) detection. *Adv Mater.* 2008; 21(36): 3674–3677.

200. Gaber BP, Ligler FS, Bredehorst R. Liposome-based immunoassays for detection of small and large molecules. *Adv Exp Med Biol.* 1988; 238: 209–214.

201. Mason JT, Xu L, Sheng ZM, O'Leary TJ. A liposome-PCR assay for the ultrasensitive detection of biological toxins. *Nat Biotechnol.* 2006; 24(5): 555–557.

202. Ruiz J, Goni FM, Alonso A. Surfactant-induced release of liposomal contents. A survey of methods and results. *Biochim Biophys Acta.* 1988; 937(1): 127–134.

203. Edwards KA, Curtis KL, Sailor JL, Baeumner AJ. Universal liposomes: Preparation and usage for the detection of mRNA. *Anal Bioanal Chem.* 2008; 391(5): 1689–1702.

204. Edwards KA, Meyers KJ, Leonard B, Baeumner AJ. Superior performance of liposomes over enzymatic amplification in a high-throughput assay for myoglobin in human serum. *Anal Bioanal Chem.* 2013; 405(12): 4017–4026.

205. Edwards KA, Baeumner AJ. Periplasmic binding protein-based detection of maltose using liposomes: A new class of biorecognition elements in competitive assays. *Anal Chem.* 2013; 85(5): 2770–2778.

206. Rongen HAH, van der Horst HM, Hugenholtz GWK, Bult A, van Bennekom WP, van der Meide PH. Development of a liposome immunosorbent assay for human interferon-γ. *Anal Chim Acta.* 1994; 287(3): 191–199.

207. Rongen HAH, van Nierop T, van der Horst HM, et al. Biotinylated and streptavidinylated liposomes as labels in cytokine immunoassays. *Anal Chim Acta.* 1995; 306(2–3): 333–341.

208. Yap WT, Locascio-Brown L, Plant AL, Choquette SJ, Horvath V, Durst RA. Liposome flow injection immunoassay: Model calculations of competitive immunoreactions involving univalent and multivalent ligands. *Anal Chem.* 1991; 63(18): 2007–2011.

209. Locascio-Brown L, Plant AL, Horvath V, Durst RA. Liposome flow injection immunoassay: Implications for sensitivity, dynamic range, and antibody regeneration. *Anal Chem.* 1990; 62(23): 2587–2593.

210. Locascio-Brown L, Plant AL, Chesler R, Kroll M, Ruddel M, Durst RA. Liposome-based flow-injection immunoassay for determining theophylline in serum. *Clin Chem.* 1993; 39(3): 386–391.

211. Ho JA, Chiu JK, Hong JC, Lin CC, Hwang KC, Hwu JR. Gold-nanostructured immunosensor for the electrochemical sensing of biotin based on liposomal competitive assay. *J Nanosci Nanotechnol.* 2009; 9(4): 2324–2329.

212. Locascio LE, Hong JS, Gaitan M. Liposomes as signal amplification reagents for bioassays in microfluidic channels. *Electrophoresis.* 2002; 23(5): 799–804.

213. Kwakye S, Baeumner A. A microfluidic biosensor based on nucleic acid sequence recognition. *Anal Bioanal Chem.* 2003; 376(7): 1062–1068.

214. Lee M, Durst RA, Wong RB. Development of flow-injection liposome immunoanalysis (FILIA) for imazethapyr. *Talanta*. 1998; 46(5): 851–859.

215. Hendrickson OD, Skopinskaya SN, Yarkov SP, Zherdev AV, Dzantiev BB. Development of liposome immune lysis assay for the herbicide atrazine. *J Immunoassay Immunochem*. 2004; 25(3): 279–294.

216. Paul A, Madan S, Vasandani VM, Ghosh PC, Bachhawat BK. Liposome immune lysis assay (LILA) for gelonin. *J Immunol Methods*. 1992; 148(1–2): 151–158.

217. Locascio-Brown L, Choquette SJ. Measuring estrogens using flow injection immunoanalysis with liposome amplification. *Talanta*. 1993; 40(12): 1899–1904.

218. Lee M, Durst RA, Wong RB. Comparison of liposome amplification and fluorophore detection in flow-injection immunoanalyses. *Anal Chim Acta*. 1997; 354: 23–28.

219. Szebeni J, Baranyi L, Savay S, et al. The interaction of liposomes with the complement system: In vitro and in vivo assays. *Methods Enzymol*. 2003; 373: 136–154.

220. Haxby JA, Gotze O, Muller-Eberhard HJ, Kinsky SC. Release of trapped marker from liposomes by the action of purified complement components. *Proc Natl Acad Sci U S A*. 1969; 64(1): 290–295.

221. Hsia JC, Tan CT. Membrane immunoassay: Principle and applications of spin membrane immunoassay. *Ann N Y Acad Sci*. 1978; 308: 139–148.

222. Haga M, Sugawara S, Itagaki H. Drug sensor: Liposome immunosensor for theophylline. *Anal Biochem*. 1981; 118(2): 286–293.

223. Chan SW, Tan CT, Hsia JC. Spin membrane immunoassay: Simplicity and specificity. *J Immunol Methods*. 1978; 21(1–2): 185–195.

224. Leute R, Ullman EF, Goldstein A. Spin immunoassay of opiate narcotics in urine and saliva. *JAMA*. 1972; 221(11): 1231–1234.

225. Leute RK, Ullman EF, Goldstein A, Herzenberg LA. Spin immunoassay technique for determination of morphine. *Nat New Biol*. 1972; 236(64): 93–94.

226. Autokit CH50. 995–40801: http://www.wakodiagnostics.com/pi/pi_autokit_ch50.pdf. Accessed February 23, 2012.

227. Shiba K, Watanabe T, Umezawa Y, Fujiwara S. Liposome immuno-electrode. *Chem Lett*. 1980; 2: 155–158.

228. Geiger B, Smolarsky M. Immunochemical determination of ganglioside GM2, by inhibition of complement-dependent liposome lysis. *J Immunol Methods*. 1977; 17(1–2): 7–19.

229. Ishimori Y, Yasuda T, Tsumita T, Notsuki M, Koyama M, Tadakuma T. Liposome immune lysis assay (LILA): A simple method to measure anti-protein antibody using protein antigen-bearing liposomes. *J Immunol Methods.* 1984; 75(2): 351–360.

230. Umeda M, Ishimori Y, Yoshikawa K, Takada M, Yasuda T. Liposome immune lysis assay (LILA). Application of sandwich method to determine a serum protein component with antibody-bearing liposomes. *J Immunol Methods.* 1986; 95(1): 15–21.

231. Six HR, Young WW, Jr., Uemura K, Kinsky SC. Effect of antibody-complement on multiple vs. single compartment liposomes. Application of a fluorometric assay for following changes in liposomal permeability. *Biochemistry.* 1974; 13(19): 4050–4058.

232. Umeda M, Ishimori Y, Yoshikawa K, Takada M, Yasuda T. Homogeneous determination of C-reactive protein in serum using liposome immune lysis assay (LILA). *Jpn J Exp Med.* 1986; 56(1): 35–42.

233. Ligler FS, Bredehorst R, Talebian A, et al. A homogeneous immunoassay for the mycotoxin T-2 utilizing liposomes, monoclonal antibodies, and complement. *Anal Biochem.* 1987; 163(2): 369–375.

234. Kobayashi K, Watarai S, Yasuda T. Sensitive detection of ganglioside GD3 on the cell surface using liposome immune lysis assay. *Acta Med Okayama.* 1992; 46(6): 435–441.

235. Litchfield WJ, Freytag JW, Adamich M. Highly sensitive immunoassays based on use of liposomes without complement. *Clin Chem.* 1984; 30(9): 1441–1445.

236. Schreier H, Valentino K, Heath BP, Kung VT. Prevention of nonspecific lysis in liposomal and erythrocyte immunoassay systems by small lipid vesicles and erythrocyte ghosts. *Life Sci.* 1989; 45(20): 1919–1930.

237. Kim CK, Park KM. Liposome immunoassay (LIA) for gentamicin using phospholipase C. *J Immunol Methods.* 1994; 170(2): 225–231.

238. Lim SJ, Kim CK. Homogeneous liposome immunoassay for insulin using phospholipase C from Clostridium perfringens. *Anal Biochem.* 1997; 247(1): 89–95.

239. Terwilliger TC, Eisenberg D. The structure of melittin. II. Interpretation of the structure. *J Biol Chem.* 1982; 257(11): 6016–6022.

240. Freytag JW, Litchfield WJ. Liposome-mediated immunoassays for small haptens (digoxin) independent of complement. *J Immunol Methods.* 1984; 70(2): 133–140.

241. Gervais C, Do F, Cantin A, et al. Development and validation of a high-throughput screening assay for the hepatitis C virus p7 viroporin. *J Biomol Screen.* 2011; 16(3): 363–369.

242. Kim HJ, Bennetto HP, Halablab MA. A novel liposome-based electrochemical biosensor for the detection of haemolytic microorganisms. *Biotechnol Tech.* 1995; 9(6): 389–394.

243. Xu D, Cheng Q. Surface-bound lipid vesicles encapsulating redox species for amperometric biosensing of pore-forming bacterial toxins. *J Am Chem Soc.* 2002; 124(48): 14314–14315.

244. Zhao J, Jedlicka SS, Lannu JD, Bhunia AK, Rickus JL. Liposome-doped nanocomposites as artificial-cell-based biosensors: Detection of listeriolysin O. *Biotechnol Prog.* 2006; 22(1): 32–37.

245. Andersen OS, Koeppe RE, 2nd, Roux B. Gramicidin channels. *IEEE Trans Nanobioscience.* 2005; 4(1): 10–20.

246. Kelkar DA, Chattopadhyay A. The gramicidin ion channel: A model membrane protein. *Biochim Biophys Acta.* 2007; 1768(9): 2011–2025.

247. Horie M, Yanagisawa H, Sugawara M. Fluorometric immunoassay based on pH-sensitive dye-encapsulating liposomes and gramicidin channels. *Anal Biochem.* 2007; 369(2): 192–201.

248. Hirano A, Wakabayashi M, Matsuno Y, Sugawara M. A single-channel sensor based on gramicidin controlled by molecular recognition at bilayer lipid membranes containing receptor. *Biosens Bioelectron.* 2003; 18(8): 973–983.

249. Reinholt SJ, Behrent A, Greene C, Kalfe A, Baeumner AJ. Isolation and Amplification of mRNA within a Simple Microfluidic Lab on a Chip. *Anal Chem.* 86(1): 849–856.

250. Zaytseva NV, Montagna RA, Baeumner AJ. Microfluidic biosensor for the serotype-specific detection of dengue virus RNA. *Anal Chem.* 2005; 77(23): 7520–7527.

251. Connelly JT, Kondapalli S, Skoupi M, Parker JS, Kirby BJ, Baeumner AJ. Micro-total analysis system for virus detection: Microfluidic pre-concentration coupled to liposome-based detection. *Anal Bioanal Chem.* 2012; 402(1): 315–323.

252. Wongkaew N, He P, Kurth V, Surareungchai W, Baeumner AJ. Multi-channel PMMA microfluidic biosensor with integrated IDUAs for electrochemical detection. *Anal Bioanal Chem.* 405(18): 5965–5974.

253. Liao WC, Ho JA. Attomole DNA electrochemical sensor for the detection of *Escherichia coli* O157. *Anal Chem.* 2009; 81(7): 2470–2476.

254. Viswanathan S, Wu LC, Huang MR, Ho JA. Electrochemical immunosensor for cholera toxin using liposomes and poly(3,4-ethylenedioxythiophene)-coated carbon nanotubes. *Anal Chem.* 2006; 78(4): 1115–1121.

255. Viswanathan S, Rani C, Vijay Anand A, Ho JA. Disposable electrochemical immunosensor for carcinoembryonic antigen using ferrocene liposomes and MWCNT screen-printed electrode. *Biosens Bioelectron.* 2009; 24(7): 1984–1989.

256. Ekong TA, McLellan K, Sesardic D. Immunological detection of Clostridium botulinum toxin type A in therapeutic preparations. *J Immunol Methods.* 1995; 180(2): 181–191.

257. Chao HY, Wang YC, Tang SS, Liu HW. A highly sensitive immuno-polymerase chain reaction assay for Clostridium botulinum neurotoxin type A. *Toxicon.* 2004; 43(1): 27–34.

258. Edwards KA, March JC. GM(1)-functionalized liposomes in a microtiter plate assay for cholera toxin in Vibrio cholerae culture samples. *Anal Biochem.* 2007; 368(1): 39–48.

259. Ahn-Yoon S, DeCory TR, Baeumner AJ, Durst RA. Ganglioside-liposome immunoassay for the ultrasensitive detection of cholera toxin. *Anal Chem.* 2003; 75(10): 2256–2261.

260. Jo SM, Lee HY, Kim JC. Glucose-sensitive liposomes incorporating hydrophobically modified glucose oxidase. *Lipids.* 2008; 43(10): 937–943.

261. Klappe K, Wilschut J, Nir S, Hoekstra D. Parameters affecting fusion between Sendai virus and liposomes. Role of viral proteins, liposome composition, and pH. *Biochemistry.* 1986; 25(25): 8252–8260.

262. Miller CR, Bondurant B, McLean SD, McGovern KA, O'Brien DF. Liposome-cell interactions in vitro: Effect of liposome surface charge on the binding and endocytosis of conventional and sterically stabilized liposomes. *Biochemistry.* 1998; 37(37): 12875–12883.

263. Dan N. Effect of liposome charge and PEG polymer layer thickness on cell-liposome electrostatic interactions. *Biochim Biophys Acta.* 2002; 1564(2): 343–348.

264. Eriksson H, Mattiasson B, Sjogren HO. Lectin-mediated binding of liposome-inserted membrane proteins to red blood cells. A method to detect binding of antibodies to purified rat histocompatibility antigen or binding of insulin to the insulin receptor. *J Immunol Methods.* 1984; 75(1): 167–179.

265. Umeda M, Kanda S, Nojima S, Wiegandt H, Inoue K. Interaction between glycophorin and ganglioside GM1 on liposomal membranes. Effect of the interaction on the susceptibility of membranes to HVJ. *J Biochem.* 1984; 96(1): 229–235.

266. Shiffer KA, Goerke J, Duzgunes N, Fedor J, Shohet SB. Interaction of erythrocyte protein 4.1 with phospholipids. A monolayer and liposome study. *Biochim Biophys Acta.* 1988; 937(2): 269–280.

267. Losey EA, Smith MD, Meng M, Best MD. Microplate-based analysis of protein-membrane binding interactions via immobilization of whole liposomes containing a biotinylated anchor. *Bioconjug Chem.* 2009; 20(2): 376–383.

268. Bilek G, Kremser L, Wruss J, Blaas D, Kenndler E. Mimicking early events of virus infection: Capillary electrophoretic analysis of virus attachment to receptor-decorated liposomes. *Anal Chem.* 2007; 79(4): 1620–1625.

269. Weiss VU, Bilek G, Pickl-Herk A, Blaas D, Kenndler E. Mimicking virus attachment to host cells employing liposomes: analysis by chip electrophoresis. *Electrophoresis.* 2009; 30(12): 2123–2128.

270. Zheng F, Wu Z, Chen Y. A quantitative method for the measurement of membrane affinity by polydiacetylene-based colorimetric assay. *Anal Biochem.* 2012; 420(2): 171–176.

271. Epand RM, Nir S, Parolin M, Flanagan TD. The role of the ganglioside GD1a as a receptor for Sendai virus. *Biochemistry.* 1995; 34(3): 1084–1089.

272. Yavin E. Gangliosides mediate association of tetanus toxin with neural cells in culture. *Arch Biochem Biophys.* 1984; 230(1): 129–137.

273. MacKenzie CR, Hirama T, Lee KK, Altman E, Young NM. Quantitative analysis of bacterial toxin affinity and specificity for glycolipid receptors by surface plasmon resonance. *J Biol Chem.* 1997; 272(9): 5533–5538.

274. Richards RL, Fishman PH, Moss J, Alving CR. Binding of choleragen and anti-ganglioside antibodies to gangliosides incorporated into preformed liposomes. *Biochim Biophys Acta.* 1983; 733(2): 249–255.

275. Guthmann MD, Bitton RJ, Carnero AJ, et al. Active specific immunotherapy of melanoma with a GM3 ganglioside-based vaccine: A report on safety and immunogenicity. 2004; 27(6): 442–451.

276. Jonah MM, Cerny EA, Rahman YE. Tissue distribution of EDTA encapsulated within liposomes containing glycolipids or brain phospholipids. *Biochim Biophys Acta.* 1978; 541(3): 321–333.

277. Arnon R, Crisp E, Kelley R, Ellison GW, Myers LW, Tourtellotte WW. Anti-ganglioside antibodies in multiple sclerosis. *J Neurol Sci.* 1980; 46(2): 179–186.

278. Poole SK, Poole CF. Separation methods for estimating octanol-water partition coefficients. *J Chromatogr B Analyt Technol Biomed Life Sci.* 2003; 797(1–2): 3–19.

279. Betageri GV, Rogers JA. Correlation of partitioning of nitroimidazoles in the n-octanol/saline and liposome systems with pharmacokinetic parameters and quantitative structure-activity relationships (QSAR). *Pharm Res.* 1989; 6(5): 399–403.

280. Choi YW, Rogers JA. The liposome as a model membrane in correlations of partitioning with alpha-adrenoceptor agonist activities. *Pharm Res.* 1990; 7(5): 508–512.

281. Esteves F, Moutinho C, Matos C. Correlation between octanol/water and liposome/water distribution coefficients and drug absorption of a set of pharmacologically active compounds. *J Liposome Res.* 2013; 23(2): 83–93.

282. Yamamoto H, Liljestrand HM. Partitioning of selected estrogenic compounds between synthetic membrane vesicles and water: Effects of lipid components. *Environ Sci Technol.* 2004; 38(4): 1139–1147.

283. van der Heijden SA, Jonker MT. Evaluation of liposome-water partitioning for predicting bioaccumulation potential of hydrophobic organic chemicals. *Environ Sci Technol.* 2009; 43(23): 8854–8859.

284. Boija E, Johansson G. Interactions between model membranes and lignin-related compounds studied by immobilized liposome chromatography. *Biochim Biophys Acta.* 2006; 1758(5): 620–626.

285. Zhang Y, Aimoto S, Lu L, Yang Q, Lundahl P. Immobilized liposome chromatography for analysis of interactions between lipid bilayers and peptides. *Anal Biochem.* 1995; 229(2): 291–298.

286. Liu XY, Nakamura C, Yang Q, Kamo N, Miyake J. Immobilized liposome chromatography to study drug–membrane interactions. Correlation with drug absorption in humans. *J Chromatogr A.* 2002; 961(1): 113–118.

287. Balaz S, Kuchar A, Drevojanek J, Adamcova J, Vrbanova A. Liposome/saline partition coefficients of low-molecular-weight solutes by gel chromatography. *J Biochem Biophys Methods.* 1988; 16(1): 75–85.

288. Beigi F, Yang Q, Lundahl P. Immobilized-liposome chromatographic analysis of drug partitioning into lipid bilayers. *J Chromatogr A.* 1995; 704(2): 315–321.

289. Carrozzino JM, Khaledi MG. Interaction of basic drugs with lipid bilayers using liposome electrokinetic chromatography. *Pharm Res.* 2004; 21(12): 2327–2335.

290. Burns ST, Khaledi MG. Rapid determination of liposome-water partition coefficients (Klw) using liposome electrokinetic chromatography (LEKC). *J Pharm Sci.* 2002; 91(7): 1601–1612.

291. Wiedmer SK, Kulovesi P, Riekkola ML. Liposome electrokinetic capillary chromatography in the study of analyte-phospholipid membrane interactions. Application to pesticides and related compounds. *J Sep Sci.* 2008; 31(14): 2714–2721.

292. Helle A, Makitalo J, Huhtanen J, Holopainen JM, Wiedmer SK. Antibiotic fusidic acid has strong interactions with negatively charged lipid membranes: An electrokinetic capillary chromatographic study. *Biochim Biophys Acta.* 2008; 1778(11): 2640–2647.

293. Muhonen J, Holopainen JM, Wiedmer SK. Interactions between local anesthetics and lipid dispersions studied with liposome electrokinetic capillary chromatography. *J Chromatogr A.* 2009; 1216(15): 3392–3397.

294. Balon K, Riebesehl BU, Muller BW. Drug liposome partitioning as a tool for the prediction of human passive intestinal absorption. *Pharm Res.* 1999; 16(6): 882–888.

295. Betageri GV, Dipali SR. Partitioning and thermodynamics of dipyridamole in the n-octanol/buffer and liposome systems. *J Pharm Pharmacol.* 1993; 45(10): 931–933.

296. Przybylo M, Borowik T, Langner M. Application of liposome based sensors in high-throughput screening systems. *Comb Chem High Throughput Screen.* 2007; 10(6): 441–450.

297. van Balen GP, Martinet C, Caron G, et al. Liposome/water lipophilicity: Methods, information content, and pharmaceutical applications. *Med Res Rev.* 2004; 24(3): 299–324.

298. Wan H, Holmen AG. High throughput screening of physicochemical properties and in vitro ADME profiling in drug discovery. *Comb Chem High Throughput Screen.* 2009; 12(3): 315–329.

299. Baird CL, Courtenay ES, Myszka DG. Surface plasmon resonance characterization of drug/liposome interactions. *Anal Biochem.* 2002; 310(1): 93–99.

300. Branden M, Dahlin S, Hook F. Label-free measurements of molecular transport across liposome membranes using evanescent-wave sensing. *Chemphyschem.* 2008; 9(17): 2480–2485.

301. Branden M, Tabaei SR, Fischer G, Neutze R, Hook F. Refractive-index-based screening of membrane-protein-mediated transfer across biological membranes. *Biophys J.* 2010; 99(1): 124–133.

302. Onishi M, Kamimori H. High-throughput and sensitive assay for amphotericin B interaction with lipid membrane on the model membrane systems by surface plasmon resonance. *Biol Pharm Bull.* 2013; 36(4): 658–663.

303. Wallner J, Lhota G, Jeschek D, Mader A, Vorauer-Uhl K. Application of Bio-Layer Interferometry for the analysis of protein/liposome interactions. *J Pharm Biomed Anal.* 2013; 72: 150–154.

304. McWhirter A. Biacore® S51 in predictive ADME studies. *Biacore Journal* 2003; https://www.biacore.com/lifesciences/technology/publications/journal/index.html?section=lifesciences&realsection=lifesciences&c=10199&d=10208&do=download&id=10224. Accessed October 1, 2012.

305. Temmerman K, Nickel W. A novel flow cytometric assay to quantify interactions between proteins and membrane lipids. *J Lipid Res.* 2009; 50(6): 1245–1254.

306. Przybylo M, Olzynska A, Han S, Ozyhar A, Langner M. A fluorescence method for determining transport of charged compounds across lipid bilayer. *Biophys Chem.* 2007; 129(2–3): 120–125.

307. Kupcu S, Sara M, Sleytr UB. Liposomes coated with crystalline bacterial cells surface protein (S-layer) as immobilization structures for macromolecules. *Biochim Biophys Acta.* 1995; 1235(2): 263–269.

308. Thanyani ST, Roberts V, Siko DG, Vrey P, Verschoor JA. A novel application of affinity biosensor technology to detect antibodies to mycolic acid in tuberculosis patients. *J Immunol Methods.* 2008; 332(1–2): 61–72.

309. Schleicher GK, Feldman C, Vermaak Y, Verschoor JA. Prevalence of anti-mycolic acid antibodies in patients with pulmonary tuberculosis co-infected with HIV. *Clin Chem Lab Med.* 2002; 40(9): 882–887.

310. Elhassan M, Elhassan O, Dirar A, Abbas E, Elmekki M. Validity of antimycolic acids antibodies in the diagnosis of pulmonary tuberculosis in TB/HIV co-infected patients in Khartoum State, Sudan *Egypt Acad J Biolog Sci.* 2011; 3(1): 27–32.

311. Lemmer Y, Thanyani ST, Vrey PJ, et al. Chapter 5: Detection of antimycolic acid antibodies by liposomal biosensors. *Methods Enzymol.* 2009; 464: 79–104.

312. Erb EM, Chen X, Allen S, et al. Characterization of the surfaces generated by liposome binding to the modified dextran matrix of a surface plasmon resonance sensor chip. *Anal Biochem.* 2000; 280(1): 29–35.

313. Graneli A, Reimhult E, Svedhem S, Pfeiffer I, Hook F, Inventors. Surface immobilised multilayer structure of vesicles. Apr 7, 2004, 2004.

314. Graneli A, Edvardsson M, Hook F. DNA-based formation of a supported, three-dimensional lipid vesicle matrix probed by QCM-D and SPR. *Chemphyschem.* 2004; 5(5): 729–733.

315. Graneli A. Incorporation of a transmembrane protein into a supported 3D-matrix of liposomes for SPR studies. *Methods Mol Biol.* 2010; 627: 237–248.

316. Wymann MP, Schneiter R. Lipid signalling in disease. *Nat Rev Mol Cell Biol.* 2008; 9(2): 162–176.

317. Connell E, Scott P, Davletov B. Real-time assay for monitoring membrane association of lipid-binding domains. *Anal Biochem.* 2008; 377(1): 83–88.

318. Demian DJ, Clugston SL, Foster MM, et al. High-throughput, cell-free, liposome-based approach for assessing in vitro activity of lipid kinases. *J Biomol Screen.* 2009; 14(7): 838–844.

319. Lundahl P, Yang Q. Liposome chromatography: Liposomes immobilized in gel beads as a stationary phase for aqueous column chromato-graphy. *J Chromatogr.* 1991; 544(1–2): 283–304.

320. Yang Q, Liu XY, Yoshimoto M, Kuboi R, Miyake J. Covalent immobilization of unilamellar liposomes in gel beads for chromatography. *Anal Biochem.* 1999; 268(2): 354–362.

321. Yang Q, Wallsten M, Lundahl P. Immobilization of phospholipid vesicles and protein–lipid vesicles containing red cell membrane proteins on octyl derivatives of large-pore gels. *Biochim Biophys Acta.* 1988; 938(2): 243–256.

322. Yang Q, Lundahl P. Immobilized proteoliposome affinity chroma-tography for quantitative analysis of specific interactions between solutes and membrane proteins. Interaction of cytochalasin B and D-glucose with the glucose transporter Glut1. *Biochemistry.* 1995; 34(22): 7289–7294.

323. Osterberg T, Svensson M, Lundahl P. Chromatographic retention of drug molecules on immobilised liposomes prepared from egg phospholipids and from chemically pure phospholipids. *Eur J Pharm Sci.* 2001; 12(4): 427–439.

324. Zhang Y, Zeng CM, Li YM, Hjerten S, Lundahl P. Immobilized liposome chromatography of drugs on capillary continuous beds for model analysis of drug–membrane interactions. *J Chromatogr A.* 1996; 749(1–2): 13–18.

325. Pidgeon C, Ong S, Liu H, et al. IAM chromatography: An in vitro screen for predicting drug–membrane permeability. *J Med Chem.* 1995; 38(4): 590–594.

326. Ong S, Liu H, Pidgeon C. Immobilized-artificial-membrane chromatography: Measurements of membrane partition coefficient and predicting drug–membrane permeability. *J Chromatogr A*. 1996; 728(1–2): 113–128.

327. IAM Chromatography. http://www.registech.com/Library/Catalog/IAM_2008.pdf. Accessed December 5, 2013.

328. Barbato F, La Rotonda MI, Quaglia F. Chromatographic indexes on immobilized artificial membranes for local anesthetics: Relationships with activity data on closed sodium channels. *Pharm Res*. 1997; 14(12): 1699–1705.

329. Barbato F, Cappello B, Miro A, La Rotonda MI, Quaglia F. Chromatographic indexes on immobilized artificial membranes for the prediction of transdermal transport of drugs. *Farmaco*. 1998; 53(10–11): 655–661.

330. Ohno M, Ikehara T, Nara T, Kamo N, Miyauchi S. The elution profile of immobilized liposome chromatography: Determination of association and dissociation rate constants. *Biochim Biophys Acta*. 2004; 1665(1–2): 167–176.

331. Mao X, Kong L, Luo Q, Li X, Zou H. Screening and analysis of permeable compounds in Radix Angelica Sinensis with immobilized liposome chromatography. *J Chromatogr B Analyt Technol Biomed Life Sci*. 2002; 779(2): 331–339.

332. Sheng LH, Li SL, Kong L, et al. Separation of compounds interacting with liposome membrane in combined prescription of traditional Chinese medicines with immobilized liposome chromatography. *J Pharm Biomed Anal*. 2005; 38(2): 216–224.

333. Wang Y, Kong L, Lei X, et al. Comprehensive two-dimensional high-performance liquid chromatography system with immobilized liposome chromatography column and reversed-phase column for separation of complex traditional Chinese medicine Longdan Xiegan Decoction. *J Chromatogr A*. 2009; 1216(11): 2185–2191.

334. Chen X, Kong L, Sheng L, Li X, Zou H. Applications of two-dimensional liquid chromatography coupled to mass spectrometry for the separation and identification of compounds in ginkgo biloba extracts. *Se Pu*. 2005; 23(1): 46–51.

335. Liu XY, Nakamura C, Tanimoto I, et al. High sensitivity detection of bisphenol A using liposome chromatography. *Anal Chim Acta*. 2006; 578(1): 43–49.

336. Suleymanoglu E. Phospholipid-nucleic acid recognition: Developing an immobilized liposome chromatography for DNA separation and analysis. *PDA J Pharm Sci Technol*. 2006; 60(4): 232–239.

337. Stewart BH, Helen Chan O. Use of immobilized artificial membrane chromatography for drug transport applications. *J Pharm Sci*. 1998; 87(12): 1471–1478.

338. Corradini D, Mancini G, Bello C. Use of liposomes as a dispersed pseudo-stationary phase in capillary electrophoresis of basic proteins. *J Chromatogr A*. 2004; 1051(1–2): 103–110.

339. Jiang J, Geng L, Qu F, Luo A, Li H, Deng Y. Application of protein-liposome conjugate as a pseudo-stationary phase in capillary electrophoresis. *J Chromatogr Sci*. 2007; 45(9): 587–592.

340. Wiedmer SK, Bo T, Riekkola ML. Phospholipid-protein coatings for chiral capillary electrochromatography. *Anal Biochem*. 2008; 373(1): 26–33.

341. Hautala JT, Wiedmer SK, Riekkola ML. Influence of pH on formation and stability of phosphatidylcholine/phosphatidylserine coatings in fused-silica capillaries. *Electrophoresis*. 2005; 26(1): 176–186.

342. Wiedmer SK, Jussila M, Hakala RM, Pystynen KH, Riekkola ML. Piperazine-based buffers for liposome coating of capillaries for electrophoresis. *Electrophoresis*. 2005; 26(10): 1920–1927.

343. Reisewitz S, Schroeder H, Tort N, Edwards KA, Baeumner AJ, Niemeyer CM. Capture and culturing of living cells on microstructured DNA substrates. *Small*. 2010; 6(19): 2162–2168.

344. Fossheim SL, Fahlvik AK, Klaveness J, Muller RN. Paramagnetic liposomes as MRI contrast agents: Influence of liposomal physicochemical properties on the in vitro relaxivity. *Magn Reson Imaging*. 1999; 17(1): 83–89.

345. Wei X, Geng F, He D, Qiu J, Xu Y. Liposomal contrast agent for CT imaging of the liver. *Conf Proc IEEE Eng Med Biol Soc*. 2005; 6: 5702–5705.

346. Grant CW, Barber KR, Florio E, Karlik S. A phospholipid spin label used as a liposome-associated MRI contrast agent. *Magn Reson Med*. 1987; 5(4): 371–376.

347. Kabalka GW, Buonocore E, Hubner K, Davis M, Huang L. Gadolinium-labeled liposomes containing paramagnetic amphipathic agents: Targeted MRI contrast agents for the liver. *Magn Reson Med*. 1988; 8(1): 89–95.

348. Jendrasiak GL, Frey GD, Heim RC, Jr. Liposomes as carriers of iodolipid radiocontrast agents for CT scanning of the liver. *Invest Radiol.* 1985; 20(9): 995–1002.

349. Balcar I, Seltzer SE, Davis S, Geller S. CT patterns of splenic infarction: A clinical and experimental study. *Radiology.* 1984; 151(3): 723–729.

350. Grant CW, Karlik S, Florio E. A liposomal MRI contrast agent: Phosphatidylethanolamine-DTPA. *Magn Reson Med.* 1989; 11(2): 236–243.

351. Csiszár A, Hersch N, Dieluweit S, Biehl R, Merkel R, Hoffmann B. Novel fusogenic liposomes for fluorescent cell labeling and membrane modification. *Bioconjug Chem.* 2010; 21(3): 537–543.

352. Kleusch C, Hersch N, Hoffmann B, Merkel R, Csiszár A. Fluorescent lipids: Functional parts of fusogenic liposomes and tools for cell membrane labeling and visualization. *Molecules.* 2012; 17(1): 1055–1073.

353. Yang K, Gitter B, Ruger R, et al. Antimicrobial peptide-modified liposomes for bacteria targeted delivery of temoporfin in photodynamic antimicrobial chemotherapy. *Photochem Photobiol Sci.* 2011; 10(10): 1593–1601.

354. Hegh DY, Mackay SM, Tan EW. CO_2-triggered release from switchable surfactant impregnated liposomes. *RSC Advances.* 2014; 4(60): 31771–31774.

355. Frisch B, Hassane FS, Schuber F. Conjugation of ligands to the surface of preformed liposomes by click chemistry. 2010; 605: 267–277.

356. Said Hassane F, Frisch B, Schuber F. Targeted liposomes: Convenient coupling of ligands to preformed vesicles using "click chemistry". *Bioconjug Chem.* 2006; 17(3): 849–854.

357. Muller A, Konig B. Vesicular aptasensor for the detection of thrombin. 2014; 50(84): 12665–12668.

358. Accardo A, Ringhieri P, Tesauro D, Morelli G. Liposomes derivatized with tetrabranched neurotensin peptides via click chemistry reactions. *New J Chem.* 2013; 37(11): 3528–3534.

359. Samoshin VV. Fliposomes: Stimuli-triggered conformational flip of novel amphiphiles causes an instant cargo release from liposomes. *Biomolecular Concepts.* 2014; 5(2): 131–141.

360. Iscla I, Eaton C, Parker J, Wray R, Kovacs Z, Blount P. Improving the design of a MscL-based triggered nanovalve. *Biosensors.* 2013; 3(1): 171–184.

361. Chen Y, Bose A, Bothun GD. Controlled release from bilayer-decorated magnetoliposomes via electromagnetic heating. *ACS Nano.* 2010; 4(6): 3215–3221.

362. Amstad E, Kohlbrecher J, Muller E, Schweizer T, Textor M, Reimhult E. Triggered release from liposomes through magnetic actuation of iron oxide nanoparticle containing membranes. *Nano Lett.* 2011; 11(4): 1664–1670.

363. Wu G, Mikhailovsky A, Khant HA, Zasadzinski JA. Chapter 14: Synthesis, characterization, and optical response of gold nanoshells used to trigger release from liposomes. *Methods Enzymol.* 2009; 464: 279–307.

364. Edwards KA, Bolduc OR, Baeumner AJ. Miniaturized bioanalytical systems: Enhanced performance through liposomes. *Curr Opin Chem Biol.* 2012; 16(3–4): 444–452.

365. Engesland A, Skalko-Basnet N, Flaten GE. Phospholipid vesicle-based permeation assay and EpiSkin in assessment of drug therapies destined for skin administration. *J Pharm Sci.* 2014.

366. Naderkhani E, Isaksson J, Ryzhakov A, Flaten GE. Development of a biomimetic phospholipid vesicle-based permeation assay for the estimation of intestinal drug permeability. *J Pharm Sci.* 2014; 103(6): 1882–1890.

Chapter 2

Applications of Liposomal Nanovesicles in Lateral Flow Assays

Hsiao-Wei Wen, Wen-Che Tsai, Pei-Tzu Chu, and Hsin-Yi Yin

Department of Food Science and Biotechnology,
National Chung-Hsing University, Taichung, Taiwan

hwwen@nhcu.edu.tw

2.1 Introduction

The lateral flow assay (LFA), also known as the immunochromato-graphic assay or the test strip assay, was developed in the late 1960s to find serum proteins.[1] This assay format has been used in home pregnancy tests to detect human chorionic gonadotropin (hCG) in the urine specimens of pregnant women, since hCG rises rapidly and predictably in the early stage of pregnancy.[2,3] With a few drops of urine sample into the round well of the cassette containing a test strip, the result can be observed based on the appearance of color bands in the observation window within 5–10 min. In 1988, the first commercial home pregnancy test was marketed by Unipath Ltd, the former owners of the Clearblue® brand. This test is a urine-based single-step LFA and is simple enough to be used by untrained consumers. Until now, LFAs have been used for the qualification, semi-quantification, or quantification of target

Liposomes in Analytical Methodologies
Edited by Katie A. Edwards
Copyright © 2016 Pan Stanford Publishing Pte. Ltd.
ISBN 978-981-4669-26-9 (Hardcover), 978-981-4669-27-6 (eBook)
www.panstanford.com

analytes, such as pathogens,[4,5] hormones,[2,6] abused drugs,[7,8] heavy metals,[9,10] pesticides,[11,12] or herbicides,[13,14] for use in clinical, veterinary, agricultural, environmental, and biodefense applications.[15,16] The LFA is widely used because it is portable, rapid, sensitive, and user friendly and so can be used for on-site detection, either as an over-the-counter or as a point-of-care product, by untrained operators, while providing reliable results.[17]

Beyond the traditional LFA, which detects one target per test in a binary fashion with a yes/no answer, barcode-style LFAs with multiple test lines per strip have been developed for either the semi-quantification of one target per strip or the simultaneous detection of multiple targets per strip, as presented in Fig. 2.1. As an example of semi-quantification (Fig. 2.1a), a barcode-style LFA was developed to estimate levels of C-reactive protein (CRP) in blood, which is an inflammation marker generated in response to bacterial infection. Since typically CRP is increased in bacterial infection, instead of viral infection, it has been used as a plasma maker to differentiate bacterial infections from viral infections.[18] Moreover, mild elevations of CRP (10 to 100 mg/L) are commonly observed in patients with infection or with bacteremia.[19] In Renneberg's study, anti-CRP-mouse IgG was used as the capture antibody for CRP on the CRP test zone; anti-mouse IgG was used for capturing anti-CRP-mouse IgG tagged colloidal gold on the control zone. With the use of anti-CRP-IgG tagged colloidal gold as the detection reagent, the intensity and number of red test lines on a strip are directly proportional to the CRP concentration due to sandwich complex formation and this assay can predict five levels of inflammation. If only one line appears, it indicates a low and mild inflammation (CRP < 10 mg/L). Two, three, and four visible lines represent moderate (≥10–25 mg/L), severe (≥25–50 mg/L), and very severe (≥50–100 mg/L) inflammation, respectively. If the visible lines become faint and the intensity of the first test line becomes weaker than the control line and even disappears, it illustrates super severe inflammation (≥100 mg/L).[20] The decline in signal in this circumstance is due to the high-dose "Hook effect" inherent with sandwich immunoassay formats. Barcode-style LFAs were developed for the semi-quantification of various targets, such as hydrogen peroxide,[21] prostate acid phosphatase,[22] and *Escherichia coli*.[23]

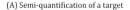

(A) Semi-quantification of a target

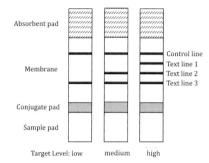

(B) Simultaneous detection of multiple targets

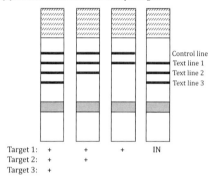

Figure 2.1   Designs of multiplex LFAs for the semi-quantification of a target per strip test (a), or for the simultaneous detection of multiple targets per strip test (b). (+) positive result; (IN) invalid result.

Another type of barcode-style LFA is focused on the simultaneous detection of various targets and is also called a multiplex LFA (Fig. 2.1b). Most barcode-style LFAs were developed to detect pathogens or abused drugs. In 2009, a nucleic acid lateral flow immunoassay (NALFIA) was developed for the simultaneous detection of *Listeria* spp. and *L. monocytogenes* in food. In a NALFIA format, antibodies are immobilized on the test strip to capture the labeled target DNA fragment; while the antibody-tagged gold nanoparticles are applied to generate a visible line reacting with the captured target DNA fragment on the test strip. Thus, this particular assay was based on a duplex polymerase chain reaction (PCR) with two labeled primer sets. One set was directed toward a specific DNA sequence that encodes 16S rRNA of *Listeria* spp., and the other was directed toward a fragment of the prfA gene that encodes the central virulence gene regulator of *L. monocytogenes*. Following the PCR reaction, the amplicons of *Listeria* spp. and *L. monocytogenes* are simultaneously analyzed on a test strip. The amplicon of 16S rRNA of *Listeria* spp. was labeled with biotin and fluorescein, while the amplicon of the prfA gene of *L. monocytogenes* was labeled with biotin and digoxigenin. These two types of amplicons were specifically captured by anti-fluorescein and anti-digoxigenin antibodies immobilized on test line 1 and test line 2 of the test strip, respectively. The captured biotin-labeled amplicons were then detected using carbon nanoparticle–NeutrAvidin conjugates. Therefore, this assay can be utilized to examine food hygiene levels and reveal dangerous contamination by *L. monocytogenes*.[24] Multiplex LFAs were also used simultaneously to screen genes that encode virulence factors (*vt1*, *vt2*, *eae*, and *ehxA*) of Shiga-toxin-producing *E. coli* with a detection limit of $\sim 10^4 - 10^5$ colony-forming units (CFU)/mL,[25] and simultaneously to detect multiple abused drugs and their metabolites in urine, including morphine, amphetamine, methamphetamine, and benzoylecgonine, with a detection limit of 2–20 ng/mL.[26] Recent developments in barcode-style LFAs, such as a multiplex chemiluminescent biosensor for detecting B-fumonisins and aflatoxin B1 in maize flour,[27] and a PCR-lateral flow assay for simultaneously identifying the *femA* of *Staphylococcus aureus,* the *mecA* for the methicillin-resistant *Staphylococcus aureus* (MRSA) with exogenous cassette DNA containing the methicillin-resistant genemecA (SCCmec), and *kdpC* for SCCmec type II,[28] have led them to provide more information in each run, improving ease of operation, time required, and cost-effectiveness.

2.2 Components of a Lateral Flow Assay

Technically, the lateral flow immunoassay is a simplified version of the western blot or enzyme-linked immunosorbent assay (ELISA), but LFA does not require as many steps (such as washing and incubation steps) as these two assays. As soon as a sample is dropped on the sample pad of a LFA strip, an assay begins by following the sample migration on the surface. Therefore, a LFA takes significantly less time (~ 10–20 min) than a western blot assay or an ELISA (2–3 h).[21,29] A standard LFA test strip has five parts:

a sample pad, a conjugate pad, a membrane, an absorbent pad, and a plastic adhesive packing card, as displayed in Fig. 2.2. The compositions and functions of these parts are discussed as follows.

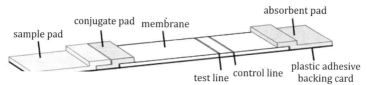

Figure 2.2   The construction of a lateral flow strip comprising a sample pad, a conjugate pad, a nitrocellulose membrane, an absorbent pad, and a plastic adhesive backing card.

The sample pad is the place where a portion of the sample (~200 µL) is applied. It is the start point of a test strip and is commonly composed of cellulose filter or woven meshes. The functions of the sample pad include filtering out unwanted particles in samples and promoting a uniform distribution of samples onto the underlying conjugate pad.[30] Proteins such as albumin or gelatin and surfactants such as Tween-20 or Triton X-100 are added to this pad during manufacturing to serve as blocking materials, which reduce nonspecific interactions between undesired molecules in the samples and the detection reagents, the capture reagents, and the membranes.[31] Moreover, treatment of the sample pad with blocking solution eliminates the need for performing the blocking procedure on the analytical membrane, simplifying the manufacturing process for the LFA strip. Furthermore, the addition of blocking materials to the sample pad can increase the viscosity of the sample and thereby reduce its flow rate, increasing the reaction time when the sample encounters the detection reagents in the conjugate pad or the capture reagents that are immobilized on the membrane. All of these modifications serve to improve the sensitivity of a LFA.[17] However, while many blocking reagent options are compatible with signaling particles such as colloidal gold or dyed latex beads, caution must be used with liposomal nanovesicle-based signaling. A low concentration of surfactants must be used in pretreating the sample pad of a LFA, which uses liposomes for signaling since such surfactants can induce the lysis of lipid bilayers. This lysis can subsequently release encapsulated dye molecules, resulting in high background noise and, therefore, reduced assay sensitivity.[32–36]

Since the sample pad is the first place with which a sample makes contact, it is the best place to modulate the properties of a sample to facilitate the detection of the target on a test strip. Typically, to modulate the pH value of a sample, a sample pad is treated with a buffer of low ionic strength, such as 50 mM borate buffer with pH 7.4,[37] 50 mM Tris-HCl with pH 8.0,[38] or 10 mM phosphate-buffered saline (PBS) with pH 7.4.[39] This sample pad pretreatment can reduce the likelihood of loss of sensitivity or specificity of detection by maintaining appropriate ionic strength and pH for optimal antibody–antigen interaction, supporting the reproducibility of the LFA for testing samples from different sources.

The detection reagents are dispensed onto the conjugate pad. When a sample passes through the sample pad and moves into the conjugate pad, the detection reagents solubilize, detach from the conjugate pad materials, react with the targets in the sample, and move with the sample into the membrane. The conjugate pad is typically composed of porous materials, such as glass filters or surface-modified polyester or polypropylene filters that are strongly hydrophilic.[40,41] The detection reagents that are dispensed into the conjugate pad are made by conjugating biomolecules (such as antibodies, antigens, or nucleic acids) to the surface of colored particles, such as liposomal nanovesicles (hereafter referred to as liposomes),[32,35,36,42] gold nanoparticles,[43] carbon nanoparticles,[25,44] or latex beads.[45,46] In a sandwich LFA, after they react with the targets in a conjugate pad, the "target-detection reagent" complexes migrate into the membrane, wherein they are captured by the immobilized capture reagents, yielding visible lines on the test strip, revealing the targets in the samples. In a study to develop a competitive LFA for detecting the major peanut allergen Ara h1, eight conjugate pads were tested to determine whether they were suitable to carry Ara h1-tagged liposomes. The best material was a non-woven 12-S, which is a cellulose rayon material, because it most effectively released liposomes. In this study, the blocking solution that was deposited on the conjugate pad was a mixture of 5 mM sodium tetraborate (pH 8.0), 4% bovine serum albumin (BSA), 3% goat serum, 1% polyvinylpyrrolidone (PVP), and 0.002% Triton X-100. Wen et al. investigated the effect of detergent

...anol reduces the stability of proteins. This partial
...tion of proteins accelerates the exposure of more
...ic parts of the proteins, resulting in an improvement in
...g of the proteins onto the membrane.[61]
...cing the size of pores in a membrane reduces its wicking
...entially increasing sensitivity of the assay by extending
...tion of the reaction by which the capture reagents trap the
...n the test line. NC membranes with different pore sizes,
...from 0.05 to 12 µm, are available.[17] In LFAs using liposomes,
...are typically on the order of 100–300 nm diameter, NC
...anes with 8 µm and 10 µm pores are preferred and have
...sed in sandwich LFAs for detecting *E. coli* O157:H7,[35,58]
...a toxin (CT),[36,59] and botulinum toxin (BT).[48] They have also
...sed in competitive LFAs for detecting potato glycoalkaloid[31]
...*ryptosporidium parvum*.[62] Recently, capillary flow time has
...in use as a descriptor instead of pore size to specify a membrane
...rial. This is the preferred parameter since pores are not
...ormly distributed in a membrane on account of the
...ufacturing process, and the estimated pore size depends on
...method used to measure it. Moreover, different manufacturers
...asure the size of the pores in their products using different
...hniques. However, capillary flow time is defined as the time for
...sample front to migrate a certain distance along a membrane.
...r example, the capillary flow time is expressed in seconds per
...ur centimeters (s/4 cm) on a Millipore or Schleicher & Schuell
...&S) product. Hence, the capillary flow time provides an easy
...nd straightforward way to describe a membrane material. The
...evelopers of one competitive liposome-based LFA for detecting
...Ara h1 tried five membrane materials: AE 99, AE 100, FF 85, Prima
...85 (S&S), and HF 120 (Millipore). The Prima 85 membrane, with
...a reported capillary flow time of 85 s across 4 cm of membrane,
...enabled the assay to be completed in the shortest time, but it yielded
...the broadest test line with the lowest signal intensity, resulting in a
...relatively low assay sensitivity. Of the other four materials, AE 100
...gave the lowest detection limit and, therefore, was the preferred
...NC membrane for the study.[42] Moreover, Shukla chose HF 240
...(Millipore) as the optimal NC membrane for detecting *Salmonella*.[
...In short, in the development of LFAs, different assay formats a
...targets require different NC membranes to balance maximal a

concentration on assay p
of Triton X-100 (0.002,
decreased as the concentr
higher concentrations (0.0
the lysis of liposomes, redu
that were captured on the
concentration of detergents
favorable performance of a LFA

As the target-detection re
conjugate pad and move into the
subjected to chromatography-lik
the immobilized capture reagent
continuously migrate and reach
detection reagents are trapped, for
indicates that the assay is complete
properly. Nitrocellulose (NC) is the
material for immune-based LFAs us
polyethersulfone (PES) is the most wi
for nucleic-acid-based LFAs using lip
membrane is used, proteins are electi
it by the interactions between the dipo
proteins and the dipoles of the nitrate e
Consequently, the pH value of a coating
capture reagents (such as the antibody,
carrier protein, avidin, or streptavidin) in
of immobilization on the NC membrane,
of a protein depends on the pH of the s
dissolved. Based on earlier studies, PBS (pH 7
used coating buffer for immobilizing pro
membrane.[34–36,48,51,58,59] Interestingly, Wen et a
phosphate buffer (PB) gave a higher immobiliz
antibodies than did PBS (which additionally conta
revealing that the presence of ions interfered wit
binding between antibodies and the NC membra
acid-based LFAs, the most common coating buffer
the mixture of streptavidin and biotin-labeled (biotil
probe onto the PES membrane is 0.4 M sodium carb
with 5% methanol.[52–54,60] Adding methanol to a
helps both rewet and reduce any static charge on tl
and improves the immobilization efficiency

since met
destabiliza
hydropho
the bindi
Redu
rate, po
the dura
targets
ranging
which
membr
been
choler
been
and (
been
mate
unifo
mar
the
me
te
a
Fo
fo
(
a

sensitivity with an acceptable assay time. Therefore, optimizing the membrane material for each developed assay is best done by testing various membranes with various capillary flow rates or materials. Additionally, in the blocking treatment used in most liposome-based LFAs, the blocking solution is applied directly to the membrane. PVP is the most frequently used "non-protein-based" blocking material, while gelatin[35,51,63] and casein[53,55,57] are the most used "protein-based" blocking materials. Still the development of every LFA depends on the optimization of the components of the blocking buffer, which depends on the unique characteristics of each assay.

After passing through the membrane, the rest of each sample is absorbed into the absorbent pad, which is placed at the end opposite that where the sample pad is located. The main purpose of the absorbent pad is to increase the total analysis volume of the sample that enters the test strip and to draw reagents across the membrane. Increasing the sample volume can wash away the unbound detection reagents, reducing the background signal and thereby enhancing the sensitivity of the assay. The absorbent pad can also modulate the sample flow over the membrane, based on its absorption efficiency[64]; it, therefore, plays an important role in providing a favorable signal intensity on the test line and the control line. Most absorbent pads are cellulose filters and cotton linters,[42] and the total volume of sample taken up by an absorbent pad can be optimized by changing its length and thickness.

Since all of the materials of a test strip are very fragile, they must be attached to a plastic adhesive backing card to increase their strength for ease of use in either a simple dipstick format or in a sophisticated plastic housing with a sample spot and a reaction window, which displays the test line and the control line.

2.3 Using Liposomes as Detection Reagents for LFAs

The principle of detection in a LFA is based on the specific biorecognition of antibody–antigen immunoreactions, biotin–avidin interactions, or DNA/RNA hybridizations, which generate visible lines on the membrane by the capture of labeled detection reagents. To form the observable lines, biomolecules are tagged onto the surface of colored particles, such as gold nanoparticles (AuNPs), latex beads, or dye-encapsulating liposomes. AuNPs are commonly used detection reagent in LFAs, because of their relatively low cost, stability in dried form, ease of conjugation with various biomolecules, and high extinction coefficient, which increases the intensity of the signals on test lines.[65,66] The diameter of AuNPs in a LFA is crucial because the color of the AuNPs, the signal intensity on the test lines, and the stability of AuNPs all depend on their size.[12] Typically, AuNPs with a diameter of 15 nm are too small to generate an easily observed signal, and those with a diameter larger than 40 nm tend to aggregate after being stored at 4°C, changing their color from wine red to blue–grey, even possibly causing them to precipitate.[67] Therefore, AuNPs with sizes from 20 to 40 nm are commonly used in LFAs. The signal intensity increases with the diameter of the AuNPs in this range, so larger AuNPs are associated with greater sensitivity of a LFA.[68]

Liposomes are spherical nanovesicles that are composed of one or more phospholipid bilayers that surround an aqueous cavity. Owing to the ease of preparation with high stability, liposomes have been applied in field-portable or point-of-care sensor systems.[69] In the 1990s, the Durst lab began to use dye-encapsulating liposomes as colorimetric detection reagents for developing LFAs.[32,33] Liposomes are effective carriers owing to their large interior cavities, which can encapsulate huge numbers of water-soluble dye molecules, such as sulforhodamine B (SRB) or carboxyfluoresceins (CF).[58,70,71] For example, when using 150 mM SRB as the rehydration solution to prepare liposomes, 1.4×10^5 SRB molecules can be trapped in each 150 nm liposome and 2.7×10^6 SRB molecules can be trapped in each 400 nm liposome.[51] This large number of encapsulated dye molecules allows the liposomes to be visually detected without further processing, satisfying the requirement for being a detection reagent of a LFA.[32,72] Additionally, various biomolecules such as peptides, hormones, antibodies, antigens, or nucleic acids can be conjugated to the liposomal surface, and these ligands make liposomes able to specifically bind to the target analytes and thereby useful as a versatile detection reagent in bioanalytical assays.[42]

2.3.1   Impact of Liposome Size

The optimization of liposomes for a LFA typically involves their diameter and the molar percentage (mol%) of biomolecules on the liposomal surface. The optimal size of liposomes for a LFA depends on the nature of the targets, the assay format, and the properties of the assay components, such as the membrane and conjugate pad. In a competitive lateral flow immunoassay for the detection of alachlor, which is a herbicide of the chloroacetanilide family, Siebert et al. used a batch of liposomes with a mean diameter of 0.68 ± 0.12 μm, prepared by the reverse-phase evaporation method and extruded through the 1.0 and 0.4 μm pore-sized polycarbonate (PC) membrane filters. After extrusion, the liposomes migrated more evenly on the NC membrane than did the unextruded liposomes, because extrusion through the PC membrane filters helped to yield a more homogeneously sized liposome population.[32] Szoka et al. also reported on the advantage of using the extrusion method for the production of liposomes, and they concluded that the size of the pores in the membrane filter strongly influenced the size of the liposomes.[73] The typical range of sizes of liposomes in LFAs is from 200 to 400 nm, as indicated in Table 2.1. For example, the optimal diameters of antibody-tagged liposomes (immunoliposomes) used for detecting *E. coli* O157:H7 in three articles were 200, 250, and 269 nm, respectively,[35,47,58] and the optimal diameter of immunoliposomes used for detecting *Salmonella enterica* Typhimurium was 236 nm in a study by Ho and 223 nm in a study by Shukla.[49,50]

Ganglioside-incorporated liposomes have been used in LFAs for detecting BT and CT, because trisialoganglioside GT1b and monosialoganglioside GM1 have been proven to be cellular receptors for these toxins, respectively.[74,75] Ganglioside GT1b is the cellular receptor for BT, which is a neurotoxin produced by *Clostridium botulinum* and poses a major threat as a bioweapon owing to its extreme lethality, ease of production, ease of transportation, possibility of misuse, and the need for prolonged intensive care of infected people.[76,77] Ganglioside GM1 has been identified as the cellular receptor for CT, which is an enterotoxin produced by *Vibrio cholera*. The binding of CT to the Gsα protein activates adenylate cyclase, resulting in cAMP accumulation in the cytoplasm and the subsequent osmotic imbalance across the membrane, which leads to diarrhea.[78] The optimal size of GT1b

Table 2.1 Biomolecule-tagged liposomes as detection reagents in immune-based LFAs

Analyte[Ref]	Lipid composition[a,b]		Sandwich assays			
		Diam. (nm)	Biomolecule on liposomes	Biomolecule modified with[c]	Liposomes modified with[c]	Tagged mol%[d]
E. coli O157:H7[35]	DPPC, Chol, DPPG, MMCC-DHPE (5:5:0.5:0.25)[RP]	200	Goat pAb anti-E. coli O157:H7	SH from 2-iminothiolane	MI from MMCC-DHPE	2.5
E. coli O157:H7[58]	DSPC, Chol, DSPG, DSPE-PEG-MI (5:5:0.5:0.25)[RP]	269	Goat pAb anti-E. coli O157:H7	SH from SATA	MI DSPE-PEG-MI	2.5
E. coli O157:H7[47]	DPPC, Chol, DPPG, DPPE, biotin-x-DHPE (5:5:0.5:0.25:0.005)[RP]	250	Goat pAb anti-E. coli O157:H7	SH from SATA	MI from sulfo-KMUS	2.5
Salmonella[49]	DPPC, Chol, DPPG, DPPE, biotin-x-DHPE (5:5:0.5:0.25:0.005)[RP]	236	Goat pAb anti-Salmonella	SH from SATA	MI from sulfo-KMUS	2.5
Salmonella[50]	DPPC, Chol, DPPG, DPPE (40.3:40.9:4.2:3.6)[RP]	223	Goat pAb anti-Salmonella	MI from sulfo-KMUS	SH from SATA	4
Staphylococcal enterotoxin B[79]	DPPC, Chol, DPPG, DPPE (5:5:0.5:0.25)[RP]	400	Mouse mAb anti-SEB	MI from SMCC	SH from SATP	2.5
Cholera toxin[36,59]	DPPC, Chol, DPPG, GM1 (40.3:40.9:4.2:1.3)[TF]	208	Ganglioside GM1	NA	Unmodified	1–2
Botulinum toxin[48]	DPPC, Chol, DPPG, GT1b (40.3:40.9:4.2:1.3)[TF]	197	Ganglioside GT1b	NA	Unmodified	1–2

		Competitive assays				
Analyte[Ref]	Lipid composition[a,b]	Diam. (nm)	Tag on liposomes	Conjugation via	Liposomes modified with[c]	Tagged mol%
Alachlor[32]	DPPC, Chol, DPPG, DPPE-alachlor (5:5:0.5:0.01)[RP]	680	Alachlor	DPPE using SATA	Unmodified	0.1
Alachlor[51]	DPPC, Chol, DPPG, DPPE-Alachlor, biotin-x-DHPE (5:5:0.5:0.01:0.01)[RP]	150	Alachlor	DPPE using SATA	Unmodified	0.1
Polychlorinated biphenyls (PCB)[33]	DPPC, Chol, DPPG, DPPE-2ClPB, biotin-x-DPPE (5:5:0.5:0.1:0.01)[RP]	610	2ClPB	DPPE using DCC/NHS	Unmodified	1
Potato glycoalkaloids[34]	DPPC, Chol, DPPG, DPPE-solanine, biotin-x-DHPE (47.2:47.8:4.9:1.0:0.1)[RP]	180	Solanine	DPPE using sodium metaperiodate	Unmodified	1
Aflatoxin B1[92]	DPPC, Chol, DPPG, DPPE (5:5:0.5:0.4)[RP]	230	Aflatoxin B1	MI from MPBH	SH from SATA	4
Ara h1[42,91]	DPPC, Chol, DPPG, DPPE-biotin, DPPE (43:45:5:4:3)[TF]	200	Ara h1	MI from sulfo-SMCC	SH from SATA	0.4
Rabbit IgG[63]	DPPC, Chol, DPPG, DPPE (45.4:46:4.5:4)[TF]	400	Goat anti-rabbit IgG	MI from sulfo-SMCC	SH from SATA	0.1
Microcystin[80]	DPPC, Chol, DPPG, DPPE (5:5:0.5:0.25)[RP]	400	Mouse mAb anti-microcystin	MI from SMCC	SH from SATP	2.5

aPreparation methods—RP: reverse-phase evaporation or TF: thin-film hydration, all followed by extrusion and gel filtration.

bLiposome Composition—Chol: cholesterol; MMCC-DHPE: N-((4-maleimidylmethyl)cyclohexane-1-carbonyl)-1,2-dihexadecanoyl-sn-glycero-3-phosphoethanolamine, triethylammonium salt; DSPE-PEG-maleimide: 1,2-distearoyl-sn-glycero-3-phosphoethanolamine-N-[maleimide(polyethylene glycol)]; biotin-x-DHPE: N-((6-(biotinoyl)amino)hexanoyl)-1,2-dihexadecanoyl-sn-glycero-3-phosphoethanolamine, triethylammonium salt.

cSATA: N-succinimidyl S-acetylthioacetate; Sulfo-KMUS: N-[κ-maleimidoundecanoyloxy] sulfo-succinimide ester; SATP: N-succinimidyl S-acetyl thiopropionate; SH: sulfhydryl; MI: maleimide; NA: not available.

dTagged mol%: the optimal mol% of the tagged biomolecules in the liposomal surface.

ganglioside liposomes for detecting BT was 197 nm,[48] while the preferred size of GM1 ganglioside liposomes for detecting CT was 208 nm.[36] Based on the results of these two studies, there was no obvious difference in the optimal sizes of GT1b and GM1 ganglioside liposomes when they were used to detect bacterial toxins BT and CT. Larger liposomes with a mean diameter of approximately 400 nm have been used in LFAs for detecting staphylococcal enterotoxin B (SEB),[79] rabbit IgG,[63] and microcystin.[80] In a very thorough study by Edwards et al., six differently sized liposomes were used to investigate the effect of liposomal diameter on the sensitivity of a sandwich hybridization LFA, and the optimal diameter for DNA-tagged liposomes was found to be 315 nm. Those authors also found that larger liposomes provided a stronger signal on the test line because their large internal cavities encapsulated more dye molecules per liposome. This strengthening of the assay signal by increasing the size of liposomes was also observed in an immunomagnetic assay with such nanovesicles.[81] Moreover, larger liposomes migrated more slowly through the membrane, providing more opportunities for them to be captured on the capture zones of the test strips. However, this advantage is sometimes diminished by the strengthening of the background signal, since larger liposomes encounter more difficulties in migrating through the membrane and are more likely to cease flowing on the membrane. Smaller liposomes can more readily migrate and thus provide a weaker background signal and more may be captured within the capture zones of the test strips. However, these advantages are insufficient to overcome the disadvantage of a weak signal on the membrane since their smaller internal cavities cannot encapsulate enough dye molecules to provide a strong signal.[55] Therefore, the size of liposome is an important parameter in the development of LFAs. This factor is optimized first by preparing various sized liposomes using the extrusion method and then evaluating their performance in terms of a signal over noise (S/N) value, where the signal is the intensity of the color on the test line and the noise is the background intensity on the membrane.[63] The batch of liposomes with the optimal size yields the highest S/N value.

2.3.2 Impact of Biorecognition Element Coverage

The mol% of biomolecules on the liposomal surface is also important in the optimization of liposome-based LFAs. Two liposome-based sandwich LFAs have been developed to detect *Salmonella* spp., and the sizes of immunoliposomes used in the two corresponding works were 220–230 nm. Interestingly, the detection limit in Shukla's study (100 CFU/mL) was significantly lower than that (1680 CFU/mL) in Ho's study.[49,50] This improvement of assay sensitivity in Shukla's study may potentially have originated in the fact that the immunoliposomes in that study had a higher antibody tag mol% (4.0%) than that (2.5%) in Ho's study, so immunoliposomes had more opportunities to capture *Salmonella* spp. in the samples.

To determine the optimal amount of gangliosides on the surface of the liposomes that are used to detect CT and BT, multiple batches of liposomes were prepared with various amounts of gangliosides in the lipid mixture. In both studies, the binding of toxin molecules to those liposomes was the strongest when gangliosides constituted 1–2 mol% of the total lipids. The authors also noted that higher amounts of gangliosides made liposomes unstable owing to the presence of the large carbohydrate moiety of the gangliosides. Accordingly, in these assays, to maximize the stability of ganglioside liposomes, the amount of ganglioside tags was maintained at less than 2 mol% of the total amount of lipids.[36,48]

Furthermore, a competitive LFA for the detection of Ara h1 was tested using four Ara h1 concentrations on the liposomal surface: 0.1, 0.4, 1.0, and 2.0 mol%. The signal intensity of the test line was directly proportional to Ara h1 tag mol%. However, when 1.0 or 2.0 mol% of Ara h1-tagged liposomes was used, a higher amount of Ara h1 was required in the sample to perform a competitive assay, so the assay sensitivity was lower. Using 0.1 mol% of Ara h1-tagged liposomes, a very weak signal on the test line resulted in the absence of Ara h1, so this batch of liposomes was not a suitable detection reagent for this assay. Therefore, 0.4 mol% was the optimal Ara h1 tag mol% for generating Ara h1-tagged liposomes in this competitive LFA.[42]

Other than the direct covalent conjugation of biomolecules to the liposomal surface, NeutrAvidin-tagged liposomes have been used in a new way as a universal detection reagent with the subsequent attachment of biotinylated ligands in LFAs.[63] Based on the stability of biotinylated ligand-tagged liposomes, 0.1 mol% of NeutrAvidin-tagged liposomes was used to develop immunoliposomes. Those tagged with 0.4 and 0.8 mol% of

NeutrAvidin formed liposomal aggregates more easily after they reacted with biotinylated antibodies and those tagged with 0.2 mol% of NeutrAvidin required a higher molar ratio of IgG/NeutrAvidin to prevent liposomal precipitation, so the cost of preparation of the IgG/NeutrAvidin-tagged liposomes was significantly higher. In short, the mol% of biomolecules that are tagged on the liposomal surface must be optimized for each assay, since it affects the stability of detection reagents and also the interaction between detection reagents and targets.

2.3.3 Lipid Composition and Modification Options

The composition of liposomes influences the stability of liposomes and determines the conjugation method that is used to tag biomolecules on liposomal surface. Commonly, one-half of the lipids of liposomes in LFAs is 1,2-dipalmitoyl-*sn*-glycero-3-phosphocholine (DPPC) and the other half is cholesterol. DPPC is an amphiphilic molecule with choline as the polar headgroup and two fatty acids as the nonpolar hydrocarbon tails (Chapter 1, Fig. 1.3); it is also a neutral molecule because it contains a positively charged choline and a negatively charged phosphate.[82] Cholesterol (Chapter 1, Fig. 1.5) is a membrane constituent that is found in many eukaryotic cells and usually added in the liposome formulation to modify the fluidity and permeability of the membrane bilayer and thereby improve the stability of the liposomes.[83,84] Additionally, to stabilize liposomes by preventing aggregation, charged lipids are included in the lipid mixture to provide a repulsive force on liposomal surface. Negatively charged 1,2-dipalmitoyl-*sn*-glycero-3-phospho-glycerol (DPPG, Chapter 1, Fig. 1.4) is the most chosen charged lipid with a working range from 4.5 mol% to 5.0 mol% in liposome-based LFAs, as indicated in Table 2.1.

To be effective detection reagents in LFAs, liposomes must be conjugated with specific biomolecules to enable them to be targeted. For covalent conjugation with ligands, 1,2-dihexadecanoyl-*sn*-glycero-3-phospho-ethanolamine (DPPE) (Chapter 1, Fig. 1.6) has been applied to provide a primary amine group from its polar headgroup, with a working range from 1.0 mol% to 4.0 mol%.[34,63] The primary amine group of DPPE can be further modified using *N*-succinimidyl S-acetylthioacetate (SATA) to form a sulfhydryl group or using *N*-[κ-maleimidoundecanoyloxy] sulfo-succinimide ester

(Sulfo-KMUS) to form a maleimide group, to provide different functional groups to conjugate with various biomolecules, discussed further in Section 2.4.1. Besides DPPE, a maleimide-modified phospholipid, MMCC-DHPE ((*N*-(4-maleimidyl-methyl) cyclohexane-1-carbonyl)-1,2-dihexadecanoyl-*sn*-glycero-3-phosphoethanolamine, triethylammonium salt) has been used in direct conjugation with a thiolated antibody for the detection of *E. coli* O157:H7.[35] Using MMCC-DHPE can simplify the conjugation process and reduce the time taken for the complete modification process. To prevent interference from the polyphenols in apple ciders, polyethylene glycol (PEG)-derivatized liposomes were produced using the commercial product DSPE-PEG-maleimide (DSPE: 1,2-distearoyl-*sn*-glycero-3-phosphoethanolamine), which is a synthetic lipid that can be incorporated into the lipid bilayer of liposomes. Thiolated antibodies were covalently conjugated to the maleimide group on the liposomal surface to form a stable thioether linkage.

Attaching an antibody to the distal end of PEG-derivatized liposomes relieved the steric hindrance that was caused by directly tagging antibodies to the lipid polar headgroups on a liposomal surface.[85] These PEG-derivatized liposomes were used to detect *E. coli* O157:H7 in apple cider with a detection limit of 7×10^3 CFU/mL without enrichment, and so they are effective detection reagent for detecting *E. coli* O157:H7 in fruit juices that contain poly-phenols. The endogenous polyphenols in fruit juices are capable of forming complexes with proteins or nucleic acids, leading to interferences in assay performance. Thus, the coating of PEG on the surface of liposomes might protect the liposomes from the nonspecific adsorption of endogenous polyphenols in apple cider.[58]

Finally, biotin molecules are sometimes tagged on the liposomal surface using biotin-DPPE or biotin-x-DHPE (*N*-((60-(biotinoyl)amino) hexanoyl)-1,2-dihexadecanoyl-*sn*-glycero-3-phosphoethanolamine). These biotinylated liposomes can be captured by immobilized avidin or streptavidin on the control line, indicating the completion of the LFA.[33,34,42,47,49,51] Surface modification with biotin molecules is very effective in antigen-tagged or DNA-tagged liposomes in LFAs because their surfaces do not have antibodies and so they cannot be captured on the control line by immobilized secondary antibodies.

2.4 Methods for Conjugating Biomolecules to Liposomal Surfaces

Numerous methods of chemical conjugation for modifying the surfaces of liposomes have been developed. With regard to immune-based LFAs, antibodies or antigens can be either covalently conjugated to the preformed liposomes using crosslinking reagents (Section 2.4.1)[32,35] or first labeled with biotin molecules and then allowed to interact with NeutrAvidin-tagged liposomes (Section 2.4.2).[63] Immunoliposomes can also be generated by mixing antibodies with "protein G-liposomes" to form "antibody-protein G-liposome" complexes through the specific binding of protein G to the Fc fragments of antibodies.[86] In the development of nucleic-acid-based LFAs, DNA-tagged liposomes are used as detection reagents and can be produced either by covalently conjugating DNA probes with the preformed liposomes[52–54,87] or by adding cholesteryl-labeled DNA probes to the initial lipid mixture to synthesize liposomes by the reverse-phase evaporation method and the extrusion method.[55–57,88] DNA-tagged liposomes can also be easily prepared by mixing the biotinylated probes with preformed NeutrAvidin or streptavidin-tagged liposomes[60,63] or by mixing dG-labeled reporter probes with generic dC probe-tagged liposomes.[89]

2.4.1 Covalent Methods

To conjugate biomolecules covalently to the liposomal surface, the appropriate crosslinking reagents must be chosen according to the available functional groups on the surfaces of the tagged molecules and the liposomes; these functional groups may be amine groups, carboxyl groups, or sulfhydryl groups, for example. The primary amine ($-NH_2$) groups of the tagged molecules are frequently used for crosslinking, and they are located in the N-terminus of each polypeptide chain or in the side chains of lysine (Lys) residues. As presented in Table 2.1, the amine group reacts with either 2-iminothiolane or SATA to generate additional sulfhydryl groups for conjugation with the maleimide groups on the liposomal surface. As displayed in Fig. 2.3, 2-iminothiolane, also called Traut's reagent, reacts with the amine group of a target molecule in a ring-opening reaction to form a sulfhydryl group. This method was utilized to conjugate polyclonal antibodies on liposomes for detecting *E. coli* O157:H7 in a sandwich immune-based LFA.[35]

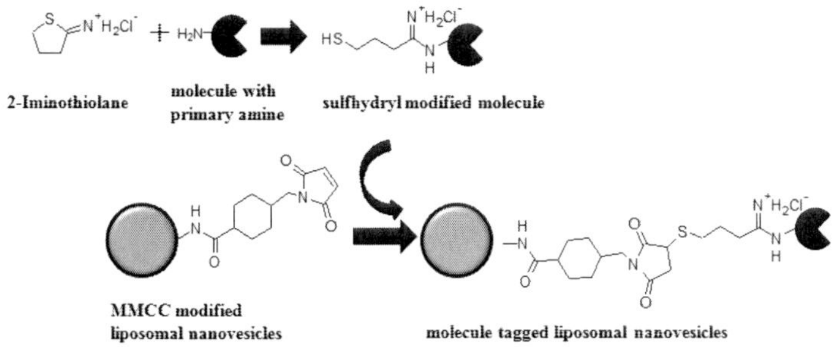

Figure 2.3   Covalent conjugation of molecules to surfaces of MMCC-modified liposomes with the use of 2-iminothiolane to react with the amine groups of the tagged molecule.

SATA is a common thiolation reagent for target molecules for making immunoliposomes that are used in LFAs.[47,49,58] In the reaction with SATA, a covalent amide bond is firstly formed by reacting the *N*-hydroxysuccinimide (NHS) ester of SATA with the primary amine group of the target molecule, with the release of an NHS group as a by-product (Fig. 2.4). Via a deprotection (deacylation) process with hydroxylamine, a free sulfhydryl group of an ATA-modified molecule is generated and further applied to bond covalently with maleimide-modified liposomes that are modified by using sulfo-KMUS. In practice, SATA is a better reagent than 2-iminothiolane for crosslinking reactions because its sulfhydryl group is introduced in the form of a protected ATA, which can be stored indefinitely before being deprotected for conjugation.[90] Additionally, immunoliposomes that are prepared using SATA retain their integrity and avidity at 4°C with double the storage time of those made with 2-iminothiolane.[58]

Thiolation using SATA has been carried out to produce immunoliposomes for detecting *E. coli* O157:H7[47,58] and *Salmonella* spp.[49] Similarly, tagged molecules can be modified with maleimide groups: sulfo-KMUS, SMCC (succinimidyl 4-[*N*-maleimidomethyl] cyclohexane-1-carboxylate), or sulfo-SMCC for generating a maleimide group, which can be covalently conjugated with the sulfhydryl groups on the liposomal surface that are produced by the addition of SATA or SATP (*N*-succinimidyl S-acetyl thiopropionate) to react with the primary amine group of the DPPE molecules in the lipid bilayers of the liposomes. This crosslinking method has been used to produce immunoliposomes for detecting *Salmonella enterica* serovar Typhimurium,[50] SEB,[79] rabbit IgG,[63] and microcystin,[80] or to generate antigen-tagged liposomes for a major peanut allergen Ara h1 in buffer[42] and in chocolate samples,[91] as displayed in Table 2.1. Since these crosslinking reactions randomly occur at the available amine groups of target molecules, the binding sites or active sites of the modified molecules may be blocked, reducing the original bioactivities of those molecules.

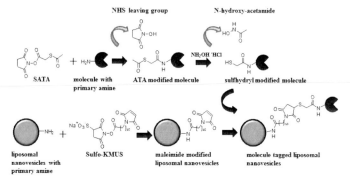

Figure 2.4   Covalent conjugation of molecules to surfaces of maleimide-modified liposomes with the use of SATA to react with the amine groups of the tagged molecule.

Besides the primary amine groups, the carboxyl groups (–COOH) of the target molecules are candidates for participating in crosslinking reactions; they are either at the C-terminus or in the side chains of the aspartate (Asp) and glutamate (Glu) residues of each polypeptide chain, or they may be functional groups of a chemical compound such as a pesticide or a herbicide. For conjugation, a carboxyl group can either be activated with dicyclohexylcarbodiimide (DCC)/NHS to link covalently with the amino groups of DPPE of liposomes,[33] or be treated with 4-[4-*N*-maleimidophenyl] butyric acid hydrazide hydrochloride (MPBH) to generate a maleimide group to conjugate covalently with the sulfhydryl groups of the deprotected ATA-liposomes.[92] As presented in Fig. 2.5a, DCC is a zero-length crosslinker, which can activate the carboxyl groups of target molecules with the use of NHS and subsequently form amide linkages with the primary amino groups of liposomes. This DCC/NHS method has been used to conjugate

2-chlorobiphenyl (2ClBP) to the liposomal surface for the detection of environmentally polluting PCBs (polychlorinated biphenyls).[33]

MPBH is a hetero-bifunctional crosslinker for conjugating sulfhydryl groups with carbonyl groups. As shown in Fig. 2.5b, the hydrazide group of MPBH conjugates to the carbonyl group of a target molecule, and the maleimide group of MPBH reacts with the sulfhydryl groups on the liposomes, which are generated by the reaction between SATA and the primary amine groups on the liposomal surface and subsequent deprotection using hydroxylamine. This method has been applied to produce aflatoxin B1-tagged liposomes for detecting aflatoxin B1, in a competitive immune-based LFA.[92]

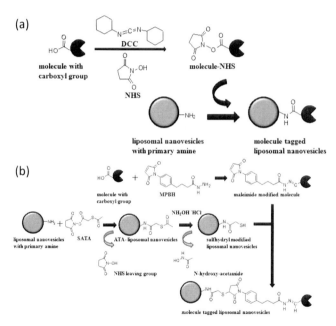

Figure 2.5 Covalent conjugation of molecules to the liposomal surface with the use of DCC/NHS (a) or MPBH (b) to react with the carboxyl groups of the tagged molecule.

2.4.2 Methods Based on Biorecognition Events

In addition to undergoing direct covalent conjugation, the target molecules can be first modified with biotin molecules and then allowed to interact with NeutrAvidin-tagged liposomes to form "target-biotin-NeutrAvidin-liposome" complexes. Since NeutrAvidin-tagged liposomes can bind to any biotinylated molecule, such as antibodies, antigens, or DNA molecules, they are also called universal liposomes as a single batch may be used in the development of various bioanalytical assays.[63] For instance, as presented in Fig. 2.6, NeutrAvidin-tagged liposomes react with biotinylated antibodies to form immunoliposomes, which can be used in a sandwich immunoassay, or react with biotinylated antigens to form antigen-tagged liposomes, which can be used in a competitive immunoassay.

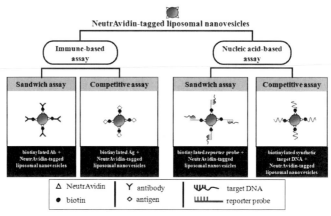

Figure 2.6 Applications of NeurAvidin-tagged liposomes as detection reagents in immune-based assay or nucleic-acid-based assay.

Moreover, to develop the DNA hybridization assay, NeutrAvidin-tagged liposomes initially react with biotinylated reporter probes for capturing target DNA molecules in a sandwich assay, or directly conjugate with biotinylated synthetic target DNA molecules, and so compete with free target DNA molecules in a competitive assay. Biotin is a small molecule with a molecular weight of 224 Da. Owing to its relatively small size, biotin can be conjugated to a variety of ligands, including carbohydrates, proteins, antibodies, or DNA/RNA molecules, without significantly altering the structure or biological functions of these biotinylated molecules.[93,94]

Three biotin-binding proteins have been used in bioassays, and they are avidin, streptavidin, and NeutrAvidin. Avidin (67 kDa) is a glycoprotein obtained from egg white with a basic isoelectric point (pI) of 10–10.5, and this basic pI of avidin easily results in nonspecific interaction with other unrelated molecules by ionic attraction.[95,96] Streptavidin (60 kDa) is originally from *Streptomyces avidinii* with a mildly acidic pI of 5.[97] Theoretically, streptavidin is less charged than avidin when both are used under neutral buffer system; thus the nonspecific interactions from streptavidin are lower than that from avidin. Furthermore, to reduce the intensity of nonspecific reactions of avidin and streptavidin, NeutrAvidin (60 kDa) is generated by the deglycosylation of avidin, which results in a near neutral pI of 6.3 as well as an improvement of the assay sensitivity.[98,99] Therefore, NeutrAvidin has been increasingly used and is selected, in particular, in generating NeutrAvidin-tagged liposomes as universal detection reagents for bioanalytical assays.[63]

Another way to produce immunoliposomes is to mix antibodies with protein A-tagged or protein G-tagged liposomes. Protein A and protein G are antibody-binding proteins, which can bind specifically to the Fc fragment of antibodies.[100] Protein A is isolated from the cell wall of *Staphylococcus aureus*, while protein G is isolated from the cell wall of group C and G of *Streptococcus* spp. Protein G can bind to antibodies from a wider variety of mammalian species (such as human, mouse, rat, bovine, goat, horse, monkey, rabbit, and sheep) than protein A, and with a stronger affinity; it also can recognize a wider range of IgG subclasses.[101,102] In bioanalytical assays, the antibody-binding ability of protein G is less pH dependent than that of protein A. The different pH dependence of these two bacterial proteins supports the notion of different molecular mechanisms for their IgG binding.[103] Hence, protein G, rather than protein A, has been used to generate immunoliposomes for the detection of *E. coli* O157:H7 in an immunomagnetic bead assay[86] and for the simultaneous detection of *E. coli* O157:H7, *Salmonella* spp., and *Listeria monocytogenes* in an array-based immunosorbent assay.[104] However, to date, protein G-liposomes have not been applied as detection reagents in any reported LFAs.

2.4.3   Direct Incorporation

To detect some specific bacterial toxins, cellular receptors, such as gangliosides, have been applied instead of antibodies in preparing liposomes as the detection reagents in LFAs.[36,48,59] Gangliosides are glycolipids that are incorporated into the cell membrane with their hydrophobic portion ceramide composed of a long-chain fatty acid and a sphingosine; their extracellular carbohydrate portion is exposed to the hydrophilic extracellular environment and is composed of hexoses, *N*-acetylated hexosamines, and sialic acids (Fig. 1.7).[105] Since gangliosides are naturally incorporated into lipid bilayers of cell membranes, ganglioside liposomes can be produced by adding gangliosides to the mixture of lipids and then applying the thin-film hydration method, followed by the extrusion method with repetitive freeze–thaw cycles.[36] GT1b-liposomes, manufactured using such a process, have been developed to detect BT in buffer systems,[48] and ganglioside GM1-liposomes have been constructed to detect CT in buffer and food samples.[36,59]

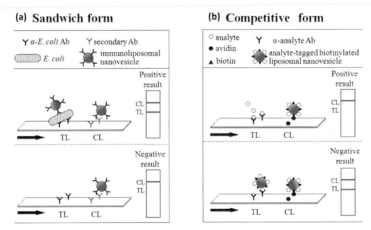

Figure 2.7 Immune-based lateral flow assay: (a) sandwich form; (b) competitive form.

2.4.4 Functionalization with DNA

DNA-tagged liposomes have been produced and used in the development of nucleic-acid-based LFAs. For detecting a specific DNA or RNA target sequence using a LFA, reporter probes must be tagged on the liposomal surface to form the detection reagents. The four different methods for producing DNA-tagged liposomes are as follows: (1) covalent conjugation with preformed liposomes, (2) direct mixing of cholesteryl-modified reporter probes with other lipids during the formation of liposomes, (3) dC-dG hybridization with generic dC probe-tagged liposomes, and (4) the interaction of biotin-NeutrAvidin/streptavidin with NeutrAvidin/streptavidin-tagged liposomes. With respect to covalent conjugation, in most previous studies, reporter probes were first modified with an internal disulfide bond at the 3'-end and reduced using dithiothreitol (DTT) to have a free sulfhydryl group, which formed a covalent linkage with maleimide-modified liposomes.[87,106] This method requires an additional step to isolate the thiol-activated probes from the DTT-containing solution and has, therefore, been often replaced by other covalent conjugation methods that involve crosslinking reagents. For example, amine-modified reporter probes are first reacted with SATA[52,53,62] or sulfo-KMUS[54,60], and then covalently conjugated to the maleimide or sulfhydryl-modified liposomes, respectively, as indicated in Table 2.2.

In 2006, an easy method for the preparation of DNA-tagged liposomes was developed using cholesteryl-modified probes.[55] Modification of the reporter probes with cholesterols enables these probes to be easily mixed with other lipids, so the lipid mixture can directly form DNA-tagged liposomes through reverse-phase evaporation methods without a complicated conjugation reaction that involves crosslinking reagents. This simplified method allows excellent control of the mol% of the DNA probes that are tagged on the liposomal surface and cuts the preparation time from two days to just 6 h. Additionally, a higher liposome concentration can be obtained from the direct incorporation method than from the multiple-step conjugation method, since the former does not require the addition of crosslinking reagents or the second gel filtration chromatography purification step. Moreover, following the normalization of their lipid concentration, the liposomes that are made by the direct incorporation method have a higher signal intensity than those made by multiple-step conjugation methods. This improvement in signal intensity might follow from the fact that the direct incorporation method more efficiently incorporates DNA probes and involves less leakage of the entrapped SRB dye molecules because it has fewer reaction steps. Owing to these advantages, direct incorporation using cholesteryl probes has been used in the manufacture of DNA-tagged liposomes for the detection of a specific DNA sequence,[55] *Streptococcus pyogenes*,[56] *Cryptosporidium* spp.,[88] and *Mycobacterium avium*,[57] as displayed in Table 2.2.

Table 2.2 Preparations of biomolecule-tagged liposomes as detection reagent in the nucleic-acid-based LFAs

Analyte[Ref]	Liposome composition[b] (molar ratio)	Biomolecule on liposomes	Biomolecule modified with	Liposomes modified with	Tagged mol%[c]
Sandwich assay					
Specific DNA sequences[87]	DPPC, Chol, DPPG, maleimide-DPPE (5:5:0.5:0.0 4)	Reporter probe	SH group from reduction of a disulfide w/DTT	Maleimide	0.4
Specific DNA sequences[106]	DPPC, Chol, DPPG, maleimide-DPPE (5:5:0.5:0.04)	Reporter probe	SH group from reduction of a disulfide w/DTT	Maleimide	0.4
Specific DNA sequences[55]	DPPC, Chol, DPPG, probe-Chol (40.3:51.7:21:0.015)	Reporter probe	Cholesteryl modification	NA	0.013
Dengue virus[52]	DPPC, Chol, DPPG, MMCC-DPPE (5:5:0.5:0.4)	Generic reporter probe	SH group from SATA	Maleimide group from MMCC	0.05–1.0
Dengue virus[54]	DPPC, Chol, DPPG, ATA-DPPE (40.3:51.7:21:7.2)	Generic reporter probe	Maleimide group from sulfo-KMUS	SH group from ATA-DPPE	NA
Astrovirus[117]	DPPC, Chol, DPPG, maleimide-DPPE (5:5:0.5:0.04)	Detection probe	NA	Maleimide	0.4
E. coli[53]	DPPC, Chol, DPPG, maleimide-DPPE (5:5:0.5:0.04)	Reporter probe	SH group from SATA	Maleimide group from MMCC	3–4

Streptococcus pyogenes[56]	DPPC, Chol, DPPG, ATA-DPPE (40.3:51.7:21.0:7.2)	Reporter probe	Cholesteryl modification	NA	NA
Cryptosporidium spp.[88]	DPPC, Chol, DPPG, probe-Chol (40.3:51.7:21:0.015)	Reporter probe	Cholesteryl modification	NA	NA
Mycobacterium avium[57]	DPPC, Chol, DPPG, probe-Chol (40.3:51.7:21:0.015)	Reporter probe	Cholesteryl modification	NA	0.013
Universal[89]	DPPC, Chol, DPPG, ATA-DPPE (40.3:51.7:21:7.2)	Generic dC probe	Maleimide group from sulfo-KMUS	SH group from ATA-DPPE	0.2
Generic[60]	DPPC, Chol, DPPG, ATA-DPPE (40.3:51.7:21.0:7.2)	Streptavidin	Maleimide group from sulfo-KMUS	SH group from ATA-DPPE	0.4
Competitive assay					
Cryptosporidium parvum[62]	DPPC, Chol, DPPG, MMCC-DPPE, biotin-DPPE (5:5:0.5:0.3:0.02)	Reporter probe	SH group from SATA	Maleimide group from MMCC	0.1

[a]All liposomes were prepared through the reverse-phase evaporation, followed by the extrusion method, and then purified by the gel filtration method.

[b]Liposomes Composition—Chol: cholesterol; probe-Chol: cholesteryl-modified probe; MMCC-DHPE: *N*-((4-maleimidylmethyl)cyclohexane-1-carbonyl)-1,2-dihexadecanoyl-*sn*-glycero-3-phosphoethanolamine, triethylammonium salt; DSPE-PEG-maleimide: 1,2-distearoyl-*sn*-glycero-3-phosphoethanolamine-*N*-[maleimide(polyethylene glycol)]; biotin-x-DHPE: *N*-((6-(biotinoyl)amino)hexanoyl)-1,2-dihexadecanoyl-*sn*-glycero-3-phosphoethanolamine, triethylammonium salt.

[c]Tagged mol%: the optimal mol% of the tagged biomolecules in the liposomal surface. NA: not available.

To simplify the conjugation of DNA probes to the liposomal surface, two types of universal liposome have been developed, and these can be transformed into DNA-tagged liposomes just by incubation with labeled reporter probes. The first type are the liposomes that are tagged with generic dC probes, which can bind to the dG-labeled reporter probes.[89] The reporter probe consists of two parts: the 3′-end is the dG fragment that is complementary to the generic dC probe on the liposomal surface and the 5′-end is complementary to the target sequence. Therefore, the reporter probe can be tagged to the liposomal surface by the dC-dG hybridization.

The developers of these types of universal liposome optimized the generic probe using four lengths of dC (17 nt, 20 nt, 25 nt, and 30 nt) to create strong binding to the reporter probe and to prevent the formation of hairpin or probe dimer structures that could block the binding to reporter probe. The optimal length was 20 nt, which gave the best signal-to-noise ratio. After the incubation of the generic liposomes with reporter probes, the target sequence and the biotinylated capture probes for 20 min in solution, a sandwich complex formed and was captured by the immobilized streptavidin on the detection zone of a LFA strip as the mixture migrated along the membrane. The other types of universal liposomes are those conjugated with NeutrAvidin or streptavidin, which can capture biotinylated DNA probes.[60,63] Therefore, a simple coupling reaction between biotin and NeutrAvidin or streptavidin can turn universal liposomes into target-specific ones that can be easily adapted to the identification or quantification of a new target in LFAs.

2.5 Immune-Based LFAs that Use Liposomes

LFAs can be classified into two groups based on their target molecules: antibody-based and nucleic-acid-based assays. Both groups can be further divided into sandwich and competitive assays, according to the assay format. Normally, sandwich immune-based LFAs are used for the detection of large molecules such as pathogens, which have multiple epitopes on their surfaces, whereas competitive immune-based LFAs are used to detect small molecules, such as pesticides, which have only a single epitope per target molecule.

In a sandwich immune-based LFA, the target molecules first react with immunoliposomes; the target-immunoliposome complexes migrate across the strip and are then trapped by the capture antibodies that are immobilized on the test line to form a visible line. The sample liquid migrates along the strip, and the excess immunoliposomes are captured by the secondary antibodies that are immobilized on the control line to form a second visible line on the strip, indicating that the sample has been properly analyzed. Thus, two lines on the membrane demonstrate a positive result, while control line alone on the membrane is a negative result. In a sandwich immune-based LFA, the intensity of the signal on the test line is directly proportional to the concentration of target molecules. Figure 2.7a displays the format of a sandwich immune-based LFA that uses immunoliposomes as the detection reagents.

LFAs with this format are applied to detect food pathogens, such as *E. coli* O157:H7 and *Salmonella* spp. With respect to the detection of *E. coli* O157:H7, the first developed LFA, which used anti-*E. coli* O157:H7 polyclonal antibody-tagged liposomes, had a detection limit of 10^4 CFU/mL in fresh cultures.[35] Subsequently, in 2003, Ho et al. developed a sandwich LFA to detect *E. coli* O157: H7 with a lower detection limit of about 2500 cells,[107] as indicated in Table 2.3. This improvement in assay sensitivity may arise from the fact that more antibodies were tagged on each liposomal surface (4800 antibodies/liposome) in Ho's study than in the earlier study (~45 antibodies/liposome), so the immunoliposomes were more likely to capture the target bacterial cells in the samples. An antibody-tagged PEG-derived liposome was developed to detect *E. coli* O157:H7 specifically in apple cider. The purpose of coating PEG on the liposomal surface was to protect liposomes from the nonspecific adsorption of endogenous polyphenols that are present in apple cider,[108] because these hydrophobic compounds may block the antibody–antigen interaction on the surface of immunoliposomes. The authors of that work diluted apple cider samples with a culture medium or buffer to eliminate other potential sources of interference from the apple cider, such as low pH (3.7) and high osmolarity (880 mmol/kg). With PEG-modified liposomes, the developed assay detected *E. coli* O157: H7 in apple cider at a concentration as low as 1 CFU/mL after an 8 h enrichment, or at 7×10^3 CFU/mL without enrichment.

Table 2.3 Summary of studies on the development of immune-based LFAs using liposomal nanovesicles

Analyte[Ref]	Capture reagent on the test line	Capture reagent on the control line	Limit of detection	Detection time[c]	Ref.
Sandwich assay					
E. coli O157:H7	Anti-*E. coli* O157:H7 pAb[a]	NA	10^4 CFU/mL (TBS)	8 min	35
E. coli O157:H7	Anti-*E. coli* O157:H7 pAb	Anti-goat Ab	7×10^3 CFU/mL (apple cider)	8 min	58
E. coli O157:H7	Anti-*E. coli* O157:H7 pAb	Anti-biotin Ab	2500 cells (PBS)	5 min	47
Salmonella	Anti-*Salmonella* pAb	Anti-biotin Ab	1680 cells (PBS)	30 min	49
Salmonella	Anti-*Salmonella* pAb	Anti-goat Ab	10^2 CFU/mL (0.1% BPW)	10–15 min	50
Staphylococcus enterotoxin B (SEB)	Anti-SEB mAb[b]	Anti-mouse Ab	0.02 ng/mL (buffer/ham extract) 0.06 ng/mL (semi-skimmed milk) 0.125 ng/mL (apple juice/tap water/surface water/cheese extract)	30 min	79
Cholera toxin (CT)	Anti-CT B subunit mAb	NA	100 fg/mL (spring water) 30 pg/mL (tap water)	20 min	36
Cholera toxin	Anti-CT B subunit mAb	NA	80 fg/mL (clam) 180 fg/mL (shrimp) 3 pg/mL (salmon)	20 min	59
Botulinum toxin (BT)	Anti-BT subtype A pAb	NA	15 pg/mL (buffer)	15–20 min	48

Competitive assay

Analyte	Reporter	Capture	Detection limit	Detection time	Ref.
Alachlor	Anti-alachlor pAb	Avidin	5–10 ppb (TBS)	8 min	32
Alachlor	Anti-alachlor pAb (as aggregation zone)	Anti-biotin Ab (as capture zone)	1 ppb (TBS)	8 min	51
Polychlorinated biphenyls (PCB)	Anti-PCB Ab	Anti-biotin Ab	0.4 nmol of PCB for an LIC assay 2.6 pmol of PCB for an LIA assay	8 min 23 min	33
Potato glycoalkaloids	Anti-solanine pAb was added to sample solution to perform a competitive assay	Anti-biotin Ab (as capture zone)	0.11 ppm TGA	23 min	34
Aflatoxin B1 (AFB1)	Anti-AFB1 pAb	NA	18 ng AFB1 (acetonitrile/methanol; 7:3; v/v)	12 min	89
Ara h1	Anti-Ara h1 pAb	Avidin	0.45 ug/mL (buffer) 158 ug peanuts per gram of chocolate	30 min 30 min	42 91
Rabbit IgG	Rabbit IgG	NA	38 pmol/mL (PBS)	30 min	63
Microcystin	MC-LR conjugated BSA	Anti-mouse Ab	0.06 ng/mL MC-LR (buffer)	30 min	80

[a]pAb: polyclonal antibody.
[b]mAb: monoclonal antibody.
[c]Detection time: only include the time for a test strip assay.

Accordingly, PEG-derived immunoliposomes are a good alternative detection reagent for detecting pathogens in fruit juices that contain polyphenols.[58] Moreover, to detect *Salmonella enterica* Typhimurium, a LFA with 2.5 mol% antibody-tagged liposomes was developed with a detection limit of 1680 cells. Another recently developed LFA with 4 mol% antibody-tagged liposomes exhibited a significantly higher assay sensitivity, with a detection limit of only 10^2 CFU/mL.[50] Therefore, optimizing the antibody-tagged mol% on the liposomal surface can effectively increase the assay sensitivity of sandwich immune-based LFAs for the detection of pathogens.

LFAs that use liposomes usually have a lower detection limit for food pathogens than do LFAs using gold nanoparticles. For instance, in detecting *E. coli* O157:H7, an immunochromatographic (IC) strip with 40 nm of colloidal gold particles had a detection limit of 1.8×10^5 CFU/mL without enrichment and 1.8 CFU/mL following enrichment.[109] Recently, a rapid and sensitive protocol was developed based on an immunochromatographic assay (ICA) with immunomagnetic nanoparticles (IMPs) for detecting *E. coli* O157:H7. In that work, the sensitivities of ICA and IMPs + ICA were 10^5 CFU/mL and 10^3 CFU/mL, respectively.[110] Furthermore, a sandwich LFA that used colloidal gold has been used to detect *Salmonella enterica* Enteritidis in eggs with a detection limit of 10^7 CFU/mL.[111] Based on the results of this research, the assay sensitivity of LFAs that use liposomes was at least one order of magnitude greater than that of those that use gold nanoparticles. Hence, liposomes are favorable detection reagents for use in LFAs for detecting pathogens, as they increase assay sensitivities.

Unlike covalently conjugating antibodies on liposomal surfaces, which depend on crosslinking reagents, gangliosides can be spontaneously incorporated into liposomes. In the detection of CT, GM1-liposomes encapsulating SRB dye molecules have been used in sandwich LFAs, yielding the limit of detection (LOD) as 0.01 pg/mL for a buffer system, 0.1 pg/mL for spring water, and 30 pg/mL for tap water.[36]

The higher LOD in tap water (pH 7.5; conductivity <400 µS; total dissolved solids 200 ppm) than that in spring wter (pH 6.7; conductivity <70 µS; total dissolved solids 50 ppm) might be due to the presence of metal ions, organic matter, and various chemicals. In addition, GM1-liposomes also have been applied to detect CT in seafood samples, providing an LOD as 0.08 pg/mL for clam, 0.18 pg/mL for shrimp, and 3 pg/mL for salmon.[59] The lower sensitivity in the detection of salmon might be due to a high content of fat in salmon samples, which could interfere with the interactions between CT and GM1 on the liposomal surface. Furthermore, GT1b-liposomes encapsulating SRB dye molecules have been used to detect BT with a detection limit of 15 pg/mL.[48] The authors of the work to develop a LFA for the detection of BT noted that the LOD of the immunoliposome assay system was slightly higher than that of the GT1b-liposome assay system (40 pg/mL versus 15 pg/mL), and its assay signal decreased with increasing BT concentration to a greater extent than that of the GT1b-liposome assay system. This weakening of the signal was possibly caused by the fact that the batch of antibodies that was used to generate immunoliposomes was also used to coat the capture zone of the test strips, resulting in competition between these antibodies for the same epitopes of toxins and the consequent weakening of assay signals. The authors suggested that this problem might be solved by using two batches of antibodies that recognize different epitopes of toxins. However, given the complexity and duration of the process for preparing immunoliposomes, the authors recommended that ganglioside liposomes were preferred to immunoliposomes for detecting BT by a sandwich LFA.[48] For detecting BT, another sandwich LFA, which used monoclonal antibodies with two distinct specificities, was developed, with one immobilized on the detection zone on an NC membrane and another tagged on the surface of colloidal gold particles, which served as the detection reagent. The detection limit of that LFA was 50 ng/mL, which was improved to 1 ng/mL with silver enhancement, which metallic ions are reduced on the surface of colloidal gold particles, resulted in increase in size and optical extinction of these particles allowing for greater visibility and better sensitivity.[112] Even though the silver enhancement significantly enhanced the sensitivity of the assay for detecting BT using gold nanoparticles, the LFA with GT1b-lipsomal nanovesicles had an even lower detection limit, perhaps because many more SRB dye molecules were encapsulated in each nanovesicle, increasing the signal intensity on the capture zone (test line) of the test strips.

Normally, dye-encapsulating liposomes are used as the colored particles in LFAs for visual observation. Interestingly, Khrecih et al. measured the intensity of the fluorescent signal of SRB-encapsulated liposomes for the first time in the development of fluorescent LFAs that use liposomes. In their study, a major cause of food poisoning, SEB, was detected using anti-SEB antibody-tagged liposomes. The detection of fluorescence increased the sensitivity by a factor of 15 over that supported by visual observation.[79] At high concentration, encapsulated SRB molecules undergo a quenching phenomenon,[113] so no fluorescence signal could be detected. In the study where that finding was presented, lipid bilayers of liposomes were destroyed by drying in air and the SRB dye molecules were released as a result and locally dispersed, producing a fluorescent signal on the strip. The detection limit of this assay was close to 20 pg/mL, which was similar to that (10 pg/mL) of a LFA with colloidal gold coupled with silver enhancement.[114] No signal could be detected when this assay was used to detect SEB in an apple juice sample owing to the low pH (~ 4) of apple juice, and a fivefold dilution yielded a detection limit of 0.125 ng/mL. The fluorescence of SRB-loaded liposomes provides an effective means of improving the assay sensitivity of LFAs. When this strategy is used in analyzing foods, the sample preparation process can be optimized by controlling the dilution factor to reduce the concentration of interfering agents.

In a competitive immune-based LFA, liposomes are normally covalently conjugated with the target molecules to form target-tagged liposomes as the detection reagent. Free target molecules in samples compete with target-tagged liposomes for binding to the limited number of anti-target antibodies that are immobilized on the test line, as shown in Fig. 2.7b. Therefore, two lines on the strip indicate a negative result, whereas a sample with a high concentration of analytes gives a positive result with only one control line on the strip. Additionally, the signal intensity of the test line is inversely proportional to the concentration of analyte in the sample, and this metric can, therefore, be used for the quantification of targets. This competitive immune-based LFA has been applied in the detection of small molecules, such as alachlor,[32,51] polychlorinated biphenyls (PCB),[33] and aflatoxin B1 (AFB1)[92]; it can also be used to detect large molecules, such as the major peanut allergen Ara h1[42,91] (Table 2.3). When used to detect alachlor or

PCB, the assay had a sensitivity in the low parts per billion[32,51]; when used to detect AFB1 or Ara h1, the detection limit was at the part per million level[42,91,92], as indicated in Table 2.3. Since AFB1 was dissolved in an acetonitrile/methanol mixture (7/3; v/v), to prevent liposomes from coming into contact with these organic solvents, the sample solution was first added and analyzed on the test strip for long enough to allow the sample solution migrate into the antibody zone, before the liposomal solution was added for analysis on the test strip. The assay sensitivity (180 ppm) of the LFA that used liposomes was not comparable to that (2.5 ppb) of a more recently developed LFA that used a colloidal gold-labeled anti-AFB1 antibody.[115] The assay sensitivity of the LFA with the liposomes may have been lower because the sample was dissolved in organic solvent, which could not only break down the membrane of the liposomes but also interfere with the antigen–antibody interaction. In the assay using colloidal gold, chemical environment was optimized and the extraction efficiency of AFB1 was maintained by first using a 60% methanol solution to extract samples, and then diluting the extraction solution with 10% methanol:PBS buffer (1:9; v/v). Moreover, the food matrix significantly influenced the assay sensitivity of the LFA. For example, the detection limit of a LFA for detecting Ara h1 in buffer was 0.45 ppm, but the detection limit increased to 158 ppm for chocolate samples.[91] To improve the assay sensitivity, poly(vinylpolypyrrolidone) (PVPP) and hexane were used to remove phenolic compounds and lipids from chocolate, respectively.[116] In Wen's study, Ara h1 was first extracted with a mixture of the extraction buffer and hexane, to extract lipid from chocolate into the hexane layer, resulting in a lower lipid content in the aqueous buffer layer, so that a higher amount of proteins can be extracted. After extraction and centrifugation, the aqueous buffer layer was further treated with 50% (w/v) insoluble PVPP to eliminate phenolic compounds from chocolate to improve the signal in LFA.[91]

Another form of competitive immune-based LFA involves coating analytes on the test line, as the anti-analyte antibodies are conjugated with liposomes to form the detection reagent. Therefore, the targets in the sample compete with the immobilized targets on the membrane for reacting with antibody-tagged liposomes. Wen et al. utilized NeutrAvidin-tagged liposomes as the universal liposomes to bind with biotinylated anti-rabbit IgG antibodies to detect rabbit IgG, achieving an assay sensitivity of 38 pmol/mL (ca. 5.7 ppm).[63] Moreover, for detecting microcystin, the anti-microcystin monoclonal antibodies were covalently conjugated to either liposomes or colloidal gold. The sensitivity of the assay with colloidal gold and visual observation was 0.8 ng/mL, while that of the assay with immunoliposomes and the measurement of fluorescence was 0.09 ng/mL. The use of immunoliposomes instead of colloidal gold transforms the detection method from one based on visual observation to one based on a fluorescence measurement, which typically allows the detection of target molecules in samples with a high sensitivity.[80]

2.6 Nucleic-Acid-Based LFAs with Liposomes

Nucleic-acid-based LFAs can be divided into sandwich and competitive assays, based on their detection mechanism. In a sandwich assay, one end of a target DNA fragment is first hybridized with a reporter probe, which is covalently conjugated on the liposomal surface to form "target-reporter probe-liposome" complexes, as displayed in Fig. 2.8a. These complexes are captured by the biotinylated capture probe, which is complementary to the second part of the target and has been immobilized on the test line of a test strip through the biotin–avidin interaction, resulting in a visible red line on the test line of the strip. As the sample solution migrates along the strip, the fluorescein isothiocyanate (FITC)-labeled liposomes are captured by the anti-FITC antibodies that are coated on the control line, forming a second visible line, which indicates that the assay is complete. Besides FITC, other small molecules, such as digoxigenin (DIG), 2,4-dinitrophenol (DNP), and Texas Red (TxR), can be conjugated on the liposomal surface for this purpose. Two lines on a strip constitute a positive result, whereas the visible control line alone constitutes a negative result. The signal intensity on the test line is directly proportional to the target concentration. This assay format has been applied to detect synthetic DNA fragments[55,87,106] and specific RNA fragments of dengue virus,[52,54] astrovirus,[117] *E. coli,*[53,60,89] *Bacillus anthracis,*[60,89] *C. parvum,*[60,88,89] *Streptococcus pyogenes,*[56] and *Mycobacterium avium* subsp. *Paratuberculosis,*[57] as indicated in Table 2.4.

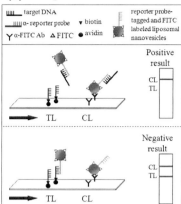

(a) Sandwich form

(b) Competitive form

Figure 2.8   Nucleic-acid-based lateral flow assay: (a) sandwich form; (b) competitive form.

The first sandwich LFA that used DNA-tagged liposomes as the detection reagent was developed in 1996 to enable specific single-stranded DNA sequences to be identified visually. In this LFA, one femtomole of the synthetic target sequence could be detected within 10 min. This high sensitivity was associated with the large number of dye molecules ($\sim 10^6$ molecules) that were encapsulated within the large cavities of the liposomes, having a signal-enhancing effect,[118] as well as the fluidity of the liposomal membranes, which provided lateral mobility of binding ligands and consequently increased the probability that tagged reporter probes could capture target sequences in the samples.[87] To increase the sensitivity and specificity above those obtained in the previous study, Rule et al. optimized various parameters for DNA hybridization, including temperature, and the concentrations of formamide, sodium dodecyl sulfate (SDS), and salts. The best detection limit obtained was 200 attomoles (in 10 µL) of target sequences, achieved using a hybridization buffer of 0.02% SDS in 3x standard saline citrate (SSC) with incubation at 40°C.[106] The results of this investigation reveal that SDS has an important influence on the behavior of liposomes in the strip assay, because liposomes did not migrate in a 3x SSC buffer alone, or in SDS at one-tenth of the aforementioned concentration (0.002%). Additionally, Rule et al. pointed out that SDS may reduce the lipid bilayer transition temperature (T_c). This reduction of liposomal membrane

Table 2.4 Summary of nucleic-acid-based LFAs using liposomes

Application	Analyte	Capture reagent on the test line	Limit of detection	Assay time[a]	Ref.
Sandwich assay					
Specific DNA sequences	Synthetic 39-mer ssDNA	CP	1 femtomole of target DNA	10 min	87
Specific DNA sequences	Synthetic 39-mer ssDNA	CP	200 attomoles of target DNA	10 min	106
Specific DNA sequences	Synthetic 43-mer ssDNA	Streptavidin + biotinylated CP	0.5 femtomole per assay	NA	55
Detection of dengue virus	RNA of dengue virus serotype 1–4	Streptavidin + biotinylated CP	10 pfu/mL	10 min	52
Detection of dengue virus	RNA of dengue virus serotype 1–4	Streptavidin + biotinylated CP	50 RNA molecules for serotype 2 500 RNA molecules for serotypes 3, 4 50000 RNA molecules for serotype 1	25 min	54
Detection of astrovirus	RNA of astrovirus	Streptavidin + biotinylated CP	NA	15 min	117
Detection of E. coli	mRNA of *E. coli* clpB gene	Streptavidin + biotinylated CP	40 CFU/mL	15–20 min	53

Detection of Streptococcus pyogenes	16S rRNA of S. pyogenes	Streptavidin + biotinylated CP	135 ng RNA	30 min	56
Detection of Cryptosporidium parvum	mRNA of C. parvum hsp70 gene	Streptavidin + biotinylated CP	5 oocysts/assay	NA	88
Detection of Mycobacterium avium	RNA of M. avium IS900	Streptavidin + biotinylated CP	10 viable cells/assay	30 min	57
Universal nucleic acid sequence biosensor	RNA of E. coli; RNA of B. anthracis; RNA of C. parvum	Streptavidin + biotinylated CP	1 femtomole/assay	30 min	89
Generic sandwich-type biosensor	RNA of E. coli; RNA of B. anthracis; RNA of C. Parvum	Anti-fluorescein Ab + fluorescein-tagged CP	5 femtomoles/assay for E. coli; 80 femtomoles/assay for B. anthracis 10 femtomoles/assay for C. parvum	30 min	60
Competitive assay					
Detection of Cryptosporidium parvum	mRNA of C. parvum hsp70 gene	Streptavidin + biotinylated antisense reporter probe	80 femtomole amplicon/test	30 min	62

CP, Capture probe.

[a]Detection time: only includes the time required for the test strip assay.

T_c by detergents has been observed elsewhere.[119] Theoretically, at a specific temperature, as the T_c of a liposome declines, its membrane becomes more fluid, resulting in more rapid DNA hybridization and improvement assay sensitivity. Accordingly, the detection limit in this study (200 attomoles) is one-fifth of that obtained in previous one published in 1996 (one femtomole). In both of these studies, DNA-tagged liposomes were produced by a covalent conjugation method using crosslinking reagents. In 2006, Edwards et al. developed a novel protocol for synthesizing DNA-tagged liposomes using cholesteryl-modified DNA probes. This new protocol can more precisely control the tagged mol% of DNA probes on the liposomal surface than can the conjugation method and can be more easily implemented with a much shorter preparation time (6 versus 16 h). The detection limit in this study was 0.5 femtomole of synthetic target sequence per assay under the optimal assay conditions of a reporter probe concentration of 0.013 mol%, a liposomal diameter of 315 nm, and a liposomal optical density of 0.4–0.6 at 532 nm.[55]

Sandwich nucleic-acid-based LFAs with liposomes have been applied for the detection of viruses, such as dengue virus[52,54] and astrovirus.[117] Both are single-stranded positive-sense RNA viruses.[120,121] For detection, their genomic RNA molecules were initially amplified by nucleic acid sequence-based amplification (NASBA) and then detected by sandwich LFAs that are based on DNA/RNA hybridization. Dengue virus is one of the major causes of arthropod-borne illness and is transmitted to humans by the *Aedes aegypti* mosquito. The virus exists as four distinct sero-types (Dengue 1–4).[122] The first assay for detecting dengue virus was based on two DNA probes. One probe was a generic reporter probe, tagged on the liposomal surface to hybridize with a generic sequence that was added to the dengue RNA amplicons during a NASBA reaction, and so could bind to every RNA amplicon. The other probe was the capture probe, immobilized on the membrane and specific toward four serotypes of the virus. Following a NASBA reaction, the RNA amplicons were first reacted with DNA reporter probes that were tagged on the dye-encapsulating liposomes and then the resultant complexes were captured by the captured probe that was immobilized on the strip. This developed assay exhibited good specificity in identifying serotypes 1, 2, and 4 from clinical human serum samples, but serotype 3 exhibited low cross-reactivity with the test strip that was designed to detect serotype 1 and 4. The detection limit of this assay was 10 plaque forming units (pfu)/mL and the results of this developed LFA correlated closely with those obtained using a laboratory-based electrochemiluminescence method.[52] In 2004, a multi-analyte LFA was developed for the simultaneous detection of four dengue serotypes on a single strip, based on the immobilization of four capture probes—each specific to one serotype in a particular location on the membrane—and generic reporter-probe-tagged liposomes for signal amplification. As in Baeumner's study in 2002,[52] RNA molecules of various dengue viruses were amplified by the NASBA reaction and then all of the RNA amplicons were conjugated with reporter-probe-tagged liposomes through DNA/RNA hybridization. The mixture was applied to the membrane and migrated along the strip. After it was captured by the specific immobilized capture probe on the membrane, the dengue virus serotype in the sample could be identified, and the viral RNA was quantified using a portable reflectometer, since the signal intensity of each test line was directly related to the amount of viral RNA. This developed multi-analyte assay exhibited 92% reliability in serotype identification with a detection limit of 500,000 RNA molecules for serotype 1500 RNA molecules for serotypes 2 and 3, and 50 RNA molecules for serotype 4. Moreover, the assay can simultaneously detect any two serotypes, and so it can be used to analyze concurrent infections of dengue viruses.[54]

A test with the same format has been used to detect astrovirus, which can cause acute gastroenteritis in children. In this study, NASBA and reverse transcriptase PCR (RT-PCR) were utilized to amplify viral RNA. The RNA amplicons from the RT-PCR reaction were analyzed by either ethidium bromide (EtBr) staining following gel electrophoresis (RT-PCR/EtBr) or liquid hybridization assay (RT-PCR/LHA); those from NASBA were identified by ether ECL detection (NASBA/ECL) or by liposome-strip assay. The agreement among the results of the assays of all four formats was good (91.0–97.2%), suggesting that the assay that combines a NASBA reaction with liposome-strip detection may be useful for field studies and environmental testing, because the two methods described herein are easy and fast to implement with no need for specialized equipment.[120]

Based on the principle described above, several sandwich LFAs have been developed for the detection of pathogens. For example, in 2003, Baeumner's group developed a highly specific and sensitive RNA biosensor for the rapid detection of viable *E. coli* in drinking water, which depended on identifying a 200 nt long target sequence from mRNA (*clp*B) coding for a heat shock protein. Their study focused on the detection of *E. coli* in drinking water, because it is often used as a fecal indicator organism in the analysis of water samples.[123] The assay exhibited a high specificity for viable *E. coli*, since no false positive result was obtained by the detection of nonviable *E. coli* and other microorganisms, including *Shigella sonnei*, *Pseudomonas aeruginosa*, *Salmonella enterica* serovar Typhimurium, and *Bacillus cereus*. The detection limit of this RNA biosensor was 40 CFU/mL and the detection time was approximately 20 min.[53]

Nugen et al. established a sandwich LFA with a new format, which was unlike the traditional sandwich assay in which a target DNA fragment was recognized by one capture probe and one reporter probe. This new sandwich LFA was developed to detect 16S rRNA of *Streptococcus pyogenes*, a food contaminant and nosocomial organism,[124] based on the optimal combination of three reporter probes and two capture probes for simultaneous hybridization with one target DNA sequence to increase the capture efficiency. Additionally, to increase assay sensitivity, 16S rRNA was used as the detection target because of its high concentration within a bacterial cell. This concept has been exploited in the detection of *E. coli*[125] and *Listeria monocytogenes*.[126,127] Without a cell culturing or a gene amplification step, this developed biosensor can detect as little as 135 ng of RNA, which corresponds to approximately 7.3×10^6 CFU/mL of *S. pyogenes*.[56] Furthermore, a biosensor was developed to identify the RNA of the IS900 element of *Mycobacterium avium* subsp. *paratuberculosis* (MAP) to detect viable MAP in fecal samples, since this IS900 gene is unique in the MAP genome and presents a high copy number.[128,129] In this study, MAP was extracted from fecal samples and then amplified using an RT-PCR. RNA amplicons were incubated first with reporter probes and then with liposomes, before being analyzed on a test strip. As they migrated along the membrane, the target-reporter probe-liposome complexes were bound by the immobilized capture probe, forming a visible line whose intensity was measured using a hand-held reflectometer. The detection limit of this assay was 10 viable cells, and the assay exhibited no cross-reaction with other mycobacteria.[57] A sandwich LFA has also been developed to detect the oocysts of the human pathogenic *Cryptosporidium* species, including *C. parvum*, *C. hominis*, and *C. meleagridis,* in bodies of natural water. In this LFA, oocysts were isolated from water samples by immunomagnetic separation (IMS) with anti-*Cryptosporidium* IMS beads, and their mRNA molecules were extracted with dT-tagged magnetic beads and further amplified by a NASBA reaction, which was specifically targeted to *hsp* 70 mRNA. The RNA amplicons were identified in a DNA/RNA hybridization LFA with reporter probes that were tagged on the liposomal surface and biotinylated capture probes that are immobilized on the membrane of a test strip. Since natural bodies of water may also be contaminated by waterborne bacteria, this developed assay was tested by detecting oocysts in the presence of *Giardia intestinalis*, *Oocystis minuta*, and *E. coli* O157:H7, and the results thus obtained revealed a high specificity to *C. parvum*. This LFA could detect as few as five oocysts, and the entire assay was complete in 4.5 h. Thus, this assay is effective for determining the safety of drinking water.[88]

To establish a universal sandwich-type nucleic-acid-based LFA, two types of liposome have been developed. One type is dC-tagged liposomes, which can hybridize any dG-labeled reporter probe, while the other is streptavidin-tagged liposomes, which can conjugate with any biotinylated reporter probe. Since universal liposomes of both types may be prepared and stored until use, the specific reporter-probe-tagged liposomes can be easily generated on demand and rapidly applied in nucleic-acid-based LFAs. The LFA that uses dC-tagged liposomes has been used to detect *hsp70* of *E. coli, atx*A of *Bacillus anthracis,* and *clpB* of *C. parvum*. The detection limit of this assay was 1 femtomole per assay (i.e., 1 nM) with dynamic ranges between 1 femtomole and at least 750 femtomoles for three targets mentioned above.[89] The other LFAs, which use streptavidin-tagged liposomes, have been used to detect pathogens with detection limits for *hsp70* from *E. coli* of 5 femtomoles, for *atxA* from *B. anthracis* of 1.5 femtomoles, and for *clpB* from *C. parvum* of 80 femtomoles.[60] Based on these detection limits, the assay with streptavidin-tagged liposomes is more sensitive than that using dC-tagged liposomes. The performance improvement of using streptavidin-tagged liposomes may be due to the fact that the affinity between streptavidin and biotin is the strongest non-covalent biological interaction known, with a dissociation constant (K_d = 4 × 10^{-14} M).[130] Moreover, the use of a biotin–streptavidin interaction to produce reporter-probe-tagged liposomes eliminates the need for the difficult coupling reaction, which is based on the hybridization between the tagged dC sequence and the dG-labeled reporter probe. Therefore, streptavidin-tagged liposomes are a better choice as the universal detection reagent in LFAs.

In a competitive nucleic-acid-based LFA, the target sequences compete with the immobilized antisense reporter probe to be hybridized with the reporter probes that are tagged on a liposomal surface. If a sample contains the target sequence, then the "target-reporter probe-liposome" complexes migrate through the test line without binding and subsequently bind to the immobilized antibodies on the control line that are against the small molecules (e.g., biotin, FITC, DIG, or DNP) also tagged on the surface of liposomes. On the other hand, reporter-probe-tagged liposomes bind to the immobilized antisense reporter probe when the sample does not contain the target sequence. Hence, in a competitive LFA, one visible control line constitutes a positive result, while the visible test line with a visible control line constitutes a negative result, as presented in Fig. 2.8b. This competitive format has been used to develop a single-use visual strip assay for rapidly detecting the *hsp70* mRNA from *C. parvum* using dye-encapsulating liposomes on which biotin molecules and reporter probes are tagged. In this study, RNA amplicons were incubated with liposomes in a 4x SSC solution that contains 20% (v/v) formamide at 40°C for 20 min, to hybridize with the reporter probe conjugated on liposomal surface. The "target-reporter prober-liposome" complexes would move through the oligonucleotide zone consisting the antisense reporter probe and then captured by the anti-biotin antibodies immobilized on the antibody zone, with the detection limit determined to be 80 femtomoles amplicons per test, as indicated in Table 2.4.[62] Therefore, this work demonstrated the applicability of a competitive nucleic-acid-based LFA that uses liposomes for the detection and quantification of nucleic acid sequences.

2.7 Conclusion

In LFAs, liposomes are used as the detection reagent in the amplification of assay signals, because their internal cavities encapsulate many dye molecules. Various biomolecules, such as antibodies, antigens, gangliosides, and DNA probes, can be tagged on the liposomal surface to make them targets. These biomolecules can be tagged on the surface of liposomes by covalent conjugation using crosslinking reagents, direct incorporation with the initial lipid mixture, or a biotin–avidin interaction with NeutrAvidin/streptavidin-tagged, preformed liposomes. To improve the sensitivity of the assay, liposomes can be optimized by controlling the diameter, lipid concentration, and the mol% of the tagged molecules. Numerous parameters can be varied to optimize the entire LFA. These include type of membrane, the compositions of the blocking buffer, coating buffer, and running buffer, and the reaction/hybridization temperature and duration. The performance of LFAs that use liposomes is generally comparable with that of LFAs that use gold nanoparticles. However, the use of liposomes is not as popular because of the instability of its dried form if they are coated and dried on the conjugate pad of a LFA test strip. On the other hand, this character can be potentially advantageous if fluorescence measurements of dried/lysed liposomes are used, as demonstrated by Volland's group. Therefore, there are still a wide range of applications of liposomes in the development of LFAs for detecting various targets.

References

1. Kohn J. An immunochromatographic technique. *Immunology,* 1968; 15(6): 863–865.

2. Vaitukaitis JL, Braunstein GD, Ross GT. A radioimmunoassay which specifically measures human chorionic gonadotropin in the presence of human luteinizing hormone. *Am J Obstet Gynecol,* 1972; 113(6): 751–758.

3. Nepomnaschy PA, Weinberg CR, Wilcox AJ, Baird DD. Urinary hCG patterns during the week following implantation. *Hum Reprod,* 2008; 23(2): 271–277.

4. Liu CC, Yeung CY, Chen PH, Yeh MK, Hou SY. *Salmonella* detection using 16S ribosomal DNA/RNA probe-gold nanoparticles and lateral flow immunoassay. *Food Chem,* 2013; 141(3): 2526–2532.

5. Terao Y, Yonekita T, Morishita N, Fujimura T, Matsumoto T, Morimatsu F. Potential rapid and simple lateral flow assay for *Escherichia coli* O111. *J Food Prot,* 2013; 76(5): 755–761.

6. You DJ, Park TS, Yoon JY. Cell-phone-based measurement of TSH using Mie scatter optimized lateral flow assays. *Biosens Bioelectron,* 2013; 40(1): 180–185.

7. Gandhi S, Caplash N, Sharma P, Raman Suri C. Strip-based immunochromatographic assay using specific egg yolk antibodies for rapid detection of morphine in urine samples. *Biosens Bioelectron,* 2009; 25(2): 502–505.

8. Shanin IA, Khan O, Petukhov AE, Smirnov AV, Eremin SA. The detection of amphetamines in urine samples using immunochromatographic test strips. *Sud Med Ekspert,* 2012; 55(4): 33–37.

9. Lopez Marzo AM, Pons J, Blake DA, Merkoci A. High sensitive gold-nanoparticle based lateral flow immunodevice for Cd^{2+} detection in drinking waters. *Biosens Bioelectron,* 2013; 47: 190–198.

10. Zhou Y, Zhang Y, Pan F, Li Y, Lu S, Ren H, Shen Q, Li Z, Zhang J, Chen Q, Liu Z. A competitive immunochromatographic assay based on a novel probe for the detection of mercury (II) ions in water samples. *Biosens Bioelectron,* 2010; 25(11): 2534–2538.

11. Guo YR, Liu SY, Gui WJ, Zhu GN. Gold immunochromatographic assay for simultaneous detection of carbofuran and triazophos in water samples. *Anal Biochem,* 2009; 389(1): 32–39.

12. Gui WJ, Wang ST, Guo YR, Zhu GN. Development of a one-step strip for the detection of triazophos residues in environmental samples. *Anal Biochem,* 2008; 377(2): 202–208.

13. Zhu J, Chen W, Lu Y, Cheng G. Development of an immunochromato-graphic assay for the rapid detection of bromoxynil in water. *Environ Pollut,* 2008; 156(1): 136–142.

14. Byzova NA, Zherdev AV, Zvereva EA, Dzantiev BB. Immunochromatographic assay with photometric detection for rapid determination of the herbicide atrazine and other triazines in foodstuffs. *J AOAC Int,* 2010; 93(1): 36–43.

15. Cui S, Zhou S, Chen C, Qi T, Zhang C, Oh J. A simple and rapid immunochromatographic strip test for detecting antibody to porcine reproductive and respiratory syndrome virus. *J Virol Methods,* 2008; 152(1–2): 38–42.

16. Anfossi L, Baggiani C, Giovannoli C, D'Arco G, Giraudi G. Lateral-flow immunoassays for mycotoxins and phycotoxins: A review. *Anal Bioanal Chem,* 2013; 405(2–3): 467–480.

17. Posthuma-Trumpie GA, Korf J, van Amerongen A. Lateral flow (immuno)assay: Its strengths, weaknesses, opportunities and threats. A literature survey. *Anal Bioanal Chem,* 2009; 393(2): 569–582.

18. Ip M, Rainer TH, Lee N, Chan C, Chau SS, Leung W, Leung MF, Tam TK, Antonio GE, Lui G, Lau TK, Hui DS, Fuchs D, Renneberg R, Chan PK. Value of serum procalcitonin, neopterin, and C-reactive protein in differentiating bacterial from viral etiologies in patients presenting with lower respiratory tract infections. *Diagn Micr Infec Dis,* 2007; 59(2): 131–136.

19. McCabe RE, Remington JS. C-reactive protein in patients with bacteremia. *J Clin Microbiol.,* 1984; 20(3): 317–319.

20. Leung W, Chan CP, Rainer TH, Ip M, Cautherley GW, Renneberg R. InfectCheck CRP barcode-style lateral flow assay for semi-quantitative detection of C-reactive protein in distinguishing between bacterial and viral infections. *J Immunol Methods,* 2008; 336(1): 30–36.

21. Fung KK, Chan CP, Renneberg R. Development of enzyme-based bar code-style lateral-flow assay for hydrogen peroxide determination. *Anal Chim Acta,* 2009; 634(1): 89–95.

22. Fang C, Chen Z, Li L, Xia J. Barcode lateral flow immunochromatographic strip for prostate acid phosphatase determination. *J Pharm Biomed Anal,* 2011; 56(5): 1035–1040.

23. Hossain SM, Ozimok C, Sicard C, Aguirre SD, Ali MM, Li Y, Brennan JD. Multiplexed paper test strip for quantitative bacterial detection. *Anal Bioanal Chem,* 2012; 403(6): 1567–1576.

24. Blazkova M, Koets M, Rauch P, van Amerongen A. Development of a nucleic acid lateral flow immunoassay for simultaneous detection of *Listeria* spp. and *Listeria monocytogenes* in food. *Eur Food Res and Technol,* 2009; 229(6): 867–874.

25. Noguera P, Posthuma-Trumpie GA, van Tuil M, van der Wal FJ, de Boer A, Moers APHA, van Amerongen A. Carbon nanoparticles in lateral flow methods to detect genes encoding virulence factors of Shiga toxin-producing *Escherichia coli. Anal Bioanal Chem,* 2011; 399(2): 831–838.

26. Taranova NA, Byzova NA, Zaiko VV, Starovoitova TA, Vengerov YY, Zherdev AV, Dzantiev BB. Integration of lateral flow and microarray technologies for multiplex immunoassay: Application to the determination of drugs of abuse. *Microchimica Acta,* 2013; 180(11–12): 1165–1172.

27. Zangheri M, Di Nardo F, Anfossi L, Giovannoli C, Baggiani C, Roda A, Mirasoli M. A multiplex chemiluminescent biosensor for type B-fumonisins and aflatoxin B1 quantitative detection in maize flour. *Analyst*, 2014; 140(1): 358–365.

28. Nihonyanagi S, Kanoh Y, Okada K, Uozumi T, Kazuyama Y, Yamaguchi T, Nakazaki N, Sakurai K, Hirata Y, Munekata S, Ohtani S, Takemoto T, Bandoh Y, Akahoshi T. Clinical usefulness of multiplex PCR lateral flow in MRSA detection: A novel, rapid genetic testing method. *Inflammation*, 2012; 35(3): 927–934.

29. Jin W, Yamada K, Ikami M, Kaji N, Tokeshi M, Atsumi Y, Mizutani M, Murai A, Okamoto A, Namikawa T, Baba Y, Ohta M. Application of IgY to sandwich enzyme-linked immunosorbent assays, lateral flow devices, and immunopillar chips for detecting staphylococcal enterotoxins in milk and dairy products. *J Microbiol Methods*, 2013; 92(3): 323–331.

30. Lee EY, Kang JH, Kim KA, Chung TW, Kim HJ, Yoon DY, Lee HG, Kwon DH, Kim JW, Kim CH, Song EY. Development of a rapid, immunochromatographic strip test for serum asialo alpha1-acid glycoprotein in patients with hepatic disease. *J Immunol Methods*, 2006; 308(1–2): 116–123.

31. Lee S, Kim G, Moon J. Performance improvement of the one-dot lateral flow immunoassay for aflatoxin B1 by using a smartphone-based reading system. *Sensors (Basel)*, 2013; 13(4): 5109–5116.

32. Siebert STA, Reeves SG, Durst RA. Liposome immunomigration field assay device for alachlor determination. *Anal Chim Acta*, 1993; 282(2): 297–305.

33. Roberts MA, Durst RA. Investigation of liposome-based immunomigration sensors for the detection of polychlorinated biphenyls. *Anal Chem*, 1995; 67(3): 482–491.

34. Glorio-Paulet P, Durst RA. Determination of potato glycoalkaloids using a liposome immunomigration, liquid-phase competition immunoassay. *J Agric Food Chem*, 2000; 48(5): 1678–1683.

35. Park S, Durst RA. Immunoliposome sandwich assay for the detection of *Escherichia coli* O157:H7. *Anal Biochem*, 2000; 280(1): 151–158.

36. Ahn-Yoon S, DeCory TR, Baeumner AJ, Durst RA. Ganglioside-liposome immunoassay for the ultrasensitive detection of cholera toxin. *Anal Chem*, 2003; 75(10): 2256–2261.

37. Weihua L, Fung DYC, Yang X, Renrong L, Yonghua X. Development of a colloidal gold strip for rapid detection of ochratoxin A with mimotope peptide. *Food Control*, 2009; 20(9): 791–795.

38. Mao X, Wang W, Du TE. Rapid quantitative immunochromatographic strip for multiple proteins test. *Sensors Actuators B-Chemical,* 2013; 186: 315–320.

39. Kim YM, Oh SW, Jeong SY, Pyo DJ, Choi EY. Development of an ultrarapid one-step fluorescence immunochromatographic assay system for the quantification of microcystins. *Environ Sci Technol,* 2003; 37(9): 1899–1904.

40. Preechakasedkit P, Pinwattana K, Dungchai W, Siangproh W, Chaicumpa W, Tongtawe P, Chailapakul O. Development of a one-step immunochromatographic strip test using gold nanoparticles for the rapid detection of *Salmonella* typhi in human serum. *Biosens Bioelectron,* 2012; 31(1): 562–566.

41. Ang GY, Yu CY, Yean CY. Ambient temperature detection of PCR amplicons with a novel sequence-specific nucleic acid lateral flow biosensor. *Biosens Bioelectron,* 2012; 38(1): 151–156.

42. Wen HW, Borejsza-Wysocki W, DeCory TR, Durst RA. Development of a competitive liposome-based lateral flow assay for the rapid detection of the allergenic peanut protein Ara h1. *Anal Bioanal Chem,* 2005; 382(5): 1217–1226.

43. Hou SY, Hsiao YL, Lin MS, Yen CC, Chang CS. MicroRNA detection using lateral flow nucleic acid strips with gold nanoparticles. *Talanta,* 2012; 99: 375–379.

44. Suarez-Pantaleon C, Wichers J, Abad-Somovilla A, van Amerongen A, Abad-Fuentes A. Development of an immunochromatographic assay based on carbon nanoparticles for the determination of the phytoregulator forchlorfenuron. *Biosens Bioelectron,* 2013; 42: 170–176.

45. Mao X, Wang W, Du TE. Dry-reagent nucleic acid biosensor based on blue dye doped latex beads and lateral flow strip. *Talanta,* 2013; 114: 248–253.

46. Nielsen K, Yu WL, Lin M, Davis SA, Elmgren C, Mackenzie R, Tanha J, Li S, Dubuc G, Brown EG, Keleta L, Pasick J. Prototype single step lateral flow technology for detection of avian influenza virus and chicken antibody to avian influenza virus. *J Immunoassay Immunochem,* 2007; 28(4): 307–318.

47. Ho JAA, Hsu HW. Procedures for preparing *Escherichia coli* O157: H7 immunoliposome and its application in liposome immunoassay. *Anal Chem,* 2003; 75(16): 4330–4334.

48. Ahn-Yoon S, DeCory TR, Durst RA. Ganglioside-liposome immunoassay for the detection of botulinum toxin. *Anal Bioanal Chem,* 2004; 378(1): 68–75.

49. Ho JA, Zeng SC, Tseng WH, Lin YJ, Chen CH. Liposome-based immunostrip for the rapid detection of *Salmonella*. *Anal Bioanal Chem*, 2008; 391(2): 479–485.

50. Shukla S, Leem H, Kim M. Development of a liposome-based immunochromatographic strip assay for the detection of *Salmonella*. *Anal Bioanal Chem*, 2011; 401(8): 2581–2590.

51. Siebert STA, Reeves SG, Roberts MA, Durst RA. Improved liposome immunomigration strip assay for alachlor determination. *Anal Chim Acta*, 1995; 311(3): 309–318.

52. Baeumner AJ, Schlesinger NA, Slutzki NS, Romano J, Lee EM, Montagna RA. Biosensor for dengue virus detection: Sensitive, rapid, and serotype specific. *Anal Chem*, 2002; 74(6): 1442–1448.

53. Baeumner AJ, Cohen RN, Miksic V, Min JH. RNA biosensor for the rapid detection of viable *Escherichia coli* in drinking water. *Biosens Bioelectron*, 2003; 18(4): 405–413.

54. Zaytseva NV, Montagna RA, Lee EM, Baeumner AJ. Multi-analyte single-membrane biosensor for the serotype-specific detection of dengue virus. *Anal Bioanal Chem*, 2004; 380(1): 46–53.

55. Edwards KA, Baeumner AJ. Optimization of DNA-tagged dye-encapsulating liposomes for lateral-flow assays based on sandwich hybridization. *Anal Bioanal Chem*, 2006; 386(5): 1335–1343.

56. Nugen SR, Leonard B, Baeumner AJ. Application of a unique server-based oligonucleotide probe selection tool toward a novel biosensor for the detection of *Streptococcus pyogenes*. *Biosens Bioelectron*, 2007; 22(11): 2442–2448.

57. Kumanan V, Nugen SR, Baeumner AJ, Chang YF. A biosensor assay for the detection of *Mycobacterium avium* subsp paratuberculosis in fecal samples. *J Vet Sci*, 2009; 10(1): 35–42.

58. Park S, Durst RA. Modified immunoliposome sandwich assay for the detection of *Escherichia coli* O157:H7 in apple cider. *J Food Prot*, 2004; 67(8): 1568–1573.

59. Ahn S, Durst RA. Detection of cholera toxin in seafood using a ganglioside-liposome immunoassay. *Anal Bioanal Chem*, 2008; 391(2): 473–478.

60. Baeumner AJ, Jones C, Wong CY, Price A. A generic sandwich-type biosensor with nanomolar detection limits. *Anal Bioanal Chem*, 2004; 378(6): 1587–1593.

61. Schneider Z. Aliphatic-alcohols improve the adsorptive performance of cellulose nitrate membranes: Application in chromatography and enzyme assays. *Anal Biochem*, 1980; 108(1): 96–103.

62. Esch MB, Baeumner AJ, Durst RA. Detection of *Cryptosporidium parvum* using oligonucleotide-tagged liposomes in a competitive assay format. *Anal Chem,* 2001; 73(13): 3162–3167.

63. Wen HW, Decory TR, Borejsza-Wysocki W, Durst RA. Investigation of NeutrAvidin-tagged liposomal nanovesicles as universal detection reagents for bioanalytical assays. *Talanta,* 2006; 68(4): 1264–1272.

64. Delmulle BS, De Saeger SMDG, Sibanda L, Barna-Vetro I, Van Peteghem CH. Development of an immunoassay-based lateral flow dipstick for the rapid detection of aflatoxin B-1 in pig feed. *J Agric Food Chem,* 2005; 53(9): 3364–3368.

65. Ching KH, Lin A, McGarvey JA, Stanker LH, Hnasko R. Rapid and selective detection of botulinum neurotoxin serotype-A and -B with a single immunochromatographic test strip. *J Immunol Methods,* 2012; 380(1–2): 23–29.

66. Huo Q. A perspective on bioconjugated nanoparticles and quantum dots. *Colloid Surface B,* 2007; 59(1): 1–10.

67. Shim WB, Yang ZY, Kim JS, Kim JY, Kang S, Gun-Jo W, Chung YC, Eremin SA, Chung DH. Development of immunochromatography strip-test using nanocolloidal gold-antibody probe for the rapid detection of aflatoxin B1 in grain and feed samples. *J Microbiol Biotechnol,* 2007; 17(10): 1629–1637.

68. Laitinen MPA, Vuento M. Affinity immunosensor for milk progesterone: Identification of critical parameters. *Biosens Bioelectron,* 1996; 11(12): 1207–1214.

69. Plant AL, Brizgys MV, Locasio-Brown L, Durst RA. Generic liposome reagent for immunoassays. *Anal Biochem,* 1989; 176(2): 420–426.

70. Park S, Oh S, Durst RA. Immunoliposomes sandwich fluorometric assay (ILSF) for detection of *Escherichia coli* O157:H7. *J Food Sci,* 2004; 69(6): M151–M156.

71. Lasic DD. Novel applications of liposomes. *Trends Biotechnol,* 1998; 16(7): 307–321.

72. Durst RA, Siebert ST, Reeves SG. Immunosensor for extra-lab measurements based on liposome amplification and capillary migration. *Biosens Bioelectron,* 1993; 8(6): xiii–xv.

73. Szoka F, Olson F, Heath T, Vail W, Mayhew E, Papahadjopoulos D. Preparation of unilamellar liposomes of intermediate size (0.1–0.2-mumm) by a combination of reverse-phase evaporation and extrusion through polycarbonate membranes. *Bioch Biophys Acta,* 1980; 601(3): 559–571.

74. Fishman PH, Pacuszka T, Orlandi PA. Gangliosides as receptors for bacterial enterotoxins. *Adv Lipid Res,* 1993; 25: 165–187.

75. Kitamura M, Iwamori M, Nagai Y. Interaction between clostridium-botulinum neurotoxin and gangliosides. *Bioch Biophys Acta,* 1980; 628(3): 328–335.

76. Franz DR, Jahrling PB, Friedlander AM, McClain DJ, Hoover DL, Bryne WR, Pavlin JA, Christopher CW, Eitzen EM. Clinical recognition and management of patients exposed to biological warfare agents. *JAMA-J Am Med Assoc,* 1997; 278(5): 399–411.

77. Arnon SS, Schechter R, Inglesby TV, Henderson DA, Bartlett JG, Ascher MS, Eitzen E, Fine AD, Hauer J, Layton M, Lillibridge S, Osterholm MT, O'Toole T, Parker G, Perl TM, Russell PK, Swerdlow DL, Tonat K. Working Group on Civilian Biodefense. Botulinum toxin as a biological weapon: Medical and public health management. *JAMA-J Am Med Assoc,* 2001; 285(8): 1059–1070.

78. Lencer WI, Delp C, Neutra MR, Madara JL. Mechanism of cholera-toxin action on a polarized human intestinal epithelial-cell line: Role of vesicular traffic. *J Cell Biol,* 1992; 117(6): 1197–1209.

79. Khreich N, Lamourette P, Boutal H, Devilliers K, Creminon C, Volland H. Detection of Staphylococcus enterotoxin B using fluorescent immunoliposomes as label for immunochromatographic testing. *Anal Biochem,* 2008; 377(2): 182–188.

80. Khreich N, Lamourette P, Lagoutte B, Ronco C, Franck X, Creminon C, Volland H. A fluorescent immunochromatographic test using immunoliposomes for detecting microcystins and nodularins. *Anal Bioanal Chem,* 2010; 397(5): 1733–1742.

81. Shin J, Kim M. Development of liposome immunoassay for *Salmonella* spp. using immunomagnetic separation and immunoliposome. *J Microbiol Biotechnol,* 2008; 18(10): 1689–1694.

82. Pasenkiewicz-Gierula M, Takaoka Y, Miyagawa H, Kitamura K, Kusumi A. Charge pairing of headgroups in phosphatidylcholine membranes: A molecular dynamics simulation study. *Biophys J,* 1999; 76(3): 1228–1240.

83. Kirby C, Gregoriadis G. The effect of the cholesterol content of small unilamellar liposomes on the fate of their lipid components in vitro. *Life Sci,* 1980; 27(23): 2223–2230.

84. Liu DZ, Chen WY, Tsai LM, Yang SP. The effects of cholesterol on the release of free lipids and the physical stability of lecithin liposomes. *J Chin Inst Chem Eng,* 2000; 31(3): 269–276.

85. Vingerhoeds MH, Storm G, Crommelin DJ. Immunoliposomes in vivo. *Immunomethods,* 1994; 4(3): 259–272.

86. Chen CS, Baeumner AJ, Durst RA. Protein G-liposomal nanovesicles as universal reagents for immunoassays. *Talanta,* 2005; 67(1): 205–211.

87. Rule GS, Montagna RA, Durst RA. Rapid method for visual identification of specific DNA sequences based on DNA-tagged liposomes. *Clin Chem,* 1996; 42(8 Pt 1): 1206–1209.

88. Connelly JT, Nugen SR, Borejsza-Wysocki W, Durst RA, Montagna RA, Baeumner AJ. Human pathogenic *Cryptosporidium* species bioanalytical detection method with single oocyst detection capability. *Anal Bioanal Chem,* 2008; 391(2): 487–495.

89. Baeumner AJ, Pretz J, Fang S. A universal nucleic acid sequence biosensor with nanomolar detection limits. *Anal Chem,* 2004; 76(4): 888–894.

90. Duncan RJS, Weston PD, Wrigglesworth R. A new reagent which may be used to introduce sulfhydryl-groups into proteins, and its use in the preparation of conjugates for immunoassay. *Anal Biochem,* 1983; 132(1): 68–73.

91. Wen HW, Borejsza-Wysocki W, DeCory TR, Baeumner AJ, Durst RA. A novel extraction method for peanut allergenic proteins in chocolate and their detection by a liposome-based lateral flow assay. *Eur Food Res Technol,* 2005; 221(3–4): 564–569.

92. Ho JAA, Wauchope RD. A strip liposome immunoassay for aflatoxin B-1. *Anal Chem,* 2002; 74(7): 1493–1496.

93. Fan YS, Davis LM, Shows TB. Mapping small DNA sequences by fluorescence in situ hybridization directly on banded metaphase chromosomes. *Proc Natl Acad Sci U S A,* 1990; 87(16): 6223–6227.

94. Wilchek M, Bayer EA. Introduction to avidin-biotin technology. *Method Enzymol,* 1990; 184: 5–13.

95. Bayer EA, Wilchek M. Application of avidin-biotin technology to affinity-based separations. *J Chromatogr,* 1990; 510: 3–11.

96. Bussolati G, Gugliotta P. Nonspecific staining of mast-cells by avidin biotin peroxidase complexes (Abc). *J Histochem Cytochemi,* 1983; 31(12): 1419–1421.

97. Sano T, Cantor CR. Expression of a cloned streptavidin gene in *Escherichia coli. Proc Natl Acad Sci U S A,* 1990; 87(1): 142–146.

98. Hiller Y, Gershoni JM, Bayer EA, Wilchek M. Biotin binding to avidin. Oligosaccharide side chain not required for ligand association. *Biochem J,* 1987; 248(1): 167–171.

99. van Roy N, Mangelschots K, Speleman F. Improved immunocytochemical detection of biotinylated probes with Neutralite avidin. *Trends Genet,* 1993; 9(3): 71–72.

100. Bjorck L, Kronvall G. Purification and some properties of streptococcal protein-G, a novel IgG-binding reagent. *J Immunol,* 1984; 133(2): 969–974.

101. Sjobring U, Bjorck L, Kastern W. Streptococcal protein G. Gene structure and protein binding properties. *J Biol Chem,* 1991; 266(1): 399–405.

102. Graille M, Stura EA, Corper AL, Sutton BJ, Taussig MJ, Charbonnier JB, Silverman GJ. Crystal structure of a *Staphylococcus aureus* protein A domain complexed with the Fab fragment of a human IgM antibody: Structural basis for recognition of B-cell receptors and superantigen activity. *Proc Natl Acad Sci U S A,* 2000; 97(10): 5399–5404.

103. Akerström B, Björck L. A physicochemical study of protein G, a molecule with unique immunoglobulin G-binding properties. *J Biol Chem,* 1986; 261(22): 10240–10247.

104. Chen CS, Durst RA. Simultaneous detection of *Escherichia coli* O157: H7, *Salmonella* spp. and *Listeria monocytogenes* with an array-based immunosorbent assay using universal protein G-liposomal nanovesicles. *Talanta,* 2006; 69(1): 232–238.

105. Eidels L, Proia RL, Hart DA. Membrane receptors for bacterial toxins. *Microbiol Rev,* 1983; 47(4): 596–620.

106. Rule GS, Montagna RA, Durst RA. Characteristics of DNA-tagged liposomes allowing their use in capillary-migration, sandwich-hybridization assays. *Anal Biochem,* 1997; 244(2): 260–269.

107. Ho JA, Durst RA. Detection of fumonisin B1: Comparison of flow-injection liposome immunoanalysis with high-performance liquid chromatography. *Anal Biochem,* 2003; 312(1): 7–13.

108. Nakayama T, Ono K, Hashimoto K. Affinity of antioxidative polyphenols for lipid bilayers evaluated with a liposome system. *Biosci Biotech Bioch,* 1998; 62(5): 1005–1007.

109. Jung BY, Jung SC, Kweon CH. Development of a rapid immunochromatographic strip for detection of *Escherichia coli* O157. *J Food Prot,* 2005; 68(10): 2140–2143.

110. Qi H, Zhong Z, Zhou HX, Deng CY, Zhu H, Li JF, Wang XL, Li FR. A rapid and highly sensitive protocol for the detection of *Escherichia coli* O157:H7 based on immunochromatography assay combined with the enrichment technique of immunomagnetic nanoparticles. *Int J Nanomed,* 2011; 6: 3033–3039.

111. Seo KH, Holt PS, Stone HD, Gast RK. Simple and rapid methods for detecting *Salmonella enteritidis* in raw eggs. *Int J Food Microbiol,* 2003; 87(1–2): 139–144.

112. Chiao DJ, Wey JJ, Shyu RH, Tang SS. Monoclonal antibody-based lateral flow assay for detection of botulinum neurotoxin type A. *Hybridoma,* 2008; 27(1): 31–35.

113. Chen RF, Knutson JR. Mechanism of fluorescence concentration quenching of carboxyfluorescein in liposomes: Energy-transfer to nonfluorescent dimers. *Anal Biochem,* 1988; 172(1): 61–77.

114. Shyu RH, Tang SS, Chiao DJ, Hung YW. Gold nanoparticle-based lateral flow assay for detection of staphylococcal enterotoxin B. *Food Chem,* 2010; 118(2): 462–466.

115. Sun XL, Zhao XL, Tang J, Gu XH, Zhou J, Chu FS. Development of an immunochromatographic assay for detection of aflatoxin B-1 in foods. *Food Control,* 2006; 17(4): 256–262.

116. Keck-Gassenmeier B, Benet S, Rosa C, Hischenhuber C. Determination of peanut traces in food by a commercially-available ELISA test. *Food and Agric Immunol,* 1999; 11(3): 243–250.

117. Tai JH, Ewert MS, Belliot G, Glass RI, Monroe SS. Development of a rapid method using nucleic acid sequence-based amplification for the detection of astrovirus. *J Virol Methods,* 2003; 110(2): 119–127.

118. Martin FJ, Kung VT. Use of liposomes as agglutination-enhancement agents in diagnostic-tests. *Method Enzymol,* 1987; 149: 200–213.

119. Frye LD, Edidin M. The rapid intermixing of cell surface antigens after formation of mouse-human heterokaryons. *J Cell Sci,* 1970; 7(2): 319–335.

120. Jiang BM, Monroe SS, Koonin EV, Stine SE, Glass RI. RNA sequence of astrovirus: Distinctive genomic organization and a putative retrovirus-like ribosomal frameshifting signal that directs the viral replicase synthesis. *Proc Natl Acad Sci U S A,* 1993; 90(22): 10539–10543.

121. Brinton MA, Fernandez AV, Dispoto JH. The 3′-nucleotides of flavivirus genomic RNA form a conserved secondary structure. *Virology,* 1986; 153(1): 113–121.

122. Chambers TJ, Hahn CS, Galler R, Rice CM. Flavivirus genome organization, expression, and replication. *Ann Rev Microbiol,* 1990; 44: 649–688.

123. Gauthier F, Archibald F. The ecology of "fecal indicator" bacteria commonly found in pulp and paper mill water systems. *Water Res,* 2001; 35(9): 2207–2218.

124. Lannigan R, Hussain Z, Austin TW. *Streptococcus pyogenes* as a cause of nosocomial infection in a critical care unit. *Diag Micr and Infec Dis,* 1985; 3(4): 337–341.

125. Fuchs BM, Glockner FO, Wulf J, Amann R. Unlabeled helper oligonucleotides increase the in situ accessibility to 16S rRNA of fluorescently labeled oligonucleotide probes. *Appl Environ Microbiol,* 2000; 66(8): 3603–3607.

126. Somer L, Kashi Y. A PCR method based on 16S rRNA sequence for simultaneous detection of the genus *Listeria* and the species *Listeria monocytogenes* in food products. *J Food Protect,* 2003; 66(9): 1658–1665.

127. Wang RF, Cao WW, Johnson MG. Development of a 16s ribosomal-RNA-based oligomer probe specific for *Listeria monocytogenes. Appl Environ Microbiol,* 1991; 57(12): 3666–3670.

128. Collins DM, Gabric DM, Delisle GW. Identification of a repetitive DNA-sequence specific to *Mycobacterium*-paratuberculosis. *Fems Microbio Lett,* 1989; 60(2): 175–178.

129. Moss MT, Green EP, Tizard ML, Malik ZP, Hermontaylor J. Specific detection of *Mycobacterium*-paratuberculosis by DNA hybridization with a fragment of the insertion element IS900. *Gut,* 1991; 32(4): 395–398.

130. Holmberg A, Blomstergren A, Nord O, Lukacs M, Lundeberg J, Uhlén M. The biotin-streptavidin interaction can be reversibly broken using water at elevated temperatures. *Electrophoresis,* 2005; 26(3): 501–510.

Chapter 3

Liposomes in Proteome Microarrays for the Study of Lipid–Protein Interactions

Kuan-Yi Lu, Guan-Da Syu, and Chien-Sheng Chen

Graduate Institute of Systems Biology and Bioinformatics,
National Central University, Jhongli 32001, Taiwan

cchen103@gmail.com

3.1 Introduction

Lipid signaling is a key regulatory system to control cell proliferation, polarization, survival, and the maintenance of many other cellular processes. The phosphoinositide-mediated signal transduction pathway is one of the representative networks that regulate physiological functions at the cellular level. Well-known examples include the IP3/DAG pathway, which is activated by G-protein-coupled receptors followed by initiating calcium signaling, and the PI3K/AKT/mTOR pathway, which is a pivotal regulator in apoptosis and senescence.[1,2] Dysregulation of lipid-signaling pathways leads to the pathogenesis of human disease and cancer, especially when key regulators are suppressed or overexpressed.[3-5] It is thus important to have a tool for better identifying lipid–protein interactions.

Typically, the bindings between protein domains and lipid head groups are reached by weak interactions, because of which

Liposomes in Analytical Methodologies
Edited by Katie A. Edwards
Copyright © 2016 Pan Stanford Publishing Pte. Ltd.
ISBN 978-981-4669-26-9 (Hardcover), 978-981-4669-27-6 (eBook)
www.panstanford.com

the high variability between experiments is imaginable. Thus far, the identification of lipid-binding proteins is mainly carried out by dot blot,[6,7] surface plasmon resonance spectroscopy,[8] and affinity chromatography coupled with mass spectrometry.[9-11] Lipid-coated beads, strips, and microtiter plates are also commercially available for binding assays.[12] However, the reproducibility, protein stability, and recovery efficiency of these assays are restricted due to their inconsistent wash stringency and low throughput. To settle these problems, a high-throughput approach is required to study protein–lipid interactions.

In modern proteomics, proteome microarrays (chips) are emerging as a robust high-throughput screening tool for protein–biomolecule interactions.[7,13-16] Proteins are simultaneously purified and printed onto a chemically modified slide surface in a high-density format that allows tens of thousands of binding tests to be examined in parallel (Fig. 3.1). Because of its strength, proteome microarrays become the antidote to the problem of high variability between experiments that individually examine protein–biomolecule interactions.

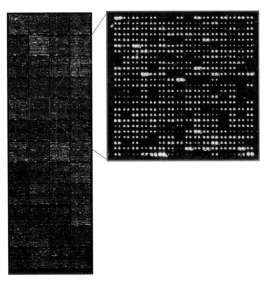

Figure 3.1   Image of a proteome microarray. A human proteome microarray was probed with 1:1000 DyLight™549-conjugated anti-GST antibody. The inset shows one of the 48 blocks in the chip. Notably, each individually purified GST-fusion protein was spotted in duplicate.

To substantiate the concept of identifying lipid–protein interactions on a chip and to mimic biological conditions, lipids of interest have to be incorporated into a model membrane that adapts to the buffer system. A fabulous model membrane would be liposomes. The lipids of interest can be easily incorporated into a phospholipid bilayer during the fabrication procedure. Those lipid head groups exposed at the outer side of liposomes can then serve as a docking site for their potential binders.

Another advantage of liposomes is their capability of encapsulating a large amount of fluorescent dye molecules so as to amplify the binding signals.[17-19] However, fluorescent liposomes that contain extremely high concentrations of fluorophores will lead to a self-quenching effect and consequently need to be lysed to detect the signals. This limitation confines the application of liposomes in real-time assays and high-density chip assays. To increase the utility of fluorescent liposomes in proteomics research, a nonquenched fluorescent (NQF) liposome has recently been developed,[20] which provides a maximal fluorescent signal without any lysis step, raising the flexibility and applicability of liposomes in proteome chip-based assays.

3.2 Proteome Microarrays

The physiological functions of living organisms are coordinated by a sophisticated and elaborate interaction network—an ensemble of signal transduction cascades. That is, the presented phenotype is the outcome of biological regulation through multiple interactions. Distinct from the study of single-molecule interactions, current biological science is developing toward systems biology, which evaluates the biological systems from a holistic point of view. This concept of systems biology is being carried out by the "omics" fields—genomics, transcriptomics, lipidomics, glycomics, and proteomics. Noticeably, the proteomics research has been in the spotlight since 1997[21] and has become more popular in contemporary molecular biology.

Proteome microarrays, or proteome chips, comprise one of the modern technologies in proteomics. As an analogue of DNA microarrays, proteome microarrays offer a miniaturized high-throughput screening tool for multiplexed bioassays such as immunoassays and protein–biomolecule binding assays (Fig. 3.2).[7,15,22,23]

In principle and based on their utilities, proteome microarrays can be divided into analytical and functional microarrays. Antibody microarrays, for example, are one of the most representative analytical proteome microarrays for antigen detection.[24–27] For identifying protein interactions, functional proteome microarrays include yeast (*Saccharomyces cerevisiae*),[7] bacteria (*Escherichia coli*),[13] plant (*Arabidopsis thaliana*),[28] virus (coronaviruses),[29] and human[16,30] proteome microarrays.

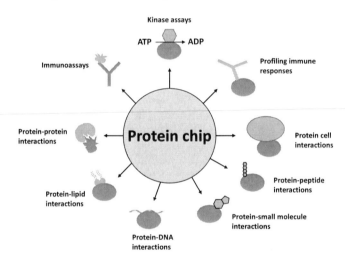

Figure 3.2   Applications of analytical and functional proteome microarrays. Analytical protein microarrays, such as antibody arrays, can be used for clinical diagnosis or environmental/food safety analysis. Functional protein arrays are mainly used to study various types of protein activity, including protein–protein, protein–lipid, protein–DNA, protein–drug, protein–peptide, protein–cell interactions, enzyme reactions, and profiling of immune responses.

3.2.1   Proteome Microarray Fabrication

Typically, proteome microarrays are fabricated by spotting small amounts of purified proteins on a glass-based microscopic slide in a high-density arrangement (ca. 16 spots per square millimeter).[28] By using this screening tool, researchers can easily identify all the possible interacting proteins of a specific biomolecule in a single experiment. The manufacturing steps consist of surface coating, protein preparation, and protein printing.

3.2.1.1   Surface coating

Above the solid support, most typically glass, is the coated material that serves as a medium for protein immobilization. In effect, the surface material is an important determinant for the quality of proteome microarrays. The protein activity and the accessibility of active sites are determined by their structural conformation and orientation, which are further influenced by the way of immobilization. Basically, three major types of immobilization strategies are physical adsorption, covalent binding, and affinity capture.[23,31]

Nitrocellulose polymers[32] and three-dimensional hydrogels[33] are common physical adsorption materials for protein capture. Both nitrocellulose and hydrogel are able to mitigate rapid evaporation and maintain the structural conformation of immobilized proteins. However, the adsorption strategy has some flaws, including random orientation, low adsorption, and difficulty in changing buffers.[23,31,34] The random orientation is suspected to block active sites of proteins sterically, thus resulting in false negative results. Low adsorption rate will, as a matter of course, largely decrease binding signals to be detected. Moreover, non-immobilized proteins may further become competitors to occupy the active binding sites, reducing the possibility to recover potential interactions.

Most of the time, protein immobilization is achieved through the covalent binding between exposed amino acid moieties and coupling groups that are modified on the surface of glass support. The amine group of lysine residue, for example, is usually exposed on the exterior side of proteins and thus becomes an excellent target for covalent crosslinking. The coupling groups that target amines include aldehydes, carboxylic esters, and epoxides. Empirically, aldehyde-modified slides have higher performance and immobilization efficiency. Similarly, the carboxyl groups of aspartic and glutamic acids are usually located on the protein surface, allowing the carboxyl side chains to react with amine substrate slides. Other accessible functional groups such as sulfhydryl and hydroxyl groups are able to form covalent bonds with maleimide and epoxy surfaces, respectively. A potential problem in using sulfhydryl and hydroxyl groups as attaching points is that these functional groups are often located in the active sites such as those of protein kinases and proteases.[35,36] The occupation of active sites can lead to the failure to detect binding interactions.

An important feature of affinity-mediated immobilization is the identical orientation of immobilized proteins. Recombinant proteins with affinity tags can be high-throughput purified and spotted on their corresponding surface materials. A famous case is that proteins expressed with 6xHis fusion tags are immobilized on a nickel-coated slide.[7] Because of the high affinity and specificity between the polyhistidine tag and nickel, the noncovalent and site-specific immobilization can be accomplished. Guo et al.[37] also reported that protein G-coated slides predominantly enhance the performance of antibody array via the strong affinity to Fc fragments of antibodies; thus the antibodies are uniformly oriented.

3.2.1.2 Protein preparation

One of the challenges in fabricating proteome microarrays is the approach required to purify thousands of individual proteins in a feasible and consistent way. Nowadays, proteins can be expressed and purified in a high-throughput manner from the open reading frame (ORF) clone libraries (Fig. 3.3). In 2005, Kitagawa et al.[38] successfully constructed a complete set of *Escherichia coli* K-12 ORF clone library, which contains 4256 individual *E. coli* genes. To extend the utility of the *E. coli* clone library to proteomic research, Chen et al.[13] developed a high-throughput protein purification protocol for *E. coli* (Fig. 3.3) and further printed all the purified proteins onto glass slides to fabricate an *E. coli* proteome microarray.

Briefly, *E. coli* cells harboring different genes were separately incubated in LB broth with an appropriate antibiotic in 96 DeepWell plates at 37°C overnight. When the optical density at 595 nm reached 0.7–0.9, the cells were induced with isopropyl β-D-thiogalactoside (IPTG) for 3.5 h to express proteins. The pellets were harvested by centrifugation and stored at −80°C. Subsequently, the frozen pellets were thawed and mixed with the lysis buffer and Ni-NTA resins, followed by 2.5 h incubation to capture each 6xHis-tagged protein. The lysate and Ni-NTA resin mixtures were transferred into 96-well filter plates for several washes. The proteins were eluted with 300 mM imidazole solution and collected into 96-well plates.

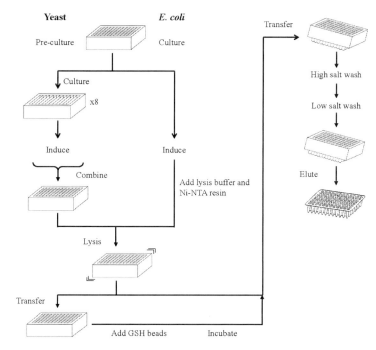

Figure 3.3 Schematic flowchart of high-throughput protein purification. *E. coli* (right) and yeast (left) that contain different ORFs are incubated in 2x LB broth with appropriate antibiotics and URA-/glucose liquid media in 96 DeepWell plates, respectively. *E. coli* cells were induced with IPTG for 3.5 h once the OD_{595} reached 0.7–0.9. Yeast cells require an additional culturing step in URA-/raffinose media in 12-channel reagent reservoirs to amplify cells and to raise the protein amounts per batch. The yeast cells were then induced with 2% galactose after the OD_{600} reached 0.6–1.0. The induced yeast cells were combined from eight 12-channel reagent reservoirs into another 96 DeepWell plates. The induced *E. coli* pellets were lysed with lysis buffer and incubated with Ni-NTA resins simultaneously to capture 6xHis-tagged proteins. The yeast pellets were lysed with lysis buffer and zirconia beads by vortexing. After centrifugation, supernatants were transferred to another 96 DeepWell plates and incubated with GSH beads to capture GST-fusion proteins. The Ni-NTA resin or GSH bead-containing mixtures were transferred to 96-well filter plates and sequentially washed with high-salt and low-salt wash buffers. Proteins were eluted with 300 mM imidazole or 40 mM reduced glutathione and collected into 96-well PCR plates.

As an example of eukaryotic systems, Zhu and his colleagues[7] established a collection of 5800 yeast ORFs into a galactose-inducible expression vector and purified the proteins in a high-throughput manner (Fig. 3.3). Briefly, yeast colonies were inoculated into 96 DeepWell plates containing URA-/glucose liquid media using a 96-pronger and cultured at 30°C with vigorous shaking. When the OD_{600} reached 4.0, the cultures were transferred to 6 mL of URA-/raffinose media in 12-channel reagent reservoirs to amplify yeast cells. Until the OD_{600} reached 0.6–1.0, the cells were induced with galactose in a final concentration of 2% and incubated at 30°C for 4 h. The pellets were harvested by centrifugation and stored at –80°C. The yeast pellets were lysed by vortexing with zirconia beads and the lysis buffer. After a centrifugation step, the supernatants were transferred to new 96 DeepWell plates and mixed with glutathione beads to capture each glutathione S-transferase (GST)-tagged fusion proteins. The mixtures were then transferred into 96-well filter plates and washed several times. Finally, the yeast proteins were eluted with 40 mM reduced glutathione and collected into 96-well plates.

Zhu and his colleagues[30,39] further extended the scope to the human proteome and enabled the first robust human proteome microarrays to come true. To make the work feasible and more efficient, they applied a high-throughput strategy throughout the gene cloning process to protein purification.[30,39] For the high-throughput gene cloning, they subcloned the human genes that were either from the Invitrogen ORF collection or from the MGC collection into a yeast expression vector pEGH-A using the Gateway cloning system. Protein expression and purification methods were the same as those for yeast.[7] By doing so, Zhu et al. successfully purified a total of approximately 17,000 full-length non-redundant human proteins.[30,39]

Thus far, high-throughput protein purification directly from mammalian cells has not been well established, presumably because of its low protein yields and more laborious handling procedures. Davies et al. has reported a protein expression and purification method for HEK293-EBNA cells in a 96-well format.[40] Although only 10 constructs of genes were handled simultaneously,[40] the 96-well format protein purification protocol would still be a foundation for mammalian systems.

3.2.1.3 Protein printing

The printing method of proteins[23,41,42] is similar to that of DNA molecules[43] except the spotting conditions. To prevent proteins from denaturing, the printing procedure is carried out in a cold room with the humidity controlled in the range of 20–40%. Purified proteins received in 96-well plates are straightforwardly rearrayed into 384-well V-bottom source plates after purification to adapt to the microarray-printing robot, to reduce sample amounts and to speed up the printing process.

Microarray-printing systems include two major types: contact spotting[44] and non-contact dispensing.[45,46] Literally, contact spotting is carried out by using capillary pins with tiny tips (ca. 80 μm diameter) to draw protein solutions and transfer proteins onto slides. A standard pinhead can hold up to 48 pins and, therefore, greatly accelerates the printing process. It is actually advantageous to use contact spotting for microarray fabrication. Because of its faster printing, proteins can better maintain their native structure and, as a result, the quality of proteome chips is improved. Furthermore, the required amount of each protein solution for printing is much lower by using contact spotting. Also the diameter of each protein spot is smaller (100–200 μm), which facilitates the fabrication of high-density proteome microarrays. However, the capillary pins are usually expensive and fragile— pins cannot function properly once their tips are damaged. Taking care of the pins' cleaning between each step is important and hard to control as well. If there are protein remnants that are not removed by wash steps, it will inevitably cross-contaminate the next protein spot. Another common problem is the so-called "missing spot" phenomenon that is due to the friction force between pins and pinhead.

The principle of non-contact dispensing is the same as that of inkjet printing: the droplets of protein solutions are ejected onto glass slides without any direct contact. Therefore, the problems of contact spotting mentioned above are obliterated. Nevertheless, the printing speed of non-contact dispensing is lower, increasing risks of protein denaturation. In addition, the non-contact dispensing method requires larger protein volume to be loaded. The size of produced protein spots (~400 μm) is larger than those produced by the contact spotting method as well. It thus limits the fabrication of high-density proteome microarrays, such as those needed to study the human proteome.[30]

3.2.1.4   Assay platforms and signal detection

The basic principle of proteome chip assays is the same as that of Western blotting or ELISA. After spotting proteins as described above, the proteome chip is typically pre-blocked with bovine serum albumin BSA and then probed with a biomolecule of interest. Researchers can either straightforwardly use a labeled sample for probing or use a specific antibody and a labeled secondary antibody to detect the binding. The labeling reagents can be fluorescent dyes, radioisotopes, and enzymes, among which fluorescent labeling is advantageous and widely used.[23,47] The incubation steps are conducted by using a cover slip that is mounted on proteome microarrays to avoid evaporation or by soaking the entire chips in the sample solution. In the case of proteome chips containing fewer spots, a multi-well glass slide will be a good choice for increasing the sample throughput. The framed glass slides with 4 to 96 wells are all commercially available for microarray format design. Probing multiple samples to each well on a single slide also abates the inter-array variation, which is a common problem in microarray data analysis.

Unbound biomolecules of interest are removed by wash steps. The wash stringency is determined by the type of samples and the assay format. Typically, proteome chips are washed three times with Tris-buffered saline (TBS; 25 mM Tris, 140 mM NaCl, pH 7.5) containing 0.05% Tween-20. To reduce non-specific binding, high-salt TBS (25 mM Tris, 500 mM NaCl, pH 7.5) containing 0.05% Tween-20 is applied in wash steps. The temperature, wash times, and shaking intensity are also adjustable factors to control the wash stringency. On the contrary, a milder wash step is required when studying weak interactions such as lipid–protein interactions. In most cases, the chips are usually dried by centrifugation; while in those of liposome-binding assays, the chips need to be air dried. Chips are scanned using a microarray scanner.

In the detection of fluorescence-based microarrays, the charge-coupled device (CCD) image sensors and laser scanners are the chief signal detection technologies, both of which have their own superiority. Generally, CCD imaging is faster, but laser-based scanning is more sensitive.[23] Most microarray scanners are two-color fluorescence (Cy5 and Cy3 channels) detection, while those equipped with four-color channels are also available. Thus far, the resolution of microarray scanners has reached the sub-micrometer level (0.5 μm), increasing the fidelity of scanning. To enhance assay throughout and to elevate inter-array consistency, a multi-slide loader allows scanners to scan up to 36 microarrays in parallel.

3.2.1.5 Microarray data analysis

To process the large dataset generated from microarrays, bioinformatics and biostatistics are surely required. In the past decade, DNA microarrays have been widely used to profile gene expressions and have become a popular tool in genetic diagnosis.[48-52] Statistical analysis and normalization approaches such as SAM,[53] the Bayesian regularization method,[54,55] CARMAweb,[56] BioMart,[57] and LIMMA[58-60] have been frequently used in DNA microarrays. However, these microarray analysis tools have difficulties to be directly applied to proteome microarrays due to some specific issues. The principle strategy of DNA microarray normalization is simple and straightforward: comparison with a reference sample and normalization against certain housekeeping genes.[43] These strategies are infeasible and cannot translate to proteome microarrays since the basic object and the assay format are different. DNA microarrays are employed to quantitatively measure mRNA levels of each gene, whereas proteome microarrays—especially functional proteome arrays—are mainly used to discover new interacting partners as a whole.

Snyder and his colleagues developed an analysis approach for proteome microarrays called ProCAT.[61] The rationale of ProCAT is to normalize the signal of each protein spot against the signals of its neighboring spots after background correction. By using ProCAT, the intra-array bias and local non-uniformity can be eliminated. Nevertheless, the problem of inter-array variation still remains unsolved. To address this issue, Sboner et al. reported a robust linear model (RLM) for proteome microarray normalization.[62] Unlike ProCAT, the RLM normalization not only strengthens the signal-to-noise ratio of each spot, but also maintains signal differences among neighboring hits. To tackle the technical variability among chips, RLM introduces multiple positive controls as a training set, against which the overall signals were normalized. Hence, the inter- and intra-array variations are minimized.

For reverse phase proteome arrays (RPPA) that contain a variety of cell lysates or biological specimens, housekeeping proteins were commonly used to estimate the total protein amounts of each spot.[63] However, the strategy of using housekeeping proteins for normalization will cause a bias when the sample-loading variation is large. To improve the RPPA data analysis, Neeley et al. proposed a variable slope normalization method,[64] which is able to exclude the sample-loading bias and to maintain good correlation between proteins. Chiechi et al. also reported an improved data normalization method for RPPA analysis, with emphasis on those arrays consisting of complex biological samples.[65]

3.3 Application of Liposomes on Proteome Microarrays

Current studies in lipid interactions with other biomolecules are chiefly conducted using liposomes as an artificial membrane model.[7,11,20,66] By using liposomes as an analyte carrier, lipids of interest can be incorporated in phospholipid bilayers and dissolved in buffers that simulate biological conditions. Lipids of interest located at the exterior side of liposomes are then allowed to bind interacting partners that are mostly proteins.

To date, proteome microarrays have been proven to be a robust technology to study protein–protein,[67–69] protein–DNA,[13] protein–RNA,[14–70] and protein–lipid interactions.[7–20] It is especially advantageous to use proteome microarrays to study weak interactions such as the protein–lipid interaction. Phosphoinositides, for example, are involved in growth and other cellular functions via interaction with proteins.[71] This interaction is facilitated by specialized lipid recognition domains, i.e., PH, PX, and FYVE domains.[72–73] Other lipids such as sphingosine and ceramide are involved in apoptosis signaling.[74] Theoretically, the bindings between protein domains and lipid head groups are mediated through electrostatic interactions and van der Waals forces. In such weak interactions, high variability between experiments and limited signal detection are imaginable. By using proteome microarrays, all of the proteins are examined on a single chip in parallel, thus minimizing the variations. The wash stringency on chips can more easily be controlled, which may better recover many potential protein–lipid interactions.

In addition to studying protein–lipid interactions, liposomal nanovesicles are an excellent signal amplifier compared to other detection methods.[75-77] Liposomes are capable of encapsulating a large amount of fluorescent molecules or signal-developing enzymes for signal enhancement.[78-82] The high sensitivity and low detection limit of fluorescent liposomes greatly facilitate the study of weak interactions and enable differentiating slight differences among experiments, especially in those cases that a minute quantity of sample expression causes a significant effect in the biological context. Taking together the advantages of liposomal nanovesicles and proteome microarrays, profiling protein–lipid interactions in a high-throughput manner with minimal variability is not far-fetched.

3.3.1 Fluorescent Liposomes on Proteome Microarrays

The use of fluorescence for detection is always an attractive strategy due to its safety, strong intensity, high sensitivity, and wide applications. A prominent benefit of liposomes is their capability of encapsulating hundreds of millions of fluorescent dye molecules, resulting in a huge signal enhancement. To date, fluorescent liposomes have been widely used in multi-well format and affinity chromatographic assays.[78-81] Whether fluorescent liposomes could directly accommodate microarray-based assays and further broaden their applications to proteomics research becomes an important and fascinating question.

3.3.2 Quenched Fluorescent Liposomes

Generally, conventional fluorescent liposomes that contain extremely high concentrations of fluorophores will lead to the so-called self-quenching effect: fluorescence intensity decreases due to the short distance between fluorescent molecules, which is exemplified when entrapped in the internal volume of liposomes. Paradoxically, the high concentration of fluorophores is both an advantage and disadvantage for proteome chip assays, contingent upon the microarray format employed. In the case of low-density protein arrays, the quenched fluorescent liposomes containing a considerable amount of fluorophores can provide greatly enhanced signals after lysing the liposomes. Given that lysis reagents such as detergents and centrifugation are not applicable to liposome-on-a-chip formats, the lysis step here is carried out by drying chips in the air. Once the chips are dried, bright fluorescent spots with a diameter of ca. 300 μm can be observed after scanning. However, the same formula cannot be directly adapted to high-density proteome microarrays. The average spot distance of current proteome microarrays is from 100 μm to 250 μm. It is thus obvious that the spot signals from the quenched fluorescent liposomes after lysis will substantially merge together and blur the chip images, giving rise to chip data that cannot be analyzed.

3.3.3 Nonquenched Fluorescent Liposomes

The self-quenching problem limits not only applications of fluorescent liposomes in high-density chip assays, but also their applications for real-time detection. To extend the scope of fluorescent liposomal nanovesicles to proteomics researches, Lu et al. developed an NQF liposome by both encapsulating sulforhodamine B (SRB) into the liposomes and incorporating lissamine rhodamine B-dipalmitoyl phosphatidylethanol (LRB-DPPE) within the liposomal bilayer.[20] Both the SRB concentration and LRB-DPPE proportion were optimized for signal amplification without lysis. The study shows that 200 μM SRB-loaded liposomes with 0.3% LRB-DPPE on the liposomal surface generate the maximal fluorescent signal without lysing the liposomes. In comparison with 200 μM SRB-loaded liposomes, the integration of 0.3% LRB-DPPE in the membrane of 200 μM SRB-loaded liposomes are able to produce stronger signals by 5.3-fold.[20] In order to demonstrate the applicability of NQF liposomes, Lu et al.[20] further constructed a phosphatidylinositol 3,5-bisphosphate (PI(3,5)P$_2$)-containing NQF liposome and applied the liposomes to yeast proteome microarrays (Fig. 3.4). Briefly, the NQF liposomes were incubated with the proteome microarrays and, after incubation, unbound liposomes were removed by a gentle wash step. The binding signals were acquired using a microarray scanner. As observed, the spot signals, or hits, were clearly identifiable and many PI(3,5)P$_2$-specific binding proteins were found (Fig. 3.5).[20] In addition to high-density proteome microarrays and real-time assays, the NQF liposomes can be directly used to low-density chip assays as well.[83]

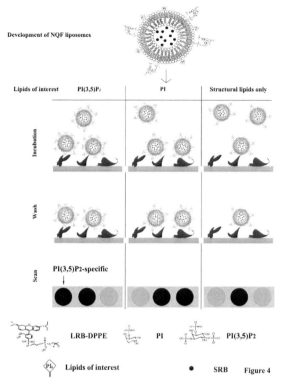

Figure 4

Figure 3.4   Schematic flowchart of NQF-liposome-binding assay using a proteome microarray. A PI(3,5)P$_2$-containing NQF liposome has been constructed and probed to a yeast proteome microarray to identify PI(3,5)P$_2$-specific binders (left).[20] The NQF liposomes were allowed to incubate with ca. 5800 individually purified yeast proteins on a chip. After a wash step, the chip was slightly air dried and scanned using a microarray scanner. To rule out non-specific bindings, PI- (middle) and structural lipids only (right) NQF liposomes were used as negative controls.

Like conventional liposomes, many modification strategies and assay platforms are also able to be applied to the NQF liposomes to improve their sensitivity and feasibility. Chen et al.

developed a protein G-liposome containing a high concentration (150 mM) SRB solution for immunosorbent or sandwich immunoassays.[79,84] The protein G-liposomes are fabricated by conjugating maleimide-modified protein G to acetylthioacetate (ATA)-tagged liposomes. Through the combination of the protein G modification and NQF liposomes, the protein G–NQF liposomes will provide an excellent tool for high-density antibody arrays and microarray-based immunoassays, allowing for more universal detection of antibody-binding events.

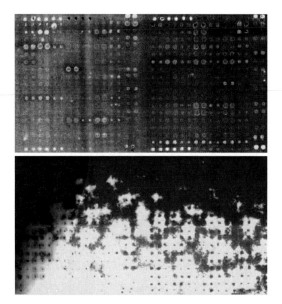

Figure 3.5 Representative images of proteome microarrays probed with quenched and NQF liposomes. The yeast proteome microarrays have been probed with NQF (upper panel) and conventional quenched liposomes (lower panel).[20] The NQF liposome can provide clear and identifiable spot signals, whereas the quenched liposome does not generate chip data that can be analyzed.

The NQF liposomes might also be applied to fluorescence polarization (FP) assays in the study of liposome–cell interactions. The principle of FP is based upon the alteration of fluorescent molecule's polarization degree after binding to a larger molecule. The most attractive features of FP include its homogeneity in solutions, which allows real-time measurement, lower limit of detection, and its tolerance to concentration variations. Notably, the design of NQF liposomes completely satisfies the format of FP assays—the optimized fluorescent signal without the need to lyse the liposomes and its nanometer size, which is 200- to 2000-fold smaller than cells. Thus, the application of NQF liposomes in FP assays might be a model platform to study lipid- or membrane protein–cell surface interactions or it could be used to study liposome-based drug delivery.

3.3.4 Nonfluorescent Liposomes on Proteome Microarrays

Other strategies to develop binding signals for detection in liposomes include conjugating bioaffinity molecules on liposomal bilayers and subsequently probing the corresponding dye-conjugated ligand to recognize the conjugated molecules on the surface of liposomes. Zhu and colleagues[7] applied biotinylated liposomes to yeast proteome microarrays and successfully identified specific binding proteins to phosphatidylinositides— PI3P, PI4P, PI(3,4)P$_2$, PI(4,5)P$_2$, and PI(3,4,5)P$_3$ (Fig. 3.6). The signal detection was carried out by probing with fluorescently labeled streptavidin. Given the extremely high affinity between biotin and streptavidin ($K_d \approx 10^{-14}$ mol/L), the bindings can be easily detected. Nevertheless, the additional wash step created by dye-labeled streptavidin probing might interfere with weak bindings between proteins and phosphatidylinositides, losing many interactions that could have biological significance. This interference could be reduced by pre-mixing the biotinylated liposomes and dye-labeled streptavidin, though the kinetics of streptavidin-bound biotinylated liposomes will be altered and the presence of this non-endogenous protein during the specificity study might interfere with the interactions under investigation.

Ruktanonchai and colleagues reported an antibody array assay using horseradish peroxidase (HRP)-encapsulated liposomes.[82] They optimized the encapsulation percentage of HRP in the antibody-conjugated liposomes and applied the liposomes to an antibody array. Three fabrication procedures of the HRP-loaded liposomes (extrusion, extrusion after a freeze–thaw step, and extrusion followed by freeze–thaw with an additional extrusion step) and two liposome sizes (200 nm and 1000 nm) were assessed.

As reported, the liposomes with 1000 nm diameter fabricated by serial steps with extrusion, freeze–thaw, and extrusion showed the highest HRP encapsulation percentage (1.6% HRP encapsulation), which apparently enhanced the signals the most. In this case, the use of 4-chloro-1-naphthol (4-CN) as a precipitating HRP substrate boosted the signal to an extent that the hits were already visible prior to scanning. Overall, the modified HRP-loaded liposomes might be a useful tool for low-density protein arrays but are not applicable for high-density chips since larger liposome size is required.

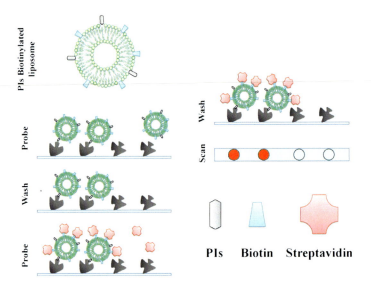

Figure 3.6   Schematic flowchart of phosphatidylinositides binding assays using biotinylated liposome and proteome microarrays. Zhu et al.[7] have reported a genome-wide screening of phosphatidylinositides—PI3P, PI4P, PI(3,4)P$_2$, PI(4,5)P$_2$, and PI(3,4,5)P$_3$—and protein interaction using the yeast proteome microarray. First, each phosphatidylinositide-containing biotinylated liposome was probed to the chips. After a wash step, the chips were incubated with dye-linked streptavidin for signal development.

3.4   Future Perspectives

Lipid-driven signaling cascades are central to maintaining the physiological functions in cells. Important lipid-signaling molecules include sphingolipids, phosphoinositides, steroid hormones, and prostaglandins.[85–89] Ceramide, for example, is one of the sphingolipid second messengers implicated in proliferation and cell death regulation.[90] It has been reported that ceramide mediates the apoptosis in differentiating embryonic stem cells via the direct binding to the PKCζ/PAR-4 complex—a paradigm for the importance of lipid–protein interactions.[91] Other sphingolipids consist of glucosylceramide, ceramide 1-phosphate, sphingosine, and sphingosine 1-phosphate, which are able to regulate the actin cytoskeleton, vesicular trafficking, inflammation, cell cycle, migration, differentiation, and survival.[92–95] Similar to ceramide, some target proteins of other lipid-signaling molecules have been found to be involved in important transduction pathways such as the G-protein coupled receptor signaling.[96,97] Still, only a limited number of lipid-binding proteins have been discovered, which is perhaps due to the weak interaction between lipids and their interacting partners.

Thus far, a cohort of $PI(3,5)P_2$-specific binding proteins and other phosphoinositide-binding proteins in yeast have been identified using the proteome microarrays and liposomes.[7,20] Through the combination of NQF liposomes and proteome microarray technology, more potential lipid–protein interactions can be high-throughput identified in the future. Given that lipid-mediated transduction pathways are tightly associated with diseases such as neurodegenerative disorders, diabetes, inflammation, and cancer, the platform can also be used to screen small molecule inhibitors of the lipid–protein interactions for drug development. As an analyte carrier, signal amplifier, or both, the NQF liposomes can be widely used in high-density proteome microarrays and real-time assays in the future.

Acknowledgments

We thank the National Science Council, Taiwan (NSC100-2627-M-008-003, NSC100-2320-B-008-001, and 101–2320-B-008-004-MY3), the National Central University and Landseed Hospital Program (NCU-LSH-101-A-024), and the National Central University and Cathay General Hospital (101CGH-NCU-A2) for financial support. We also thank Yu-Chieh Wang for figure editing.

References

1. Huang YH, Sauer K. Lipid signaling in T-cell development and function. *Cold Spring Harb Perspect Biol.* 2010; 2(11): a002428.

2. Wymann MP, Zvelebil M, Laffargue M. Phosphoinositide 3-kinase signalling—which way to target? *Trends Pharmacol Sci.* 2003; 24(7): 366–376.

3. Wymann MP, Schneiter R. Lipid signalling in disease. *Nat Rev Mol Cell Biol.* 2008; 9(2): 162–176.

4. Croce CM. Oncogenes and cancer. *N Engl J Med.* 2008; 358(5): 502–511.

5. Chen Z, Trotman LC, Shaffer D, et al. Crucial role of p53-dependent cellular senescence in suppression of Pten-deficient tumorigenesis. *Nature.* 2005; 436(7051): 725–730.

6. Bakrac B, Gutierrez-Aguirre I, Podlesek Z, et al. Molecular determinants of sphingomyelin specificity of a eukaryotic pore-forming toxin. *J Biol Chem.* 2008; 283(27): 18665–18677.

7. Zhu H, Bilgin M, Bangham R, et al. Global analysis of protein activities using proteome chips. *Science.* 2001; 293(5537): 2101–2105.

8. Mozsolits H, Aguilar MI. Surface plasmon resonance spectroscopy: An emerging tool for the study of peptide-membrane interactions. *Biopolymers.* 2002; 66(1): 3–18.

9. Catimel B, Schieber C, Condron M, et al. The PI(3,5)P2 and PI(4,5)P2 interactomes. *J Proteome Res.* 2008; 7(12): 5295–5313.

10. Catimel B, Yin MX, Schieber C, et al. PI(3,4,5)P3 Interactome. *J Proteome Res.* 2009; 8(7): 3712–3726.

11. Bieberich E. Lipid vesicle-mediated affinity chromatography using magnetic activated cell sorting (LIMACS): A novel method to analyze protein-lipid interaction. *J Vis Exp.* 2011; (50).

12. Zhang P, Wang Y, Sesaki H, Iijima M. Proteomic identification of phosphatidylinositol (3,4,5) triphosphate-binding proteins in *Dictyostelium discoideum. Proc Natl Acad Sci U S A.* 2010; 107(26): 11829–11834.

13. Chen CS, Korobkova E, Chen H, et al. A proteome chip approach reveals new DNA damage recognition activities in *Escherichia coli. Nat Methods.* 2008; 5(1): 69–74.

14. Fan B, Lu KY, Reymond Sutandy FX, et al. A human proteome microarray identifies that the heterogeneous nuclear ribonucleo-

protein K (hnRNP K) recognizes the 5′ terminal sequence of the hepatitis C virus RNA. *Mol Cell Proteomics.* 2014; 13(1): 84–92.

15. Kung LA, Tao SC, Qian J, Smith MG, Snyder M, Zhu H. Global analysis of the glycoproteome in Saccharomyces cerevisiae reveals new roles for protein glycosylation in eukaryotes. *Mol Syst Biol.* 2009; 5: 308.

16. Lueking A, Possling A, Huber O, et al. A nonredundant human protein chip for antibody screening and serum profiling. *Mol Cell Proteomics.* 2003; 2(12): 1342–1349.

17. Ahn-Yoon S, DeCory TR, Durst RA. Ganglioside-liposome immunoassay for the detection of botulinum toxin. *Anal Bioanal Chem.* 2004; 378(1): 68–75.

18. DeCory TR, Durst RA, Zimmerman SJ, et al. Development of an immunomagnetic bead-immunoliposome fluorescence assay for rapid detection of *Escherichia coli* O157:H7 in aqueous samples and comparison of the assay with a standard microbiological method. *Appl Environ Microbiol.* 2005; 71(4): 1856–1864.

19. Wen HW, Borejsza-Wysocki W, DeCory TR, Durst RA. Development of a competitive liposome-based lateral flow assay for the rapid detection of the allergenic peanut protein Ara h1. *Anal Bioanal Chem.* 2005; 382(5): 1217–1226.

20. Lu KY, Tao SC, Yang TC, et al. Profiling lipid–protein interactions using nonquenched fluorescent liposomal nanovesicles and proteome microarrays. *Mol Cell Proteomics.* 2012; 11(11): 1177–1190.

21. James P. Protein identification in the post-genome era: The rapid rise of proteomics. *Q Rev Biophys.* 1997; 30(4): 279–331.

22. Kusnezow W, Jacob A, Walijew A, Diehl F, Hoheisel JD. Antibody microarrays: An evaluation of production parameters. *Proteomics.* 2003; 3(3): 254–264.

23. Tao SC, Chen CS, Zhu H. Applications of protein microarray technology. *Comb Chem High Throughput Screen.* 2007; 10(8): 706–718.

24. Angenendt P. Progress in protein and antibody microarray technology. *Drug Discov Today.* 2005; 10(7): 503–511.

25. Haab BB. Methods and applications of antibody microarrays in cancer research. *Proteomics.* 2003; 3(11): 2116–2122.

26. Lv LL, Liu BC. High-throughput antibody microarrays for quantitative proteomic analysis. *Expert Rev Proteomics.* 2007; 4(4): 505–513.

27. Wingren C, Borrebaeck CA. Antibody microarrays: Current status and key technological advances. *OMICS.* 2006; 10(3): 411–427.

28. Popescu SC, Popescu GV, Bachan S, et al. Differential binding of calmodulin-related proteins to their targets revealed through high-density Arabidopsis protein microarrays. *Proc Natl Acad Sci U S A.* 2007; 104(11): 4730–4735.

29. Zhu H, Hu S, Jona G, et al. Severe acute respiratory syndrome diagnostics using a coronavirus protein microarray. *Proc Natl Acad Sci U S A.* 2006; 103(11): 4011–4016.

30. Jeong JS, Jiang L, Albino E, et al. Rapid identification of monospecific monoclonal antibodies using a human proteome microarray. *Mol Cell Proteomics.* 2012; 11(6): O111.016253.

31. Rusmini F, Zhong Z, Feijen J. Protein immobilization strategies for protein biochips. *Biomacromolecules.* 2007; 8(6): 1775–1789.

32. Stillman BA, Tonkinson JL. FAST slides: A novel surface for microarrays. *BioTechniques.* 2000; 29(3): 630–635.

33. Charles PT, Goldman ER, Rangasammy JG, Schauer CL, Chen MS, Taitt CR. Fabrication and characterization of 3D hydrogel microarrays to measure antigenicity and antibody functionality for biosensor applications. *Biosens Bioelectron.* 2004; 20(4): 753–764.

34. Zhu H, Snyder M. Protein chip technology. *Curr Opin Chem Biol.* 2003; 7(1): 55–63.

35. Edelman AM, Blumenthal DK, Krebs EG. Protein serine/threonine kinases. *Annu Rev Biochem.* 1987; 56: 567–613.

36. Van Wart HE, Birkedal-Hansen H. The cysteine switch: A principle of regulation of metalloproteinase activity with potential applicability to the entire matrix metalloproteinase gene family. *Proc Natl Acad Sci U S A.* 1990; 87(14): 5578–5582.

37. Guo SL, Chen PC, Chen MS, et al. A fast universal immobilization of immunoglobulin G at 4 degrees C for the development of array-based immunoassays. *PLoS One.* 2012; 7(12): e51370.

38. Kitagawa M, Ara T, Arifuzzaman M, et al. Complete set of ORF clones of *Escherichia coli* ASKA library (a complete set of *E. coli* K-12 ORF archive): Unique resources for biological research. *DNA Res.* 2005; 12(5): 291–299.

39. Hu S, Xie Z, Onishi A, et al. Profiling the human protein-DNA interactome reveals ERK2 as a transcriptional repressor of interferon signaling. *Cell.* 2009; 139(3): 610–622.

40. Davies A, Greene A, Lullau E, Abbott WM. Optimisation and evaluation of a high-throughput mammalian protein expression system. *Protein Expr Purif.* 2005; 42(1): 111–121.

41. Sutandy FX, Qian J, Chen CS, Zhu H. Overview of protein microarrays. *Curr Protoc Protein Sci.* 2013; Chapter 27: Unit 27.21.

42. Chen CS, Zhu H. Protein microarrays. *BioTechniques.* 2006; 40(4): 423, 425, 427 passim.

43. Schena M, Shalon D, Davis RW, Brown PO. Quantitative monitoring of gene expression patterns with a complementary DNA microarray. *Science.* 1995; 270(5235): 467–470.

44. Austin J, Holway AH. Contact printing of protein microarrays. *Methods Mol Biol.* 2011; 785: 379–394.

45. Gutmann O, Niekrawietz R, Kuehlewein R, et al. Non-contact production of oligonucleotide microarrays using the highly integrated TopSpot nanoliter dispenser. *Analyst.* 2004; 129(9): 835–840.

46. Hartmann M, Sjodahl J, Stjernstrom M, Redeby J, Joos T, Roeraade J. Non-contact protein microarray fabrication using a procedure based on liquid bridge formation. *Anal Bioanal Chem.* 2009; 393(2): 591–598.

47. Templin MF, Stoll D, Schrenk M, Traub PC, Vohringer CF, Joos TO. Protein microarray technology. *Trends Biotechnol.* 2002; 20(4): 160–166.

48. Budovskaya YV, Wu K, Southworth LK, et al. An elt-3/elt-5/elt-6 GATA transcription circuit guides aging in *C. elegans. Cell.* 2008; 134(2): 291–303.

49. Coser KR, Chesnes J, Hur J, Ray S, Isselbacher KJ, Shioda T. Global analysis of ligand sensitivity of estrogen inducible and suppressible genes in MCF7/BUS breast cancer cells by DNA microarray. *Proc Natl Acad Sci U S A.* 2003; 100(24): 13994–13999.

50. Pomeroy SL, Tamayo P, Gaasenbeek M, et al. Prediction of central nervous system embryonal tumour outcome based on gene expression. *Nature.* 2002; 415(6870): 436–442.

51. Song YJ, Stinski MF. Effect of the human cytomegalovirus IE86 protein on expression of E2F-responsive genes: A DNA microarray analysis. *Proc Natl Acad Sci U S A.* 2002; 99(5): 2836–2841.

52. van't Veer LJ, Dai H, van de Vijver MJ, et al. Gene expression profiling predicts clinical outcome of breast cancer. *Nature.* 2002; 415(6871): 530–536.

53. Tusher VG, Tibshirani R, Chu G. Significance analysis of microarrays applied to the ionizing radiation response. *Proc Natl Acad Sci U S A.* 2001; 98(9): 5116–5121.

54. Baldi P, Long AD. A Bayesian framework for the analysis of microarray expression data: Regularized t-test and statistical inferences of gene changes. *Bioinformatics.* 2001; 17(6): 509–519.

55. Kayala MA, Baldi P. Cyber-T web server: Differential analysis of high-throughput data. *Nucleic Acids Res.* 2012; 40(Web Server issue): W553–559.

56. Rainer J, Sanchez-Cabo F, Stocker G, Sturn A, Trajanoski Z. CARMAweb: Comprehensive R- and bioconductor-based web service for microarray data analysis. *Nucleic Acids Res.* 2006; 34(Web Server issue): W498–503.

57. Durinck S, Moreau Y, Kasprzyk A, et al. BioMart and bioconductor: A powerful link between biological databases and microarray data analysis. *Bioinformatics.* 2005; 21(16): 3439–3440.

58. Smyth GK, Speed T. Normalization of cDNA microarray data. *Methods.* 2003; 31(4): 265–273.

59. Smyth GK. Linear models and empirical bayes methods for assessing differential expression in microarray experiments. *Stat Appl Genet Mol Biol.* 2004; 3: Article3.

60. Ritchie ME, Silver J, Oshlack A, et al. A comparison of background correction methods for two-colour microarrays. *Bioinformatics.* 2007; 23(20): 2700–2707.

61. Zhu X, Gerstein M, Snyder M. ProCAT: A data analysis approach for protein microarrays. *Genome Biol.* 2006; 7(11): R110.

62. Sboner A, Karpikov A, Chen G, et al. Robust-linear-model normalization to reduce technical variability in functional protein microarrays. *J Proteome Res.* 2009; 8(12): 5451–5464.

63. Spurrier B, Ramalingam S, Nishizuka S. Reverse-phase protein lysate microarrays for cell signaling analysis. *Nat Protoc.* 2008; 3(11): 1796–1808.

64. Neeley ES, Kornblau SM, Coombes KR, Baggerly KA. Variable slope normalization of reverse phase protein arrays. *Bioinformatics.* 2009; 25(11): 1384–1389.

65. Chiechi A, Mueller C, Boehm KM, et al. Improved data normalization methods for reverse phase protein microarray analysis of complex biological samples. *BioTechniques.* 2012; 0(0): 1–7.

66. Xu X, Costa A, Burgess DJ. Protein encapsulation in unilamellar liposomes: High encapsulation efficiency and a novel technique to assess lipid–protein interaction. *Pharm Res.* 2012; 29(7): 1919–1931.

67. Chen Y, Yang LN, Cheng L, et al. Bcl2-associated athanogene 3 interactome analysis reveals a new role in modulating proteasome activity. *Mol Cell Proteomics.* 2013; 12(10): 2804–2819.

68. Huang Y, Jeong JS, Okamura J, et al. Global tumor protein p53/p63 interactome: Making a case for cisplatin chemoresistance. *Cell Cycle.* 2012; 11(12): 2367–2379.

69. Ho YH, Sung TC, Chen CS. Lactoferricin B inhibits the phosphorylation of the two-component system response regulators BasR and CreB. *Mol Cell Proteomics.* 2012; 11(4): M111 014720.

70. Zhu J, Gopinath K, Murali A, et al. RNA-binding proteins that inhibit RNA virus infection. *Proc Natl Acad Sci U S A.* 2007; 104(9): 3129–3134.

71. Lemmon MA, Ferguson KM. Signal-dependent membrane targeting by pleckstrin homology (PH) domains. *Biochem J.* 2000; 350 Pt 1: 1–18.

72. Balla T. Inositol-lipid binding motifs: Signal integrators through protein–lipid and protein–protein interactions. *J Cell Sci.* 2005; 118 (Pt 10): 2093–2104.

73. Lemmon MA. Phosphoinositide recognition domains. *Traffic.* 2003; 4(4): 201–213.

74. Woodcock J. Sphingosine and ceramide signalling in apoptosis. *IUBMB Life.* 2006; 58(8): 462–466.

75. Park S, Durst RA. Immunoliposome sandwich assay for the detection of *Escherichia coli* O157:H7. *Anal Biochem.* 2000; 280(1): 151–158.

76. Baeumner AJ, Pretz J, Fang S. A universal nucleic acid sequence biosensor with nanomolar detection limits. *Anal Chem.* 2004; 76(4): 888–894.

77. Ho JA, Hsu HW, Huang MR. Liposome-based microcapillary immuno-sensor for detection of *Escherichia coli* O157:H7. *Anal Biochem.* 2004; 330(2): 342–349.

78. Ho JA, Wu LC, Chang LH, Hwang KC, Reuben Hwu JR. Liposome-based immunoaffinity chromatographic assay for the quantitation of immunoglobulin E in human serum. *J Chromatogr B Analyt Technol Biomed Life Sci.* 2010; 878(2): 172–176.

79. Chen CS, Baeumner AJ, Durst RA. Protein G-liposomal nanovesicles as universal reagents for immunoassays. *Talanta.* 2005; 67(1): 205–211.

80. Edwards KA, Wang Y, Baeumner AJ. Aptamer sandwich assays: Human alpha-thrombin detection using liposome enhancement. *Anal Bioanal Chem.* 2010; 398(6): 2645–2654.

81. Ho JA, Wu LC, Huang MR, Lin YJ, Baeumner AJ, Durst RA. Application of ganglioside-sensitized liposomes in a flow injection immunoanalytical system for the determination of cholera toxin. *Anal Chem.* 2007; 79(1): 246–250.

82. Ruktanonchai U, Nuchuchua O, Charlermroj R, Pattarakankul T, Karoonuthaisiri N. Signal amplification of microarray-based immunoassay by optimization of nanoliposome formulations. *Anal Biochem.* 2012; 429(2): 142–147.

83. Su WH, Ho TY, Tsou TS, et al. Development of a chip-based multiplexed immunoassay using liposomal nanovesicles and its application in the detection of pathogens causing female lower genital tract infections. *Taiwan J Obstet Gynecol.* 2013; 52(1): 25–32.

84. Chen CS, Durst RA. Simultaneous detection of *Escherichia coli* O157: H7, *Salmonella* spp. and *Listeria monocytogenes* with an array-based immunosorbent assay using universal protein G-liposomal nanovesicles. *Talanta.* 2006; 69(1): 232–238.

85. Liscovitch M, Cantley LC. Lipid second messengers. *Cell.* 1994; 77(3): 329–334.

86. Spiegel S, Milstien S. Sphingolipid metabolites: Members of a new class of lipid second messengers. *J Membr Biol.* 1995; 146(3): 225–237.

87. Spiegel S, Foster D, Kolesnick R. Signal transduction through lipid second messengers. *Curr Opin Cell Biol.* 1996; 8(2): 159–167.

88. Delmas P, Coste B, Gamper N, Shapiro MS. Phosphoinositide lipid second messengers: New paradigms for calcium channel modulation. *Neuron.* 2005; 47(2): 179–182.

89. Farach-Carson MC, Davis PJ. Steroid hormone interactions with target cells: Cross talk between membrane and nuclear pathways. *J Pharmacol Exp Ther.* 2003; 307(3): 839–845.

90. Saddoughi SA, Ogretmen B. Diverse functions of ceramide in cancer cell death and proliferation. *Adv Cancer Res.* 2013; 117: 37–58.

91. Wang G, Silva J, Krishnamurthy K, Tran E, Condie BG, Bieberich E. Direct binding to ceramide activates protein kinase Czeta before the formation of a pro-apoptotic complex with PAR-4 in differentiating stem cells. *J Biol Chem.* 2005; 280(28): 26415–26424.

92. Smith ER, Merrill AH, Obeid LM, Hannun YA. Effects of sphingosine and other sphingolipids on protein kinase C. *Methods Enzymol.* 2000; 312: 361–373.

93. Peters SL, Alewijnse AE. Sphingosine-1-phosphate signaling in the cardiovascular system. *Curr Opin Pharmacol.* 2007; 7(2): 186–192.

94. Gomez-Munoz A, Kong JY, Parhar K, et al. Ceramide-1-phosphate promotes cell survival through activation of the phosphatidylinositol 3-kinase/protein kinase B pathway. *FEBS Lett.* 2005; 579(17): 3744–3750.

95. Watanabe R, Wu K, Paul P, et al. Up-regulation of glucosylceramide synthase expression and activity during human keratinocyte differentiation. *J Biol Chem.* 1998; 273(16): 9651–9655.

96. Hla T, Lee MJ, Ancellin N, Paik JH, Kluk MJ. Lysophospholipids: Receptor revelations. *Science.* 2001; 294(5548): 1875–1878.

97. Lee MJ, Van Brocklyn JR, Thangada S, et al. Sphingosine-1-phosphate as a ligand for the G protein-coupled receptor EDG-1. *Science.* 1998; 279(5356): 1552–1555.

Chapter 4

Functional Polydiacetylene Liposomes as a Self-Signaling and Signal-Amplifying Bio- and Chemical Sensor and Sensor Array

Sungbaek Seo, Apoorv Shanker, Min Sang Kwon, and Jinsang Kim

Macromolecular Science and Engineering and Materials Science and Engineering, University of Michigan, Ann Arbor, Michigan 48109-2136, USA

jinsang@umich.edu

4.1 General Background of Polydiacetylene Liposomes and Sensory Properties

Conjugated polymers (CPs) are macromolecules having alternating saturated and unsaturated bonds, i.e., their conjugated backbones are sp^1- or sp^2-hybridized.[1] The consequent p-orbital overlap along the conjugated backbone provides unique optoelectronic properties to CPs. Changes of intramolecular conformation and/or intermolecular packing of CPs are the parameters largely affecting the effective conjugation length, which triggers changes in absorption, emission, and conductive properties of CPs.[2-7] Accordingly, this responsive mechanism originating from intra- and intermolecular rearrangement can be adapted to a rational sensor design as a signaling mechanism. Moreover, CP-based

Liposomes in Analytical Methodologies

Edited by Katie A. Edwards

Copyright © 2016 Pan Stanford Publishing Pte. Ltd.

ISBN 978-981-4669-26-9 (Hardcover), 978-981-4669-27-6 (eBook)

www.panstanford.com

sensors can provide signal amplification and consequently more sensitive detection than small molecular analogues because the aforementioned property changes of CPs are a collective response as a macromolecule to a local event even at a single unit of CPs.[8-10] While any binding event on a small molecular fluorophore only triggers a single chromophore to change its optical property, the recognition event along the CP backbone causes optical property changes of an entire chain of macromolecular chromophores, inducing large signal amplification. Polydiacetylene (PDA) is a CP consisting of alternating double and triple bonds (ene–yne) along its main chain. PDA has colorimetric and fluorometric changes, i.e., dual-mode response to environmental effects (pH,[11,12] temperature,[13,14] mechanical pressure,[15] and ligand–receptor interactions[16-18]) and easy formation into a self-assembled structure. In this chapter, we will review the overall background of PDA-liposome-based sensors and their bio- and chemical analyte detection applications.

4.1.1 PDA Liposomes for Sensor Applications

PDA is a unique material in terms of colorimetric/fluorescence dual detection capability, convenient preparation through self-assembly, and subsequent photopolymerization. Separately, liposomes have been used for a sensory platform with the following benefits: (1) easy preparation via a self-assembly procedure, (2) protecting compounds inside liposomes from their exterior surroundings, and (3) providing loading spaces for various hydrophilic or/and hydrophobic agents. Therefore, PDA liposomes have integrated features of both PDA material and liposome platform together, i.e., label-free detection, sufficient colloidal stability, and tunable sensory signalization (Fig. 4.1).

Since the PDA material itself generates its own sensory signal (colorimetric and fluorometric) upon exposure to external stimuli, it does not need fluorophores or dye labeling. This saves time and cost for encapsulating such fluorophores into carriers. Generally, phospholipid-based liposome structures are unstable at room temperature and finally either disassemble or aggregate.[19] For example, liposomes of 1,2-dimyristoyl-*sn*-glycero-3-phosphocholine, a phospholipid, aggregate within a few days. However, diacetylene (DA)-incorporated or -composed liposomes have a longer shelf life, usually stable for months because the DA monomers within them are chemically bonded to form polymeric PDA. Lastly, another benefit of using liposome carriers is the flexible accommodation of various hydrophilic or hydrophobic dyes in the liposome, which allows a sensor design incorporating energy transfer between the encapsulated fluorophore and the fluorescent PDA backbone.[20]

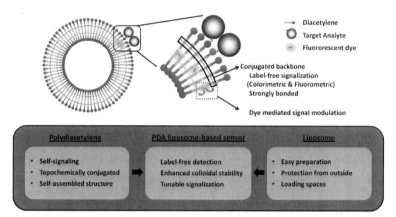

Figure 4.1   Illustration of the benefits of PDA liposome-based sensors.

4.2   Properties of PDA Liposomes

4.2.1   Self-Assembled Structure

DA is an amphiphilic monomer consisting of two moieties: (1) a polar headgroup and (2) a hydrophobic tail having a DA group. This amphiphilic nature of DA produces a self-assembled structure in an aqueous medium. Each tail is further divided into three segments: the DA group, a spacer between the headgroup and the DA, and the terminal alkyl chain. Each unit of a DA amphiphile is a key parameter to determine if the amphiphile will form a self-assembled structure and what kinds of assembled structures are formed. For example, headgroup chirality affects colloidal structure; DAs with achiral headgroups usually form spherical liposomes, while chiral DAs often form nonspherical structures such as helices and tubules.[21] Moreover, there exists intermolecular (between DA monomers) packing in aqueous medium with hydrophobic–hydrophobic interactions of the adjacent tails of

DAs. The hydrophilic headgroups such as carboxylic acid or amide groups in DAs also have chances of intermolecular hydrogen bonding and/or aromatic headgroups of DAs can promote π-π stacking interactions, stabilizing the self-assembled structure of DAs.[22]

At low concentrations, the DAs are individually dispersed in an aqueous medium. However, above the critical concentration, they are likely to form bilayered liposome structures to minimize their surface energy (Fig. 4.2a). This critical concentration is defined as critical bilayer concentration (CBC). For example, one of the representative DA monomers, 10,12-pentacosadiynoic acid (PCDA), can be dispersed in water (usually by probe sonication) to form self-assembled liposome particles above its CBC (Fig. 4.2b).

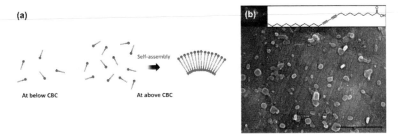

Figure 4.2 (a) Procedure of self-assembled liposome formation using diacetylenes; (b) SEM image of 10,12-pentacosadiynoic acid (PCDA) liposomes. Scale bar is 1 μm. Chemical structure of monomer PCDA (*inset*).

4.2.2 Topochemical Polymerization

PDA is formed by 1,4-photopolymerization between intermolecular DA packing along the liposome structure, resulting in a conjugated backbone with side alkyl chains (Fig. 4.3). The polymerization occurs only when the DAs are arranged in a lattice within the liposome structure. This topochemical constraint indicates that polymerization can happen only in a highly ordered packing structure. Accordingly, polymerization of DA monomers leads to physical stabilization of the liposome structure, increasing its thermal stability and mechanical strength.[21] By contrast, bulky receptor-functionalized DAs hardly form a stable liposome structure, which subsequently inhibits topochemical polymerization.

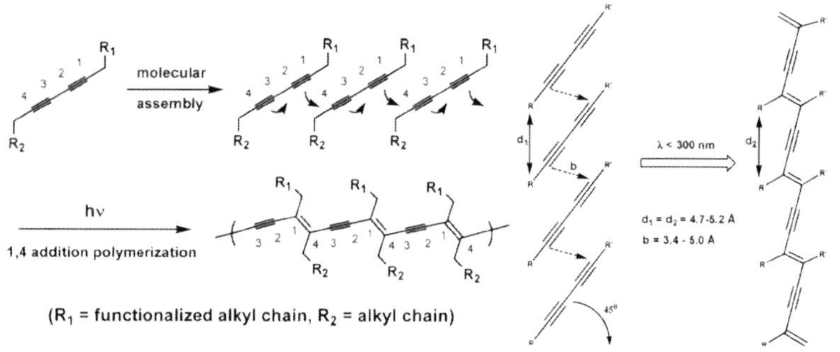

Figure 4.3   Schematic representation of topochemical photopolymerization of assembled diacetylenes. Reproduced with permission
from Ref. [22] (left), Copyright 2005, American Chemical
Society   (http://pubs.acs.org/doi/abs/10.1021/ma051551i)
and Ref. [23] (right), Copyright 2008, American Chemical
Society (http://pubs.acs.org/doi/abs/10.1021/ja076553s).

Moreover, it is known that the arrangement of DA monomers
is necessary in such topochemical reactions of DA, i.e., there
must be 4.9 Å of intermolecular distance between the DA units
and an inclination angle of 45° between the DA axes[24,25] when
aligned as liposome structures in aqueous solution. Shinkai group
demonstrated that the photopolymerizable unit with flexible
linkers is expected to be strongly stabilized by intermolecular
hydrogen bonds between two amide linkages that are surrounded
by the gel-forming segments.[26] The amide groups are widely
used to fix DA in a suitable orientation because the distance
between them (about 4.8 Å) is comparable to that of the DA units
(about 4.9 Å).

4.2.3   Self-Signaling (Colorimetric and Fluorometric Transition)

4.2.3.1   Colorimetric transition

A solution of self-assembled DA monomers before polymerization
is transparent and does not have absorption in the visible
region. Through photopolymerization, conjugation is formed by
the overlap of the p-orbitals of the adjacent double and triple
bonds and generates planar overlap (Fig. 4.4).

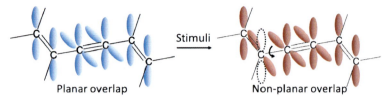

Figure 4.4   Schematic diagram of π-orbital overlap in the conjugated PDA backbone. By stimuli, the planar overlap is twisted by rotation about one of the C–C bonds in the backbone. The red phase consists of a non-planar backbone with rotated alkyl side chains.

Heating these films of p-orbital overlap determines the effective conjugation length, implying how much the backbone planarity is continued.[27] The longer the conjugation length, the smaller the energy band gap between the valence and conduction bands. After polymerization, PDA has its absorption maximum at 650 nm and is blue in color (Fig. 4.5a, inset).

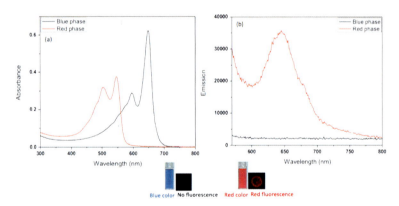

Figure 4.5   (a) Absorption and (b) emission spectra of poly(10,12-PCDA) liposome solution.

When the blue-phase PDAs are subjected to external stimuli, e.g., pH, temperature, mechanical stress, and receptor–ligand interactions, the conjugated backbone becomes twisted and non-planar p-orbital overlap occurs (Fig. 4.4). Eventually, this decreases the conjugation length and broadens the energy band gap. As a consequence, the twisted PDAs absorb maximum at 550 nm and become red.

4.2.3.2   Emission

The red-phase PDA is emissive in fluorescence, while the blue phase is not. It can be described by energy shifts based on symmetry from excited state to ground state. The lowest excited state in the blue phase has the same symmetry as the ground state, so called, A_g symmetry. While, in the red phase, the lowest excited state has B_u symmetry, generating radiative decay. Hence, the red fluorescence can be detected at 650 nm, while no fluorescence is observed in the blue phase (Fig. 4.5b, inset).

4.2.3.3   Mechanisms of color and emission change

The mechanisms of color and fluorescence change continue to be studied. A major theory that describes the mechanism is as follows: polymerization changes the hybridization of the terminal alkyne carbons from sp to sp^2 and, therefore, alters the preferred bond angle from 180° to 120°, but the packing of the side chains does not allow the polymer backbone to re-orient and relieve strain, resulting in the accumulation of stress in the material as polymerization ensues (Fig. 4.4).[28] The way to induce color change can be thought of as overcoming the barrier to reorganization of the polymer backbone created by the packing of the side chains. For example, thermal energy at high temperatures increases motion of the side chains and allows changes in the packing of the chains and increases the overall stress of the system, thereby effectively reducing the energy required for backbone reorientation.

4.3   Sensory Platforms Using PDA Liposomes

4.3.1   Liquid-Phase-Based Sensing

The most studied system using PDA liposomes is the solution-based tests. Liposome suspensions are freely mobile in an aqueous medium. The target analytes are also freely mobile and are randomly captured by the receptor moieties of the PDA liposome. Liquid-phase-based sensors are easily prepared and more readily scaled to larger volume production and tested with analyte solution. They are also more easily used as reagents in assays than films or coatings as they can be readily distributed in controlled amounts.

However, the solution-based platform is not suitable for portable applications and has limited long-term storage stability. Also the post-preparation modification of the colloids, e.g., conjugation of reactive or binding sites to the liposome surface, requires size exclusion column chromatography or dialysis purification steps to separate unreacted moieties from the liposome solution.[21]

4.3.2 Gel-Phase-Based Sensing

Polymer gels have been utilized as matrices for PDA liposomes incorporated in a hybrid sensory system. These systems are potentially useful for portable kits such as gel patches or films. Alginate or agarose are the most well-known polymer gel materials. These gel matrices maintain PDA-liposome structures as well as their sensory efficacy. Moreover, these have relatively longer stability than liquid-based sensory systems. However, unlike solution-phase assays, in gel-based formats, as the system loses mobility of the PDA liposomes and analytes, the response generally decreases. Protein kits that capture target proteins using protein receptors on PDA liposomes would fall under this sensor category.[29,30] The hydrogel matrix in such protein kits can potentially keep the proteins from denaturing.

4.3.3 Solid-Phase-Based Sensing

Solid-phase-based sensing is the most easy-to-carry system and is more desirable as a simple kit. For example, pregnancy testing strips and lateral flow assays are the most standard commercial systems. When applied as a PDA-liposome-based system, the liposomes are immobilized onto a solid support, such as filter paper. For example, our group developed a strip-type PDA sensor for nerve agent detection using PDA liposomes immobilized onto cellulose acetate membrane filter paper.[31] Another example of an immobilized PDA-liposome system is a microarray. We developed PDA-liposome-immobilized array systems for potassium, mercury, melamine, and influenza A virus detection. This kind of system maintains the stability of PDA liposomes most among the three sensor categories mentioned here. However, in some cases, they need complex surface treatment to make them compatible with target analyte solutions.

4.4 Sensor Applications of Polydiacetylene Liposomes

The fascinating blue-to-red color transition of PDA liposomes has been extensively used for sensor applications for the colorimetric detection of environmental, chemical, and biological analytes. The chromism, or color transition, as exhibited by these liposomes can be classified according to the stimulating agent—thermochromism (temperature),[13,14] solvatochromism (solvent),[32,33] mechanochromism (mechanical stress),[15] halochromism (pH),[11,12] and affinochromism (affinity based).[16-18] Among the aforementioned chromisms of PDA liposomes, the first four can be attributed to "environmental" stimulations while affinochromism is effected by the interaction of the liposomes with biological or chemical analytes. While most of the research effort in PDA-liposome-based sensors has been directed toward the development of affinity-based sensor applications, the development of sensors for environmental analytes has not been as robust.[34] The different types of chromisms in PDA liposomes will be discussed in this section, with special emphasis on affinochromism. Selected sensor and colorimetric display applications of the liposomes will be discussed in detail.

4.4.1 Thermochromism

Perhaps the most extensively studied chromic transition of PDA liposomes is the thermally induced blue-to-red color transition. However, in spite of the efforts of a number of investigators, the exact mechanism of the thermally induced color transition is not well understood.[35] The color transition can be attributed to the change in the effective conjugation length of the PDA-conjugated backbone. While the blue phase with its longer effective conjugation length shows an absorbance maximum at around 640 nm, the red phase with its shorter conjugation length has an absorbance maximum at 540 nm (Fig. 4.5). This change in effective conjugation length is widely accepted to be related to the conformation of the PDA side chain.[36-38] While the blue form of PDA is believed to have well-ordered conformation of the side chains, the red form is supposed to have a distorted confirmation. However, recent studies by Lee et al.[39] and Kim et al.[40] attributed the color transition to the release of the mechanical strain developed on the side chains during the polymerization of DA monomers. PDA liposomes can be made to undergo reversible or irreversible thermally induced colorimetric transition by rationally designing the DA monomer. Inclusion of strongly interacting moieties such as aromatic groups (π-π interaction),[41] ionic groups (coloumbic interaction),[42] covalent bonds,[43,44] H-bonding,[40,45,46] or multiple bonds[47–49] can restore the original blue phase effective conjugation length upon cooling. Absence of such mutually interactive groups impairs the restoring force resulting in an irreversible blue-to-red colorimetric transition. Likewise, the colorimetric response temperature of PDA liposomes can also be modulated by changing the size of the headgroup and hence the stability of the liposomes.[50]

Many researchers have made use of the thermally induced colorimetric transition in PDA liposomes for developing temperature sensors or patterned color and fluorescent imaging. Chen et al. reported a reversible temperature sensor based on DA monomer 2,2,2-trifluoro-N-(4-hydroxyphenyl)acetamide with a phenylacetamide head in which the π-π stacking between the aromatic benzene rings and H-bonding between the acetamide units resulted in a close-packed self-assembly and enhanced thermal stability.[34] However, this system did not show perfectly reversible blue-to-red transition. After the first heating from 30°C to 70°C, the blue-phase liposomes change to red phase but subsequent cooling to lower temperature does not restore the blue phase. Instead, a purple phase is obtained, which undergoes reversible thermally induced phase transition to red phase on all subsequent heating–cooling cycles. The authors attributed this phenomenon to the relaxation of steric hindrance during the first heating and slight reorganization of the aliphatic side chains to give a somewhat less effective conjugation resulting in the purple phase. Ryu et al.[51] demonstrated the use of PDA liposomes as a temperature sensor in microfluidic devices where accurate temperature measurement and control are desired for several applications such as polymerase chain reaction for amplification of DNA, enzyme-activated reactions, and chemical reactions. As the blue-phase non-fluorescent 10,12-PCDA-2,2′-(ethylenedioxy)bis(ethyl-amine) (EDEA), (structure shown in Fig. 4.6) droplets travel along the microfluidic device heated by a film microheater, they experience a temperature gradient and emit red fluorescence at higher temperatures. The peak emission intensities of the PDA liposomes were found to be linearly proportional to temperature in the range 40–60°C. This finding verified that the flow temperature in a microchannel can be determined by measuring the fluorescence intensities of PDA liposomes. Also, they expected that the applicable temperature range can be extended by utilizing structurally diverse DA monomers.

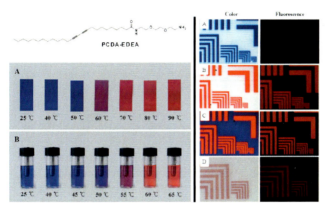

Figure 4.6   **Left panel:** Chemical structure of monomer 10,12-pentacosadiynoic acid-2,2′-(ethylenedioxy)bis(ethylamine) (PCDA-EDEA) (*top*) and photographs of (a) the PDA-incorporated poly(vinyl alcohol) (PVA) film and (b) the PDA-liposome solution at varied temperature according to the heating process (*bottom*). **Right panel:** patterned color (left) and fluorescence (right) images of the PDA-incorporated PVA film (a) after 254 nm UV polymerization for 1 min through a photomask; (b) after heating film A at 100°C for 10 s; (c) irradiation of 254 nm UV light on film B for 1 min without using a photomask; and (d) magnified images of prepared film B. The narrowest linewidth in these images is 6 μm. Adapted from Ref. [52], Copyright 2006, with permission from John Wiley and Sons. http://onlinelibrary.wiley.com/doi/10.1002/adfm.200600039/abstract.

Kim et al.[52] reported patterned color and fluorescence imaging in polymers based on PDA liposomes formed from the amine-terminated DA monomer PCDA-EDEA. Pre-polymerized PDA supramolecules were embedded in a poly(vinyl alcohol) (PVA) film by a mixing–drying process to give a blue-colored transparent film. The PDA-embedded film showed thermally induced colorimetric transition from blue phase at 25°C to red phase at above 70°C. This color transition in the film state required higher temperature as compared to similar transition in the solution state owing to the hindered mobility of the liposomes in the film. Patterned color and fluorescent images were made by a photo-lithographic method wherein un-polymerized self-assembled PDA supramolecules were embedded in PVA film and the film was UV irradiated through a photomask to yield blue patterned images (Fig. 4.6). Heating these films at 120°C for 10 s produced the fluorescent red phase. Development of blue phase only in the UV-irradiated portions of the film indicated that the PDA supramol-ecules are quite stable and their integrity is not adversely affected by the PVA matrix. Such robustness of PDA supramolecules and the ease of making such a PDA-embedded polymer matrix open up an exciting avenue for micro-patterned functional images without employing wet developing processes.[52] Yarimaga et al.[53] demonstrated a multicolor thermochromic display device based on PCDA-EDEA liposomes, which underwent colorimetric transi-tion from blue to red phase at 70°C and further to yellow phase at 180°C. By modulating the temperature of PDA-PVA film through a microheater array, a whole range of colorimetric transition starting from blue to red, orange, yellow, and green was achieved.

4.4.2 Halochromism

PDA liposomes with pH-sensitive moieties such as amines and carboxylic acids in the headgroup undergo colorimetric transition with the change in the solution pH. Cheng and Stevens[11] studied halochromic transitions in a series of amino-acid-derivatized PDA liposomes with glutamic acid (GLU), glutamine (GLN), and histidine (HIS) headgroups and found that all three underwent blue-to-red phase transition with an increase in the pH. The 50% colorimetric response (pH required to attain 50% of maximum color transition), CR_{50}, was found to be 6.3, 8.1, and 9.0 for GLU-PDA, HIS-PDA, and GLN-PDA, respectively. The authors attributed this colorimetric transition to the ionization-induced coulombic repulsion resulting in conformational change of the side chain and concomitant perturbation of the CP backbone. Interestingly, only PDA with HIS headgroup exhibited blue-to-red halochromism at lower pH as well due to the charge-induced perturbation resulting from the protonation of imidazole ring of the amino acid. A similar study of carboxy-terminated-10,12 tricosadiynoic acid (TRCDA) liposomes by Kew and Hall showed the same results.[54] The color transition was observed in the pH range of 9.0–10.1, which is in accordance with the pK_a of 9.5–9.9 for the liposome. No chromism was observed at lower pH (<4). In fact, neutralization of surface charges at lower pH resulted in the aggregation and subsequent precipitation of the liposomes. In addition to deprotonation and surface-charge-induced perturbation of the conjugated backbone resulting in colorimetric transition, the authors also identified subsequent binding of a proper cationic species to the liposome surface as a causative agent. In a more recent investigation, Seo et al.[55] argued that the halochromatic transition in PDA liposomes is not only dependent on pH but also on the size of the acids. Studying colorimetric transition in polymerized liposomes of *N*-(2-aminoalkyl)-10,12-pentacosadiynamide (APCDA2) with a series of alkanoic acids—formic, acetic, propionic, and butyric acids—they observed that the larger sized acid showed higher colorimetric response. They concluded that molecular size of the acid analyte is the dominant factor for pH chromism of PDA, though acidity was necessary as the driving force for salt formation. Furthermore, they developed a PDA sensor to distinguish larger sized diethyl phosphate (DEP) from general acids (Fig. 4.7). DEP was produced by the hydrolysis of diethyl chlorophosphate (DCP), a nerve gas stimulant, and was used as a model compound for indirect detection of nerve agents. This can open up avenues for simple, reliable, and low-cost optical biosensors for the detection of toxic organophosphorus chemicals.

Since the fluorescence intensity of the red-phase PDA liposomes is very low, they have also been used with fluorescent molecules to increase the sensitivity via fluorescence resonance energy transfer (FRET). Lee et al.[56] reported one such pH sensor based on mixed PDA liposomes of PCDA and phospholipid, 1,2-dimyristoyl-*sn*-glycero-3-phophocholine and benzoxazole derivatives as fluorescent donor dye for FRET embedded within the liposome bilayer. The integrity of mixed liposome as well as molecular characteristic of benzoxazole changed with pH. When the benzoxazole molecules were entrapped by hydrophobic interactions within the liposome bilayer, there was effective

FRET, resulting in more intense PDA emission. The fluorescence intensity remained unchanged in pH range 4–10. At lower pH, the intramolecular tautomerization of benzoxazole is prevented resulting in ineffective FRET with the liposome and decrease in emission intensity. Destruction of liposome to release benzoxazole and latter's tautomerization at basic pH resulted in a color change, as schematically shown in Fig. 4.8.

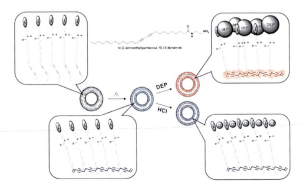

Figure 4.7   Schematic illustration of PDA's chromatic transition reliant on the molecular size of acid analytes (diethyl phosphate vs HCl). Reproduced from Ref. [55], Copyright 2010, with permission from John Wiley and Sons. http://onlinelibrary. wiley.com/doi/10.1002/adfm.201000262/abstract.

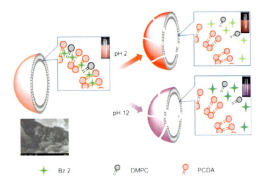

Figure 4.8   Schematic illustration of FRET change in PDA-liposome structures by pH changes (pH 2 vs pH 12). Reprinted from Ref. [56], Copyright 2013, with permission from Elsevier Science. http://www.sciencedirect.com/science/article/pii/ S1381514812002982.

4.4.3 Solvatochromism

The colorimetric transition in PDA vesicles induced by organic solvents has been used for the detection and differentiation of solvents such as different alcohols and chlorine compounds. Pires et al.[32] did extensive thermodynamic studies of colorimetric transition in PCDA liposomes and mixed liposomes of PCDA, cholesterol, and sphingomyelin induced by different chlorine-containing solvents such as methylene chloride (CH_2Cl_2), chloroform ($CHCl_3$), and carbon tetrachloride (CCl_4). Both the PCDA and mixed liposomes showed colorimetric transition for each of the three solvents, and the response for PCDA liposomes was better in all the three cases. Inclusion of cholesterol and sphingomyelin in the liposome's structure resulted in different intermolecular interactions and higher stability resulting in lower solvent-induced chromism. Among the three solvents, $CHCl_3$ showed the maximum colorimetric response, but CCl_4 induced the quickest response. This chromism behavior depends on the interplay between solvent–water and solvent–vesicle interactions. When the solvent is added to the aqueous suspension of the liposomes, it gets partitioned between the two phases—water and vesicles; and within the vesicle, the solvent molecule can reside either on the hydrophilic interface or the inner hydrophobic region of the bilayer. Such distribution of the added solvent leads to their different behavior. The solubility of the solvent in water decides its relative concentration in the two phases. CCl_4, because of its very low solubility in water, gets partitioned in the vesicle, resulting in the disruption of the conjugated backbone at lower concentration and hence quicker colorimetric response compared to CH_2Cl_2 and $CHCl_3$. Through microcalorimetric studies, the authors established that the solvatochromism is enthalpically driven in the case of $CHCl_3$ and it is entropically driven for the other two solvents.

Several reports show that addition of alcohol to aqueous suspensions of PDA liposomes causes solvatochromic transition from blue phase to red.[33,57,58] Traiphol et al.[59] systematically investigated the effect of linear alkyl chain length, position of hydroxyl group, and size of alkyl branch of alcohol on its capability to induce chromism in three types of PDA liposomes—PCDA, 10,12-tricosadiynoic acid (TCDA), and N-(2-aminoethyl)pentacosap-10,12-diynamide (AEPCDA). While PCDA and TCDA have a single H-bonding moiety in the headgroup, AEPCDA has one amine and one amide group, which can form H-bonds. This difference in headgroup interactions in the liposome resulted in different behavior of AEPCDA vesicles compared to PCDA and TCDA. The colorimetric transition in PDA liposomes is induced by the swelling of alcohol into the inner layer of the liposomes and hence disruption of the inter-chain and intra-chain H-bonding interactions and the subsequent conformational change of the side chain and twisting of the conjugated PDA backbone. While the hydrophobic alkyl chain of the alcohol interacts with the inner layer of the liposome, the hydroxyl group interacts with the hydrophilic headgroup of the liposome. As such, alcohols with longer alkyl chain are expected to show easier colorimetric response. It was found that 1-pentanol resulted in blue-to-red phase transition at the lowest concentration, which was nearly 20 times smaller than that for methanol. While PCDA and TCDA liposomes with single H-bonding moieties in their headgroups showed one-step transition for all alcohols, AEPCDA with two H-bonding moieties showed a two-step transition for methanol and ethanol corresponding to sequential disruption of the two H-bonds. More hydrophobic alcohols with longer alkyl chains resulted in one-step transition in AEPCDA liposomes as they penetrated and disrupted both H-bonds in a single step. The increase in liposome size and reduction in surface charge density upon addition of alcohol (up to 50% (v/v)) support the chromic transition explained by swelling of alcohol molecules into PDA vesicles. In the case of propanol, the position of the hydroxyl group affected the colorimetric response. 2-propanol showed lower response than 1-propanol and this difference was found to be more prominent in AEPCDA liposomes than PCDA liposomes. However, swelling of differently substituted pentanols into the PDA vesicle was more driven by their hydrophobicity and hence the effect of the position of hydroxyl group seemed negligible. The size of alkyl branch and hydrophobicity also affect the penetration of alcohol molecule in the PDA vesicle. Depending on the actual chemical structure, one factor dominates over the other.

Potisatityuenyong et al.[60] developed a colorimetric ethanol sensor through layer-by-layer deposition of polycationic polymer chains of chitosan or poly(diallyldimethylammonium chloride) (PDADMAC) and negatively charged polymerized PCDA vesicles.

While the polyelectrolyte membrane (PEM) prepared with PDADMAC resulted in inadvertent red phase of the liposome, chitosan-based PEM maintained the liposomes in the blue phase. Immersion of PEM films in ethanol solution resulted in a colorimetric response, which increased with the concentration of ethanol and achieved 100% response at 62% (w/w) ethanol. This value was higher than that for PDA-liposome suspension (47% (w/w) ethanol), which may be due to the repulsion of more hydrophobic ethanol by the polyelectrolyte film.

The varied colorimetric response of different PDA liposomes to different solvents due to the hydrophobicity or chemical structure of the latter can be used to develop low-cost, yet sensitive, optical sensors for organic solvents.

4.4.4 Mechanochromism

Mechanical stress or shear can cause colorimetric transition in PDAs.[13,38,61] Most of the research in this field has involved PDAs prepared as elastomers[61] or Langmuir–Blodgett films.[38] Recently, Lee et al.[62] investigated mechanochromatic transition in PDA liposomes. The PDA liposomes were dispersed in a polymer solution of PVA, hyaluronic acid (HA), or PVA/sodium borate (PVA/B) in 1:20 volume ratio, and the zero shear viscosities of the solutions were maintained constant at 40 Pas. When these solutions were subjected to increasing shear stress controlled by a stress control rheometer at a temperature of 47°C, only PVA/B showed colorimetric transition. Figure 4.9 shows the absorbance spectrum and visible colorimetric transition for PVA/B solution as a function of shear stress. However, it did not show any color transition when subjected to shear below 40°C. At 47°C, PDA liposomes can be assumed to be in the meta-stable state just below the thermochromic transition temperature of 50°C and the applied shear results in the chromatic transition. Such transition cannot be induced at 40°C as PDA liposomes are in the stable blue phase at that temperature. The mechanochromatic behavior of PDA only in PVA/B solution was explained by the shear-thickening nature of PVA/B, which results in higher stress development in the solution. HA and PVA solutions were found to be shear thinning and, therefore, did not show mechanochromism. Given the advantages of PDA liposomes, such as easy dispersion in target materials and high sensitivity, such PDA/polymer systems can be used to visualize shear stress distribution in flow devices.[62] However, much effort is required to fully understand the mechanochromatic behavior of PDA liposomes and develop sensitive sensors.

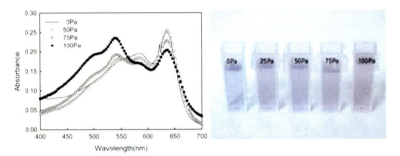

Figure 4.9 Shear-dependent colorimetric transition of PDA in PVA/ sodium borate solution (left) and photograph of color-tuned PDAs (right). Adapted with permission from Ref. [62], Copyright 2007, The Korean Society of Rheology. http://infosys.korea. ac.kr/PDF/KARJ/KR19/KR19-1-0043.pdf.

4.4.5 Affinochromism

PDA liposomes functionalized with specific receptors provide a recognition function (receptor) as well as a signaling element (PDA backbone) within a single supramolecular assembly.[21,63–68] Receptor–ligand interactions on the liposome surface cause the disorder and tangling in the lipid chain and concomitant perturbation of the CP backbone, resulting in colorimetric/ fluorometric transition. This affinochromic feature of PDA liposomes offers a general method for the direct detection of receptor–ligand interactions, employing to a wide range of sensing applications such as viruses,[69–72] toxins,[73] bacteria,[74] oligonucleotides,[75,76] enzymes,[77,78] antibiotics,[79,80] glucose,[81] metal ions,[16,17,82,83] harmful chemicals,[18,31,84] surfactants,[85] and CO_2 gas,[86] as illustrated in Fig. 4.10.

In an early experiment, Charych et al.[69–71] investigated affinochromic transitions in PDA liposomes for the first time. In order to detect influenza virus, they prepared PDA liposomes from cleverly designed sialic-acid-functionalized DA monomers and 12-

pentacosadiynoic acids (Fig. 4.11a). Sialic acid was introduced as a specific receptor unit because terminal α-glycosides of sialic acid bind to hemagglutinin (HA), which is anchored to a lipid bilayer of influenza virus. The 87% of color response (CR) was achieved for 60 hemagglutinating units (HAUs) of virus and as little as 11 HAUs could be detected. They hypothesized that specific interaction of the viral hemagglutinin to the sialic acid residues on the liposome surface affected the lipid chain conformations in a similar manner to thermal annealing, resulting in a blue-to-red color transition. In a following work, they developed a cholera toxin detection system in a very similar way by incorporating ganglioside-functionalized DA monomers into PDA liposomes (Fig. 4.11b).[73] Recognition of cholera toxin was achieved through a specific interaction between the ganglioside and cholera toxin at the interface of liposome, resulting in a colorimetric transition due to conformational changes in the conjugated ene–yne backbone.

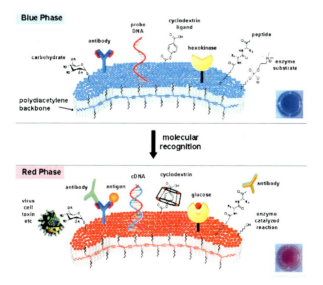

Figure 4.10 A schematic illustration of PDA liposomes functionalized with specific receptors. Receptor–ligand interactions cause a colorimetric transition in PDA liposomes owing to conformational changes in conjugated ene–yne backbone.[65] Reprinted with permission from Ref. [65], Copyright 2008, American Chemical Society. http://pubs.acs.org/doi/abs/10.1021/ar7002489.

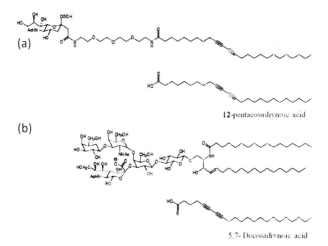

12-pentacosadiynoic acid

5,7-Docosadiynoic acid

Figure 4.11 Chemical structures of (a) sialic-acid-functionalized diacetylene monomer (*upper*) and 12-pentacosadiynoic acids (*lower*), (b) ganglioside-functionalized diacetylene monomer (*upper*) and 5,7-docosadiynoic acid (*lower*).[71] Adapted with permission from Ref. [71], Copyright 1995, American Chemical Society. http://pubs.acs.org/doi/abs/10.1021/ja00107a032.

Ma et al. developed novel PDA vesicles for the detection of *E. coli*.[74] Interestingly, they introduced the receptor molecules into PDA matrix by using a glycolipid, dioctadecyl glycerylether-β-glucoside (DGG), instead of a glucoside-functionalized DA monomer (Fig. 4.12), which is more generally available and easily obtained without difficult synthesis. In this study, two types of diacetylenic acid, tricosa-2,4-diynoic acid (TCDA), and 10,12-PCDA were compared as the matrix lipids. While TCDA/DGG system showed distinct blue-to-red transition after exposure to *E. coli* within several seconds, there was no color change in PDCA/DGG system. The authors attributed this difference to the strong interaction and good miscibility between TCDA/DGG.

In a more recent study, Kang et al. incorporated a natural lipid of phosphatidylinostiol-4,5-bisphosphate (PIP$_2$) as a receptor into a PDA liposome to detect aminoglycosidic antibiotic, neomycin.[79,80] PIP$_2$/PCDA co-assembled liposome showed a sharp color change and concomitant fluorescence development upon treatment with a neomycin solution (Fig. 4.12b). More sensitive detection was attained by introducing 1,2-dimyristoyl-*sn*-glycero-3-phosphate (DMPA) into PIP$_2$/PCDA liposome. They ascribed the enhanced sensitivity to the role of DMPA that makes PDA backbone in the liposome more mobile.

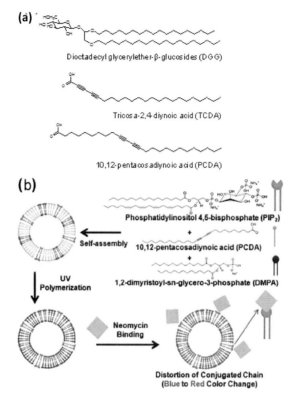

Figure 4.12 (a) Chemical structures of dioctadecyl glycerylether-β-glucosides (DGG), tricosa-2,4-diynoic acid (TCDA), and 10,12-pentacosadiynoic acid.[74] Adapted with permission from Ref. [74], Copyright 1998, American Chemical Society (http://pubs.acs.org/doi/abs/10.1021/ja982663a). (b) Schematic representation of antibiotic detection based on PIP2-PDA co-assembled liposome reported by Kang et al. Reproduced from Ref. [79], Copyright 2012, with permission from The Royal Society of Chemistry (http://dx.doi.org/10.1039/C2CC31466E).

Kolusheva et al. reported a cation-selective colorimetric sensor based on PDA-mixed vesicles.[82] They prepared supramolecular assemblies of PDA vesicles, comprising natural phospholipids and PDA lipids, to which ionophore molecules were added. The resulting mixed vesicles showed blue-to-red color transition upon exposure to ions such as Li$^+$, Na$^+$, K$^+$, Rb$^+$, and Cs$^+$, caused through interaction between the ionophore–ion complexes and PDA-mixed vesicles.

The quantitative and selective detection of a cation was recently accomplished by our group (Fig. 4.13).[17]

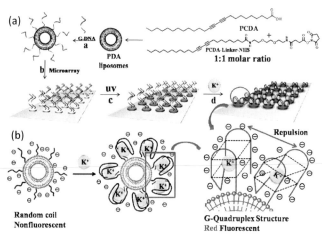

Figure 4.13 (a) The chemical structure of the diacetylene monomers and a schematic representation of the PDA-liposome-based microarray for potassium detection. (b) Diagram of the G-quadruplex formation and the subsequent steric repulsion between G-quadraplexes.[17] Reprinted with permission from Ref. [17], Copyright 2008, American Chemical Society. http://pubs.acs.org/doi/abs/10.1021/ja709996c.

We developed the highly selective and quantitative detection of K$^+$ based on PDA liposomes functionalized with a single-strand DNA (ssDNA) having a guanine-rich (G-rich) sequence. When the G-rich ssDNA probe recognized K$^+$ on the liposome surface, it could fold into a G-quadruplex through Hoogsteen hydrogen bonding wrapping around the K$^+$. The authors reasoned that the steric repulsion of the resulting bulky G-quadruplex perturbed the PDA backbone conformation and triggered the blue-to-red color transition and the fluorescence development. The quantitative analysis of K$^+$ concentration was also demonstrated by our group in the practically useful PDA-liposome-based microarrays.[17]

In a following study, our group developed PDA-liposome microarrays for sensitive and selective detection of Hg^{2+} (Fig. 4.14).[16] We incorporated a specific ssDNA aptamer as a selective receptor for Hg^{2+} onto the PDA-liposome surface. The ssDNA aptamers recognized Hg^{2+} and subsequently formed T-Hg^{2+}-T complexes. The authors postulated that the resulting bulky T-Hg^{2+}-T complexes repel each other owing to steric hindrance and induce the color change and the fluorescence development in a way similar to the previous report. In this study, our group focused more on the development of a universal PDA platform, which can be generally applicable to microarrays. The unique design included the development of epoxy-functionalized PDA liposomes. Such liposomes offered both enhanced stability as well as the efficient tethering of probes and immobilization on a glass substrate compared to generally used N-hydroxysuccinimide (NHS)-activated carboxylic acid functionalized liposome. This allows for convenient user-prepared microarrays.

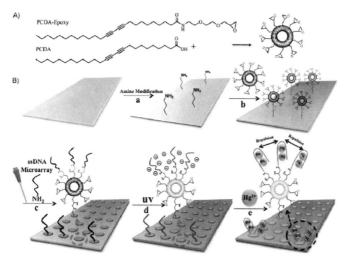

Figure 4.14 (A) Chemical structure of the diacetylene monomers, PCDA, and PCDA-epoxy. (B) Schematic design of the PDA-liposome-based microarray for mercury detection: (a) surface modification of the glass substrate with amine functionality, (b) immobilization of the epoxy liposomes onto the amine glass slide through epoxy–amine coupling, (c) post-tethering of the ssDNA aptamer by means of a microarrayer, (d) photopolymerization of the PDA liposomes using a 254 nm UV lamp, and (e) recognition of the target mercury ions results in red fluorescent emission. Reproduced from Ref. [16], Copyright 2009, with permission from John Wiley and Sons. http://onlinelibrary.wiley.com/doi/10.1002/adma.200900639/abstract.

The detection of harmful chemicals has also been successfully achieved through rationally designed PDA liposomes. Lee et al. reported the sensitive and selective detection of melamine by PDA liposomes prepared from a cyanuric acid (CA)-functionalized DA monomer and a PCDA (Fig. 4.15).[18]

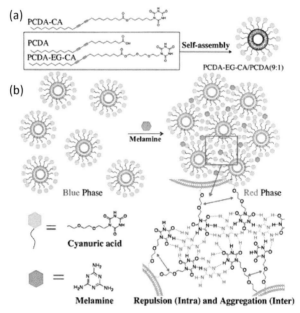

Figure 4.15 (a) Chemical structure of the studied diacetylene monomers, PCDA, PCDA-CA, and PCDA-EG-CA for melamine detection. (b) Schematic illustration of colorimetric transition in CA-derived PDA liposome by intra/intermolecular hydrogen bond and consequential steric aggregation and repulsion. Reproduced from Ref. [18], Copyright 2010, with permission from The Royal Society of Chemistry. http://dx.doi.org/10.1039/C0CC02183K.

They found that the intra-liposomal repulsion and inter-liposomal aggregation mediated by strong hydrogen bonding between melamine and CA at the PDA-liposome surfaces perturbed the PDA backbone and triggered the sensitive and rapid color/fluorescence change.

The detection of warfare gases has recently been attained by our group (Fig. 4.16).[31] Oxime (OX) functional groups were introduced into the system to utilize their strong affinity to nerve agents. PDA liposomes were prepared from OX-functionalized DA monomers (PCDA-HBO) and matrix monomers (PCDA-pBA). Sharp blue-to-red color transition was observed upon exposure to the nerve agent diisopropylfluorophosphate (DFP). We postulated that the color change originated from the covalent bond formation between OX and DFP, which induces intra-liposomal steric repulsion as well as inter-liposomal aggregation caused by increased hydrophobicity of liposome surfaces through OX-DFP complex formation. Our group further developed liposome-coated cellulose acetate membranes showing selective and rapid colorimetric detection down to 160 ppb of DFP. This development opens up a way for simple label-free detection of nerve gases.

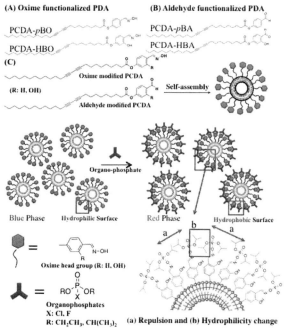

Figure 4.16 Chemical structure of the considered (A) oxime-functionalized and (B) aldehyde-functionalized PDA monomers for warfare gas detection. (C) Schematic drawing of the PDA-liposome-based organophosphate detection strategy in terms of (a) intra-liposomal repulsion and (b) inter-liposomal aggregation due to the hydrophobic surface property. Reproduced from Ref. [31], Copyright 2012, with permission from John Wiley and Sons. http://onlinelibrary.wiley.com/doi/10.1002/adfm.201102486/abstract.

Multitarget detection was developed by embedding sensory PDA liposomes into multiphasic alginate microparticles (Fig. 4.17). Lee et al. realized the biphasic alginate microparticles by co-injecting two different PDA liposome/alginate mixtures into an aqueous solution of CaCl$_2$ using a simple needle injection system.[87] They could manipulate the size and constituent of alginate particles by regulating centrifugal force and controlling the composition of PDA-liposome solution, respectively. This system offers the potential for multitarget detection with the enhanced stability and sensitivity compared to conventional PDA-liposome solution. For example, within bi- and tri-phasic alginate microparticles, two target molecules such as melamine and avidin-FITC can be discriminatively detected. The microparticles make integration with microfluidic devices to achieve facile detection of biological targets possible.

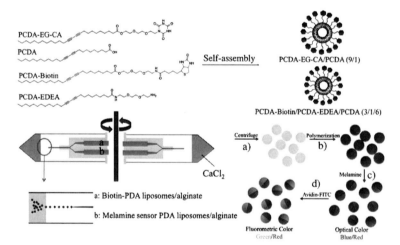

Figure 4.17   (a) Chemical structures of the PDA monomers and (b) the schematic design of the fabrication of biphasic alginate particle having embedded PDA liposomes demonstrating a potential multitargeting capability.[87] Reprinted with permission from Ref. [87], Copyright 2012, American Chemical Society. http://pubs.acs.org/doi/abs/10.1021/cm3015012.

Although a variety of affinochromic PDA liposomes were investigated since the pioneering work of Charych et al., the exact mechanism of the affinity-induced color/fluorescence transition is not fully understood. Very recently, Seo et al. systematically studied the analyte size effect on the sensory mechanism of PDA liposomes (Fig. 4.18).[72] The researchers selected influenza A virus M1 peptide and M1 antibody as a probe–target pair. They could not observe blue-to-red color transition when they used a larger M1 antibody as a probe and smaller M1 peptide as a target. However, interestingly, distinct color/fluorescence transition was observed when they used an M1 peptide as a probe and M1 antibody as a target. They argued that these results clearly indicated that the steric repulsion between probe and target mainly contributed to the sensory signal intensity of PDA liposomes rather than the probe–target binding force.

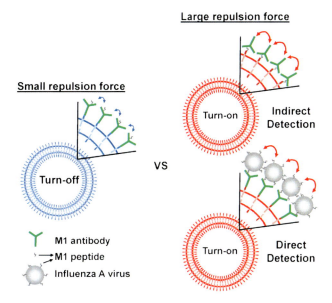

Figure 4.18 Molecular size effect on colorimetric PDA liposomes for influenza A virus sensor. Reproduced from Ref. [72], Copyright 2013, with permission from John Wiley and Sons. http://onlinelibrary.wiley.com/doi/10.1002/marc.201200819/abstract.

4.5 Conclusion

With an ever-increasing emphasis on efficient and robust chemical sensors and biosensors in recent times, much scientific research has been expended to develop sensors that are simple and sensitive, yet cost effective. Owing to their properties of environmentally sensitive fluorescence and signal amplification, CPs have proved to be the material of choice for the development of optical chemical sensors and biosensors. PDAs with their colorimetric and fluorometric dual detection capability and ease of liposome formation have been one of the most studied CP systems. In this chapter, we have discussed the self-assembled structure, topochemical polymerization, and colorimetric transitions in PDA systems with focus on their sensory applications. Although the exact mechanism of color change in PDA liposomes is far from being definitively clear and still is one of the most heatedly contested research areas, it has not hindered the application and development of PDA-liposome-based sensors for the detection of environmental, chemical, and biological analytes. While PDA-liposome-based temperature, solvent, pH, and mechanical stress sensing have been demonstrated, affinity-based sensing has been the most actively and successfully researched area for sensor development.

With a better understanding of the mechanism of color transition in PDA liposomes, the effect of liposome composition and analyte size on color transition, and the development of newer methods to enhance the colorimetric response through a clever design of FRET-based or turn-off systems, PDA-liposome-based chemical sensors and biosensors will continue to be one of the prime research areas in the foreseeable future.

Acknowledgments

We acknowledge financial supports from the National Science Foundation (BES 0428010), NSF CAREER Award (DMR 0644864), Animal, Plant and Fisheries Quarantine and Inspection Agency of Korea (I-AD14-2011-13-11), and Converging Research Center Program funded by the Ministry of Science, ICT and Future Planning (Project No. 2014M3C1A8048791).

References

1. Shirakawa H, Louis EJ, MacDiarmid AG, Chiang CK, Heeger AJ. Synthesis of electrically conducting organic polymers: Halogen derivatives of polyacetylene. *J Chem Soc, Chem Commun.* 1977; 16: 578–580.

2. Kim J, Swager M. Control of conformational and interpolymer effects in conjugated polymers. *Nature.* 2001; 6855: 548–548.

3. Kim J, Levitsky IA, McQuade DT, Swager TM. Structural control in thin layers of poly(p-phenyleneethynylene)s: Photophysical studies of Langmuir and Langmuir–Blodgett films. *JACS.* 2002; 124: 7710–7718.

4. Wang Y, Zappas AJ, Wilson JN, Kim I-B, Solntsev KM, Tolbert LM, Bunz UHF. Optical spectroscopy of grafted poly(p-phenyleneethynylene)s in water and water–DMF mixtures. *Macromolecules.* 2008; 41: 1112–1117.

5. Lebouch N, Garreau S, Louarn G, Belletête M, Durocher G, Leclerc M. Structural study of the thermochromic transition in poly(2,5-dialkyl-p-phenyleneethynylene)s. *Macromolecules.* 2005; 38: 9631–9637.

6. Zhao X, Pinto MR, Hardison LM, Mwaura J, Müller J, Jiang H, Witker D, Kleiman VD, Reynolds JR, Schanze KS. Variable band gap poly(arylene ethynylene) conjugated polyelectrolytes. *Macromolecules.* 2006; 39: 6355–6366.

7. Bunz UHF, Imhof JM, Bly RK, Bangcuyo CG, Rozanski L, Vanden Bout DA. Photophysics of poly[p-(2,5-didodecylphenylene)ethynylene] in thin films. *Macromolecules.* 2005; 38: 5892–5896.

8. McQuade DT, Pullen AE, Swager TM. Conjugated polymer-based chemical sensors. *Chem Rev.* 2000; 100: 2537–2574.

9. Zhou Q, Swager TM. Conjugated polymer-based chemical sensors. Fluorescent chemosensors based on energy migration in conjugated polymers: The molecular wire approach to increased sensitivity. *JACS.* 1995; 117: 12593–12602.

10. Swager TM. The molecular wire approach to sensory signal amplification. *Acc Chem Res.* 1998; 31: 201–207.

11. Cheng Q, Stevens RC. Charge-induced chromatic transition of amino acid-derivatized polydiacetylene liposomes. *Langmuir.* 1998; 14: 1974–1976.

12. Jonas U, Shah K, Norvez S, Charych DH. Reversible color switching and unusual solution polymerization of hydrazide-modified diacetylene lipids. *JACS.* 1999; 121: 4580–4588.

13. Carpick RW, Sasaki DY, Burns AR. First observation of mechano-chromism at the nanometer scale. *Langmuir.* 2000; 16: 1270–1278.

14. Chance RR, Patel GN, Witt JD. Thermal effects on the optical properties of single crystals and solution-cast films of urethane substituted polydiacetylenes. *J Chem Phys.* 1979; 71: 206–211.

15. Tashiro K, Nishimura H, Kobayashi M. First success in direct analysis of microscopic deformation mechanism of polydiacetylene single crystal by the X-ray imaging-plate system. *Macromolecules.* 1996; 29: 8188–8196.

16. Lee J, Jun H, Kim J. Polydiacetylene–liposome microarrays for selective and sensitive mercury(ii) detection. *Adv Mater.* 2009; 21: 3674–3677.

17. Lee J, Kim H-J, Kim J. Polydiacetylene liposome arrays for selective potassium detection. *JACS.* 2008; 130: 5010–5011.

18. Lee J, Jeong EJ, Kim J. Selective and sensitive detection of melamine by intra/inter-liposomal interaction of polydiacetylene liposomes. *Chem Commun.* 2011; 47: 358–360.

19. Malcolm NJ. The surface properties of phospholipid liposome systems and their characterization. *Adv Colloid Interface Sci.* 1995; 54: 93–128.

20. Yue X, Guo C, Jing Y, Ma F. Free-standing liposomal nanohybrid cerasomes as ideal materials for sensing of cupric ions. *Analyst.* 2012; 137: 2027–2031.

21. Reppy MA, Pindzola BA. Biosensing with polydiacetylene materials: Structures, optical properties and applications. *Chem Commun.* 2007; 42: 4317–4338.

22. Kim J-M, Lee J-S, Choi H, Sohn D, Ahn DJ. Rational design and in-situ FTIR analyses of colorimetrically reversibe polydiacetylene supramolecules. *Macromolecules.* 2005; 38: 9366–9376.

23. Hsu L, Cvetanovich GL, Stupp SI. Peptide amphiphile nanofibers with conjugated polydiacetylene backbones in their core. *JACS.* 2008; 130: 3892–3899.

24. Baughman RH, Yee KC. Solid-state polymerization of linear and cyclic acetylenes. *J Polym Sci Macromol Rev.* 1978; 13: 219–239.

25. Enkelmann V. Structural aspects of the topochemical polymerization of diacetylenes. In *Polydiacetylenes*; Cantow, H-J, Ed.; Springer Berlin Heidelberg: 1984; 63: 91–136.

26. Fujita N, Sakamoto Y, Shirakawa M, Ojima M, Fujii A, Ozaki M, Shinkai S. Polydiacetylene nanofibers created in low-molecular-weight gels by post modification: Control of blue and red phases by the odd–even effect in alkyl chains. *JACS.* 2007; 129: 4134–4135.

27. Shand ML, Chance RR, LePostollec M, Schott M. Raman photoselection and conjugation-length dispersion in conjugated polymer solutions. *Phys Rev B.* 1982; 25: 4431–4436.

28. Dobrosavljević V, Stratt RM. Role of conformational disorder in the electronic structure of conjugated polymers: Substituted polydiacetylenes. *Phys Rev B.* 1987; 35: 2781–2794.

29. Kolusheva S, Shahal T, Jelinek R. Peptide-membrane interactions studied by a new phospholipid/polydiacetylene colorimetric vesicle assay. *Biochemistry.* 2000; 39: 15851–15859.

30. Gou M, Qu X, Zhu W, Xiang M, Yang J, Zhang K, Wei Y, Chen S. Bio-inspired detoxification using 3D-printed hydrogel nanocomposites. *Nat Commun.* 2014; 5: 1–9.

31. Lee J, Seo S, Kim J. Colorimetric detection of warfare gases by polydiacetylenes toward equipment-free detection. *Adv Funct Mater.* 2012; 22: 1632–1638.

32. Pires ACS, Soares NdFF, da Silva LHM, da Silva MCH, Mageste AB, Soares RF, Teixeira AVNC, Andrade NJ. Thermodynamic study of colorimetric transitions in polydiacetylene vesciles induced by the solvent effect. *J Phys Chem B.* 2010; 114: 13365–13371.

33. Su Y-L, Li J-R, Jiang L. Effect of amphiphilic molecules upon chromatic transitions of polydiacetylene vesicles in aqueous solutions. *Colloids Surf B.* 2004; 39(3): 113–118.

34. Chen X, Yoon J. A thermally reversible temperature sensor based on polydiacetylene: Synthesis and thermochromic properties. *Dyes Pigments.* 2011; 89: 194–198.

35. Ahn DJ, Lee S, Kim J-M. Rational design of conjugated polymer supramolecules with tunable colorimetric responses. *Adv Funct Mater.* 2009; 19: 1483–1496.

36. Huo Q, Russell KC, Leblanc RM. Chromatic studies of a polymerizable diacetylene hydrogen bonding self-assembly: A "self-folding" process to explain the chromatic changes of polydiacetylenes. *Langmuir.* 1999; 15: 3972–3980.

37. Eckhardt H, Bourdeaux DS, Chance RR. Effects of substituent-induced strain on the electronic structure of polydiacetylenes. *J Chem Phys.* 1986; 85: 4116–4119.

38. Tomioka Y, Tanaka N, Imazeki S. Surface-pressure-induced reversible color change of a polydiacetylene monolayer at a gas water interface, *J Chem Phys.* 1989; 91: 5694–5700.

39. Lee DC, Sahoo SK, Cholli L, Sandman DJ. Structural aspects of the thermochromic transition in urethane-substituted polydiacetylenes. *Macromolecules.* 2002; 35: 4347–4355.

40. Kim J-M, Lee J-S, Choi H, Sohn D, Ahn DJ. Rational design and in-situ FTIR analyses of colorimetrically reversible polydiacetylene supramolecules. *Macromolecules.* 2005; 38: 9366–9376.

41. Hammond PT, Rubner MF. Thermochromism in liquid crystalline polydiacetylenes. *Macromolecules.* 1997; 30: 5773–5782.

42. Huang X, Jiang S, Liu M. Metal ion modulated organization and function of the Langmuir–Blodgett films of amphiphilic diacetylene: Photopolymerization, thermochromism and supramolecular chirality. *J Phys Chem B.* 2004; 109: 114–119.

43. Peng H, Tang J, Pang J, Chen D, Yang L, Ashbaugh HS, Brinker CJ, Yang Z, Lu Y. Polydiacetylene/silica nanocomposites with tunable mesostructure and thermochromatism from diacetylenic assembling molecules. *J Am Chem Soc.* 2005; 127: 12782–12783.

44. Peng H, Tang J, Yang L, Pang J, Ashbaugh HS, Brinker CJ, Yang Z, Lu Y. Responsive periodic mesoporous polydiacetylene/silica nanocomposites. *J Am Chem Soc.* 2006; 128: 5304–5305.

45. Ahn DJ, Chae EH, Lee GS, Shim HY, Chang TE, Ahn KD, Kim, J-M. Colorimetric reversibility of polydiacetylene supramolecules having enhanced hydrogen-bonding under thermal and pH stimuli. *J Am Chem Soc.* 2003; 125: 8976–8977.

46. Lee S, Kim JM. Alpha-cyclodextrin: A molecule for testing colorimetric reversibility of polydiacetylene supramolecules. *Macromolecules.* 2007; 40: 9201–9204.

47. Song J, Cisar JS, Bertozzi CR. Functional self-assembling bolaamphiphilic polydiacetylenes as colorimetric sensor scaffolds. *J Am Chem Soc.* 2004; 126: 8459–8465.

48. Li LS, Stupp S. I Two-dimensional supramolecular assemblies of a polydiacetylene. 2. Morphology, structure, and chromic transitions. *Macromolecules.* 1997; 30: 5313–5320.

49. Yang Y, Lu Y, Lu M, Huang J, Haddad R, Xomeritakis G, Liu N, Malanoski AP, Sturmayr D, Fan H, Sasaki DY, Assink RA, Shelnutt JA, van Swol F, Lopez GP, Burns AR, Brinker CJ. Functional nanocomposites prepared by self-assembly and polymerization of diacetylene surfactants and silicic acid. *J Am Chem Soc.* 2003; 125: 1269–1277.

50. Kim JW, Lee CH, Yoo HO, Kim J-M. Thermochromic polydiacetylene supramoleculesw with oligo(ethylene oxide) headgroups for tunable colorimetric response. *Macromol Res.* 2009; 17(6): 441–444.

51. Ryu S, Yoo I, Song S, Yoon B, Kim J-M. A thermoresponsive fluorogenic conjugated polymer for temperature sensor in microfluidic devices. *J Am Chem Soc.* 2009; 131(11): 3800–3801.

52. Kim J-M, Lee YB, Chae SY, Ahn DJ. Patterned color and fluorescent images with polydiacetylene supramolecules embedded in poly(vinyl alcohol) films. *Adv Funct Mater.* 2006; 16: 2103–2109.

53. Yarimaga O, Im M, Choi Y-K, Kim TW, Jung YK, Park HG, Lee S, Kim J-M. A color display system based on thermochromic conjugated polydiacetylene supramolecules. *Macromol Res.* 2010; 18(40): 404–407.

54. Kew SJ, Hall EAH. pH response of carboxy-terminated colorimetric polydiacetylene vesicles. *Anal Chem.* 2006; 78: 2231–2238.

55. Seo D, Kim J. Effect of molecular size of analytes on polydiacetylene liposome chromism. *Adv Funct Mat.* 2010; 20: 1397–1403.

56. Seo S, Kim D, Jang G, Kim D-M, Kim DW, Seo B-K, Lee K-W, Lee TS. Fluorescence resonance energy transfer between polydiacetylene vesicles and embedded benzoxazole molecules for pH sensing. *React Funct Polym.* 2013; 73: 451–456.

57. Jiang H, Wang Y, Ye Q, Zou G, Su W, Zhang Q. Polydiacetylene-based colorimetric sensor microarray for volatile organic compounds. *Sens Actuators B Chem.* 2010; 143: 789.

58. Potisatityuenyong A, Rojanathanes R, Tumcharern G, Sukwattanasinitt M. Electronic absorption spectroscopy probed side-chain movement in chromic transitions of polydiacetylene vesicles. *Langmuir.* 2008; 24: 4461.

59. Pattanatornchai T, Charoenthai N, Wacharasindhu S, Sukwattanasinitt M, Traiphol R. Control over the color transition behavior of polydiacetylene vesicles using different alcohols. *J. Colloid Interface Sci.* 2013; 391: 45–53.

60. Potisatityuenyong A, Dubas ST, Sukwattanasinitt M. Layer-by-layer deposition of chitosan/polydiacetylene vesicles for convenient preparation of colorimetric sensing film. *NSTI Nanotech.* 2006; 1: 27–30.

61. Nallicheri RA, Rubner MF. Investigations of the mechanochromic behavior of poly(urethane diacetylene) segmented copolymers, *Macromolecules.* 1991; 24: 517–525.

62. Lee SS, Chae EH, Ahn DJ, Ahn KH, Yeo J-K. Shear induced color transition of PDA(polydiacetylene) liposome in polymeric solutions. *Korea-Aust Rheol J.* 2007; 19(1): 43–47.

63. Sarkar A, Okada S, Matsuzawa H, Matsuda H, Nakanishi H. Novel polydiacetylenes for optical materials: Beyond the conventional polydiacetylenes. *J Mater Chem.* 2000; 10: 819–828.

64. Jelinek R, Kolusheva S. Polymerized lipid vesicles as colorimetric biosensors for biotechnological applications. *Biotechnol Adv.* 2001; 19: 109–118.

65. Ahn DJ, Kim JM. Fluorogenic polydiacetylene supramolecules: Immobilization, micropatterning, and application to label-free chemosensors. *Acc Chem Res.* 2008; 41: 805–816.

66. Sun X, Chen T, Huang S, Li L, Peng H. Chromatic polydiacetylene with novel sensitivity. *Chem Soc Rev.* 2010; 39: 4244–4257.

67. Lee K, Povlich LK, Kim J. Recent advances in fluorescent and colorimetric conjugated polymer-based biosensors. *Analyst.* 2010; 135: 2179–2189.

68. Chen X, Zhou G, Peng X, Yoon J. Biosensors and chemosensors based on the optical responses of polydiacetylenes. *Chem Soc Rev.* 2012; 41: 4610–4630.

69. Charych DH, Nagy JO, Spevak W, Bdenarski MD. Direct colorimetric detection of a receptor-ligand interaction by a polymerized bilayer assembly. *Science.* 1993; 261: 585–588.

70. Spevak W, Nagy JO, Charych DH, Schaefer ME, Gilbert JH, Bednarski MD. Polymerized liposomes containing c-glycosides of sialic acid: Potent inhibitors of influenza virus in vitro infectivity. *J Am Chem Soc.* 1993; 115: 1146–1147.

71. Reichert A, Nagy JO, Spevak W, Charych D. Polydiacetylene liposomes functionalized with sialic acid bind and colorimetrically detect influenza virus. *J Am Chem Soc.* 1995; 117: 829–830.

72. Seo S, Lee J, Choi EJ, Kim EJ, Song JY, Kim J. Polydiacetylene liposome microarray toward influenza A virus detection: Effect of target size on turn-on signaling. *Macromol Rapid Commun.* 2013; 34: 743–748.

73. Pan JJ, Charych D. Molecular recognition and colorimetric detection of cholera toxin by poly(diacetylene) liposomes incorporating G_{M1} Ganglioside. *Langmuir.* 1997; 13: 1365–1367.

74. Ma Z, Li J, Liu M, Cao J, Zou Z, Tu J, Jiang L. Colorimetric detection of *Escherichia coli* by polydiacetylene vesicles functionalized with glycolipid. *J Am Chem Soc.* 1998; 120: 12678–12679.

75. Wang C, Ma Z. Colorimetric detection of oligonucleotides using a polydiacetylene vesicle sensor. *Anal Bioanal Chem.* 2005; 382: 1708–1710.

76. Jung YK, Kim TW, Kim J, Kim JM, Park HG. Universal colorimetric detection of nucleic acids based on polydiacetylene (PDA) liposomes. *Adv Funct Mater.* 2008; 18: 701–708.

77. Okada SY, Jelinek R, Charych D. Induced color change of conjugated polymeric vesicles by interfacial catalysis of phospholipase A_2. *Angew Chem Int Ed.* 1999; 38: 655–659.

78. Nie Q, Zhang Y, Zhang J, Zhang M. Immobilization of polydiacetylene onto microbeads for colorimetric detection. *J Mater Chem.* 2006; 16: 546–549.

79. Kang DH, Jung HS, Ahn N, Lee J, Seo S, Suh KY, Kim J, Kim K. Biomimetic detection of aminoglycosidic anitibiotics using polydiacetylene-phospholipids supramolecules. *Chem Commun.* 2012; 48: 5313–5315.

80. Kang DH, Jung HS, Lee J, Seo S, Kim J, Kim K, Suh KY. Design of polydiacetylene-phospholipid supramolecules for enhanced stability and sensitivity. *Langmuir.* 2012; 28: 7551–7556.

81. Cheng Q, Stevens RC. Coupling of an induced fit enzyme to polydiacetylene thin films: Colorimetric detection of glucose. *Adv Mater.* 2009; 21: 481–483.

82. Kolusheva S, Shahal T, Jelinek R. Cation-selective color sensors composed of ionophore-phopholipid-polydiacetylene mixed vesicles. *J Am Chem Soc.* 2000; 122: 776–780.

83. Xu Q, Lee KM, Wang F, Yoon J. Visual detection of copper ions based on azide- and alkyne-functionalized polydiacetylene vesicles. *J Mater Chem.* 2011; 21: 15214–15217.

84. Xia H, Li J, Zou G, Zhang Q, Jia C. A highly sensitive and reusable cyanide anion sensor based on spiropyran functionalized polydiacetylene vesicular receptors. *J Mater Chem. A.* 2013; 1: 10713–10719.

85. Chen X, Lee J, Jou MJ, Kim JM, Yoon J. Colorimetric and fluorometric detection of cationic surfactants based on conjugated polydiacetylene supramolecules. *Chem Commun.* 2009; 23: 3434–3436.

86. Xu Q, Lee S, Cho Y, Kim MH, Bouffard J, Yoon J. Polydiacetylene-based colorimetric and fluorescent chemosensor for the detection of carbon dioxide. *J Am Chem Soc.* 2013; 135: 17751–17754.

87. Lee J, Kim J. Multiphasic sensory alginate particle having poly-diacetylene liposome for selective and more sensitive multitargeting detection. *Chem Mater.* 2012; 24: 2817–2822.

Chapter 5

Taking Advantage of Liposomes in Microfluidic Systems

Nongnoot Wongkaew,[a] John T. Connelly,[b] and Antje J. Baeumner[a]

[a]*Institute of Analytical Chemistry, Chemo- and Biosensors,
University of Regensburg, University Street 31, Regensburg 93053, Germany*
[b]*Diagnostics for All, 840 Memorial Drive, Cambridge, Massachusetts 02139, USA*

antje.baeumner@chemie.uni-regensburg.de

This chapter reviews the use of liposomes in microfluidic systems. It highlights improved performance of analytical systems, describes the formation of liposomes using microfluidic channel devices, and concludes with the characterization of liposomes with the help of miniaturized systems and their use in separation processes.

The development of miniaturized sensors with liposomes as signal amplification means requires the study of aspects ranging from the detection strategy, transduction principle to nonspecific binding. These aspects will be thoroughly described here based on published research.

Regardless of the liposomes' application, an efficient method for liposome production with control over size and polydispersity is critical. Microfluidic technology developed for these purposes will be highlighted. Microfluidic systems also have a great potential as efficient tools for the characterization and study of

Liposomes in Analytical Methodologies
Edited by Katie A. Edwards
Copyright © 2016 Pan Stanford Publishing Pte. Ltd.
ISBN 978-981-4669-26-9 (Hardcover), 978-981-4669-27-6 (eBook)
www.panstanford.com

liposomes. Precise control and manipulation, as well as high-throughput capability, can be realized through microscale systems and will be the topic of the third section of this chapter.

Finally, liposomes are able to assist with separation processes in microfluidic systems, particularly those in which their surface properties play a major role. Alternatively, microstructures in microfluidic systems are capable of separating liposomes from unwanted species by size selection.

In the end, our goal is to demonstrate with this chapter the rich scientific field of research on liposomes in conjunction with microfluidic systems.

5.1   Introduction

A liposome is an artificial spherical vesicle formed by amphiphilic molecules, e.g., phospholipids, which undergo self-assembly establishing colloidal structures in aqueous solution. Hydrophobic chains are organized within the bilayer, while hydrophilic heads are oriented toward the inner cavity and vesicle exterior. Liposomes emerged in the 1960s when Bangham et al., who were interested in cell membranes, observed the spontaneous formation of phospholipids into closed membranes in aqueous negative stain. Bangham et al. initially studied the diffusion of univalent cations and anions across the lipid bilayer of liposomes as a model for cell membranes.[1]

Liposomes exhibit several distinctive properties such as encapsulation capabilities, versatile surface chemistry, adjustable hydrophobic and hydrophilic nature, tunable size, and chemical composition flexibility. Unlike almost all other nanobeads, liposomes possess the ability to release their encapsulants in response to various changes in a controlled environment. Also the semipermeability of the membrane allows for reactions to take place across the membrane without lysis. These make liposomes highly attractive for a wide range of applications, in particular for analytical purposes.

A recent article by Liu and Boyd provides an extensive review of liposomes in the field of biosensors and bioanalyses with a major emphasis on using liposomes to amplify signals as well as progress toward commercialization of liposome-based diagnostics.[2] In addition, more reviews regarding liposomes in analytical applications were written by the authors Gómez-Hens and Fernández-Romero[3] as well as Edwards and Baeumner.[4] The former describes the advantages and the limitations of the most recent applications of liposomes in chromatography, capillary electrophoresis, immunoassays, and sensors, while the latter discusses the use of liposomes as analytical reagents for signal amplification and compares their performance with conventional techniques, especially in terms of sensitivity. Furthermore, Bally and Vörös described liposomes as nanoscale labels in high-performance biosensors.[5]

Microfluidics is the field of science focusing on systems that manipulate small volumes of fluid in the range of 10^{-9} to 10^{-18} L employing channels with dimensions between tens to hundreds of micrometers.[6] Once the technology is implemented with analytical systems, it offers a great number of advantages, including the reduction in reagent and sample consumption, the ability to conduct separation and detection with high resolution and sensitivity, low cost, short analysis time, and promising portable analytical devices. The combination of liposomes and microfluidic systems can provide mutual benefits leading to a wide variety of useful applications. Our research group reviewed recently research describing the enhanced performance of miniaturized bioanalytical systems through liposomes as well as proposed handling strategies that could be implemented in analytical microfluidic devices.[7] Here, we provide an in-depth review with a focus on synergistic advantages from combining liposomes and microfluidic systems not only limited to analytical applications. The advantages of liposomes have been extensively exploited in microfluidic systems, for instance, as a signal amplification reagent in analytical systems, as a tool for analyte separation by an electric field, as a tool for studying the flow profile in a microchannel, or for enhanced mixing in microchannels. On the other hand, microfluidic systems also permit several interesting benefits for liposomes in different aspects, e.g., liposome synthesis, characterizations and studies of liposomes, and separation of liposome from undesired species. In this chapter, we discuss liposome-based microfluidic systems according to the areas in which liposomes and microfluidic systems are combined, as illustrated in Fig. 5.1. We focus on current research and indicate areas of growth and opportunity.

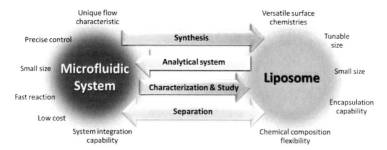

Figure 5.1   Schematic overview of synergistic characteristics expected from the combination of liposomes and microfluidic systems.

5.2   Liposomes in Analytical Microfluidic Systems

5.2.1   Enhanced Analytical Performance

Liposome-based microfluidic analytical systems benefit from all the positive aspects of miniaturization. Namely, lower reagent consumption, lower limits of detection, and rapid binding between analyte and biorecognition element due to the alleviation of diffusion limitations. In addition, microfluidic designs enable direct and indirect assay formats, integration of multiple process steps, as well as internal calibration through their ability to perform highly parallelized multichannel structures leading to enhanced assay reliability.

A major driving force in the development of new analytical methods is the detection of analytes at very low concentration levels. Due to, in general, small sample volumes applied to analytical microfluidic systems, the development of sensitive detection schemes is especially important as the sheer number of analyte molecules is limited. Consequently, the amplification of an obtainable signal is of great interest, which can be achieved through biological, chemical, and physical strategies. At the chemical level, increases in signal-to-noise levels can take advantage of signal amplification strategies and, therefore, it is not surprising that highly sensitive immunoassays and nucleic acid biosensors have been described using the liposome amplification strategy. In comparison to single-label tags, nanoparticles, and bead-based systems, their lysis-triggered signal response and biological membrane surface make them valuable analytical tools in microfluidic systems. In return, microfluidic systems can minimize diffusion limitations observed with liposomes in bulk phase assays determined by their low diffusion coefficients.[8] In fact, this is similar to the advantage described for lateral-flow assays (LFAs) provided through their capillary-driven flow through pores, avoiding diffusion limitations (Chapter 2).[9,10]

Early microfluidic assays with liposome-based amplification simply translated the LFA concept found to be so successful previously into a microfluidic environment.[11] Through consecutive improvements of assay formats, detection strategies, and assay elements, limits of detection were significantly improved from 5 fmol to 50 amol detection, which is 100 times better than those obtained through an LFA approach.[9] Figure 5.2 shows the general layout of these microfluidic systems. First, test systems used directly immobilized probes on gold surfaces (Fig. 5.2a),[11] whereas more advanced systems took advantage of superparamagnetic beads enabling quasi-homogenous assay conditions, enhanced mixing and washing capabilities as well as providing larger surface areas for binding reactions to occur (Fig. 5.2b).[12]

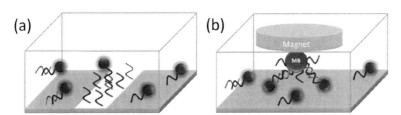

Figure 5.2   Liposome-based microfluidic analytical systems: (a) immobilized capture probe and (b) superparamagnetic bead (MB)-based assay.

Continued development of this microfluidic biosensor module with fluorescent-dye-encapsulating liposomes focused on improvements to the fluidic network, optimization of flow rates, and implementation of detergent lysis of liposomes to release the self-quenched dye from the core, improving the signal-to-noise ratio.[13] This optimized system was then applied to the detection of four serotypes-specific sequences of dengue virus RNA.[14] A detection limit as low as 50 amol could be achieved from the lysed liposome detection system with the entire analysis taking only

20 min. The developments here accomplished the translation of complicated bench-top assays into a portable device. Also, through different detection approaches, namely, fluorescence and electrochemical detection, flexible formats were developed that are further described below.

Combining the laminar flow regime and small volumes of microfluidics with the phospholipid bilayer of liposomes can enable analytical systems that mimic conditions as they may appear within the human body. Recently, liposomes encapsulating europium were immobilized onto the glass bottom of a microfluidic channel to determine the permeation rate of tetracycline.[15] As the drug crossed the membrane of the liposomes, it would bind the europium generating a fluorescent signal measurable by total internal reflection fluorescence microscopy. The impacts of varying concentrations and flow rates on the permeation kinetics could be studied with this system. Here, the implementation of these technologies in tandem eliminated experimental uncertainties associated with standard methods that commonly utilize animal cells as a studied model.

5.2.2   Signal Generation

5.2.2.1   Intact versus lysed liposomes

Upon hybridization to targets, liposome reporter probes can be monitored from either intact or lysed liposomes. Intact liposome measurement enables a simpler design of microfluidic systems as no additional reagents need to be introduced, eliminating the potential need for additional channels and switching of flow rates.[13] Self-quenching of organic fluorescent dyes inside liposomes could be overcome by simply decreasing the concentration, thus allowing a higher signal for intact liposomes. In addition, there are a variety of detection techniques that utilize the intrinsic properties of liposomes, e.g., surface charge or size, to indicate the presence of analytes, surface plasmon resonance,[16] quartz crystal microbalance,[17,18] and micro-cantilever biosensors[19] have been described.

Prior detection of liposome lysis is highly desirable in some systems, as it leverages the capacity of the aqueous core to provide greater assay sensitivity in microfluidic systems (as also exploited in LFA and microtiter plate liposome-based assays).

A number of liposome lysis techniques can be implemented into microfluidic systems. Thermally induced liposome rupture is an efficient lysis technique that can avoid interference resulting from other additional reagents.[20] This is especially attractive, as the integration of a heating system in microfluidic chip is feasible and has been successfully demonstrated.[21] However, this strategy really makes sense only if heating elements are otherwise also needed for chip operation, such as for controlled binding reactions, sample preparation, or alike. In contrast, (bio)chemically triggered liposome lysis can be realized through enzymes such as phospholipase[22] or trypsin,[23] natural cell lysis agents such as mellitin,[24] and surfactants.[25] Surfactant-mediated liposome lysis is most widely employed since it requires inexpensive and simple reagents and, most importantly, is a time-independent approach, thus allowing instantaneous signal generation. However, in some assays, surfactants may be detrimental to the reaction or binding event being detected.[7]

A nonionic surfactant, n-octyl-β-D-glucopyranoside (OG), has been commonly used in our lab. At concentrations lower than the critical micellar concentration (CMC), the detergent molecules intercalate into the lipid bilayer causing its perturbation and allowing leakage of the molecules entrapped in the liposomes. At or above the CMC, a complete restructuring of the phospholipid bilayer into micelles occurs leading to a rapid release of the encapsulated markers.[13] Zaytseva et al. found a significant increase in fluorescence upon lysis of sulforhodamine B (SRB)-containing liposomes with 30 mM OG since the release diluted the previously self-quenched dye; here, lysed liposomes yielded a single signal approximately six times higher than intact liposomes, as shown in Fig. 5.3,[13] and when integrated over time and fluid flow to thousands of times higher signal levels. Thus, the improvement could have been much greater if the fluorescence measurement integrated the signal intensity over time instead of using a single image analysis; as the system is operated under continuous flow, some of the freed dye will trail the peak intensity resulting from the initial burst. Though this type of measurement can be easily carried out with bench-top equipment using fluorescence, an electrochemical detection strategy can make the integration of the result simple, for example, by detecting Coulombs. In fact, electrochemical signals will also substantially increase upon release of electroactive species from liposomes. Goral et al. found that intact liposomes gave background signals of 92 nA and liposomes lysed using a final concentration of 50 mM OG had signals more than 100 times higher, i.e., 9,470 nA.[26] These examples demonstrate that the integration of signals generated in the flow system, much like with any chromatography technique, provides interesting variables to tune the sensitivity of an assay. High flow rates result in lower signal generation.[27,28] Particularly for amperometric transducers, a combination of surfactant contact time resulting in liposome lysis, diffusion of the redox couple away from the electrode, and length of the time spent over the electrode area are the main factors of the flow rate dependency.

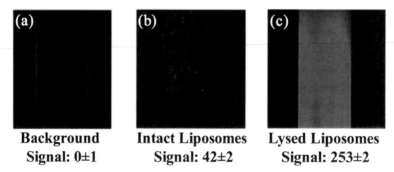

Background	**Intact Liposomes**	**Lysed Liposomes**
Signal: 0±1	**Signal: 42±2**	**Signal: 253±2**

Figure 5.3   Fluorescence images of the capture zone with immobilized superparamagnetic beads: (a) no RNA present in a sample (background), (b) intact liposomes bound in specific complexes with the target RNA, (c) fluorescence de-quenching of liposomes upon addition of the surfactant. All analyses were done in triplicate and representative images are shown here.[13] Reproduced in part from Ref. [13] with permission of The Royal Society of Chemistry. http://dx.doi.org/10.1039/B503856A.

5.2.2.2   Detection strategies

As described earlier, fluorescence-based and electrochemical detection techniques have been successfully implemented to liposome-based microfluidic analytical systems. The detection limits for both signal transductions in microfluidic chips were comparable as shown in our earlier study.[27] Moreover, the required total assay times for both detection strategies were found to be roughly the same.

Fluorescence detection relies, simply put, on a molecular light absorption that triggers the emission of fluorescence signal with longer wavelengths. The technique is commonly employed in analytical microfluidic systems due to its superior sensitivity and selectivity. In addition, similar to other optical techniques, fluorescence detection simplifies multiplexed analysis system in which several analytes can be monitored simultaneously.[29,30]

However, the readout of the fluorescent signal often requires a complicated hardware setup through optical fibers, excitation sources, and camera systems. Advances in the general field of fluorescence detection and bioimaging provide here important assistance to overcome these disadvantages.[31,32]

Electrochemical detection is an alternative means that ideally suit incorporation into analytical microfluidic devices owing to the simplicity of system miniaturization. Moreover, high sensitivity, rapid generation of stable signals, low power consumption, and cost effectiveness are additional advantages. The technique relies mainly on the measurement of electrical property changes at an electrode surface upon analyte introduction. Coulometric detection, the method of integrating current over time, is commonly employed with liposome-based analytical microfluidic devices as it simplifies the integration means of output signals. As the entrapped electrochemical markers are shielded from contact with the electrode, signals occur only after liposome lysis. It is also attractive that existing background signals can be recorded prior to liposome lysis and be subtracted from post-lysis signals leading to very high signal-to-noise ratios.

Our research group has investigated some parameters relevant to the improvement of electrochemical detection systems for liposome-based microfluidic chips. In addition to liposome optimization and the optimization of buffer and flow conditions, we focused on electrode and microfluidic channel design. For example, advanced electrode structures were used to enable a simple two-electrode setup and a highly sensitive marker detection. Here, signal amplification of redox couples, e.g., potassium ferri/ ferro hexacyanide, can be realized through the utilization of interdigitated ultramicroelectrode (IDUA). A small gap size between adjacent IDUA fingers enables the increase in the diffusion flux of redox species, which consequently leads to an enhanced redox cycling, a decreased equilibrium time, and an increased collection efficiency.[26] Apart from this two-electrode configuration, we also developed a three-electrode system with a stable reference electrode in the microfluidic device to support the measurement of liposomes that encapsulate other redox species.[33]

Since the liposomes contain a set concentration of the redox couple, lysing the same number of liposomes in a smaller volume will produce a higher overall concentration of the electroactive species, as depicted in Fig. 5.4.

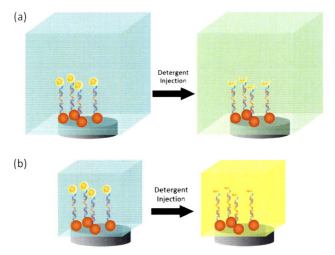

Figure 5.4   When a set number of liposomes containing an electroactive species are lysed into a confined volume, the overall concentration of the electroactive species is dependent on that volume, i.e., when that volume is relatively large (a), the concentration of the species will be relatively dilute, and when the volume is reduced (b), the concentration will be increased. As the current generated at the IDUA just downstream is dependent on the concentration of the electoactive species (and the sandwich hybridization complexes they indicate), channel volume reduction can generate signal enhancements.[34] Pictured as described in reference [34].

Using a nucleic acid sandwich hybridization assay as a model, the detection limit decreased from 0.1 fmol to 0.01 fmol per assay by simply decreasing the channel height from 50 μm to 20 μm. Further reductions in the channel dimensions should further enhance the sensitivity of the assay. However, to maintain similar linear flow rates in the smaller channel dimensions, the volumetric flow rates needed to be lowered. This, in turn, resulted in superparamagnetic beads settling and clogging the device. At higher volumetric flow rates, capture of beads on magnets became insufficient. Thus, a careful balance between optimal volume and optimal flow rate needed to be found. Nonetheless, this strategy is promising and unique to electrochemical detection, as in a fluorescence-based system, the resulting high concentration of dye would likely self-quench.[34]

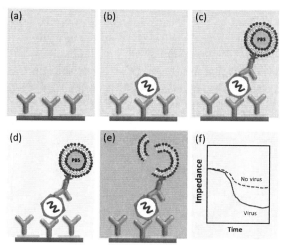

Figure 5.5   Schematic illustration of virus sensing with liposomes and ion-release impedance spectroscopy. (a) Antibodies are immobilized on the surface of the microfluidic device; (b) virus is captured by immobilized antibody; (c) liposomes, functionalized with protein A (PrA) and anti-HIV IgG, bind specifically to immobilized virus; (d) background medium is replaced by deionized water to decrease the conductivity of the solution; (e) device is heated to release encapsulated ions (10x PBS); and (f) presence of virus results in the increase in solution conductivity, which consequently reduces the impedance, and vice versa (pictured as described in Ref. [28]).

The extension of this microfluidic system using a single IDUA to multi-analyte detection is feasible. Using multiple parallel detection channels flowing over the IDUA, one can lyse the liposomes in a time-dependent manner by altering the length of each channel's associated surfactant introduction channel. Thus, the currents resulting from liposome lysis can be discriminated.[28]

Apart from coulometric-based detection, impedance detection was also employed in liposome-based microfluidic biosensor. Impedance measurements are typically conducted by applying a constant small alternating current to an electrochemical cell and measuring the change in the circuits' resistance resulting from the assay. This method is sensitive and particularly appropriate for detecting changes on the electrode surface upon biomolecule interactions.[35] Recently, Damhorst et al. proposed an enzyme-linked immunosorbent assay (ELISA)-inspired lab-on-a-chip device using liposome tags and ion-release impedance spectroscopy to detect human immunodeficiency virus (HIV) as shown in Fig. 5.5a–f.[36] The release of liposome-encapsulating phosphate-buffer saline (PBS) increased the conductivity of the solution exposed to the electrodes, thus resulting in the reduction of impedance (Fig. 5.5e,f).

5.2.3 Nonspecific Binding of Liposomes ...

5.2.3.1 ... to microfluidic devices

As in any bioanalytical assay nonspecific interactions between the various assay components must be overcome to achieve optimal sensitivity and specificity, the use of liposomes in microfluidic devices is no exception. The adsorption of liposomes either to native or modified microchannel surfaces can result in significant background noise, especially when used as a signal amplification reagent. The problem can be overcome by modifying microfluidic channel surfaces to repel the liposomes. For example, Durst et al. reported that negatively charged liposomes adhered to gold surfaces where DNA capture probes were immobilized, producing a signal from negative controls indistinguishable from positive samples.[11] In order to passivate the gold layer, the authors created a blocking layer using mercaptohexane and untagged, buffer-filled liposomes, termed blocking liposomes. The authors suggested that the capture probes and mercaptohexane generated a mixed monolayer, which could repel the negatively charged liposomes, reducing nonspecific adsorption, and the blocking liposomes saturated any potentially remaining nonspecific binding sites.

Nonspecific adsorption of liposomes that generated high background signals was also a major problem in a microfluidic competitive assay in microchannel modified with charged proteins investigated by Locascio et al.[8] The platform relied on competitive binding between free biotin and biotin-bound liposomes to the microchannel modified with biotin. In this study, positively charged avidin molecules at neutral pH generated a high background fluorescence signal as they electrostatically attracted negatively charged biotinylated liposomes. Streptavidin is a non-glycosylated derivative of avidin that is relatively uncharged at neutral pH, which makes it a proper choice to reduce the liposome nonspecific adsorption in the modified microchannels. As expected, the signal associated with nonspecific liposome binding was reduced significantly in the streptavidin-coated channels. With streptavidin, the resulting nonspecific signal was less than 2% of the specific signal.

Surface treatments of microchannels for device fabrication might enable the repulsion between liposomes and microchannel surfaces. For example, UV treatment causes polymer chain scission at the very surface of poly(methyl methacrylate) (PMMA) substrates. This is routinely exploited to lower the glass transition temperature of the PMMA facilitating low temperature bonding. Concurrently, this treatment produces negatively charged carboxylic acid residues on the surface that assisted in repelling the liposomes.[37]

5.2.3.2   … to superparamagnetic beads

When using superparamagnetic beads, nonspecific adsorption of liposomes can be an added concern due to the significant surface area additionally available. Our group evaluated suitable blocking solutions and beads.[12] It was found that blocking solutions containing bovine serum albumin (BSA) generated high background fluorescence, which increased with increasing BSA concentration. Casein was investigated as an alternative blocking reagent, and although it did reduce nonspecific binding between liposome and magnetic beads, it also introduced considerable variability in resulting detection signals. It was found that by simply selecting a negatively charged superparamagnetic bead, e.g., M270 streptavidin Dynabeads® (ThermoFisher), no blocking reagent was required as the electrostatic charge was sufficient to eliminate nonspecific binding.

5.3 Synthesis of Liposomes in Microfluidic Systems

In most applications for which liposomes may be useful, production methods yielding uniform particle sizes are important. In analytical applications where liposomes serve as marker carriers, small diameters and monodisperse populations are desirable, as variability in size can cause variability in signal generation and, therefore, poor assay reproducibility. Particularly, the monodispersity of the labeling agent in miniaturized analytical systems becomes more relevant as fewer labels contribute to an averaged system. When used in drug-delivery systems, liposome size plays a significant role in drug dosage and rate of clearance from the body. The size of the liposome does not just impact the volume of material encapsulated or the amount bound to its membrane, it also affects stability, rate of surfactant disruption, and membrane curvature, which influences reporter probe conjugation capacity. Therefore, efficient methods for liposome production with control over size have been developed using microfluidic technology.

Traditionally, liposomes are formed in bulk-scale systems by several different techniques, including lipid film hydration,[38] reverse phase evaporation,[13] detergent dialysis,[39] and alcohol injection.[40] Additional post-formation processing steps, such as sonication or extrusion through a porous track-etch membrane, are often used to obtain smaller and uniform size distributions. These bulk production methods can suffer from localized chemical fluctuations or mechanical perturbations, resulting in large polydispersity with respect to size and lamellarity. These issues can further result in significant batch-to-batch variation and inefficient use of materials and reagents.

Microfluidic systems for highly reproducible and controllable liposome synthesis have been demonstrated to have efficient and controllable mixing under continuous flow conditions, providing the necessary homogenous reaction environment for formation. Moreover, these systems allow temporal control of reactions by the addition of reagents at precise time intervals during the process. Liposome characteristics, such as size, can be precisely controlled through the kinetics of the process. Furthermore, synthesis of liposomes in microfluidic systems offers an excellent opportunity to integrate post-synthesis processes, like biorecognition molecule conjugation, and measurement systems on a single technology platform.

In this part of the chapter, we will demonstrate the advancements of microfluidic systems in liposome synthesis. The strategies described here allow the formation of small to large unilamellar vesicles as they are widely used in analytical and drug-delivery applications.

5.3.1 Electroformation

First proposed by Angelova and Dimitrov in 1986, electroformation is widely employed for unilamellar liposome production.[41] The method consists of three major steps: creation of a dry lipid film on a planar electrode surface, immersion of the coated electrode in an aqueous solution, and the application of an electric field across the lipid and surrounding buffer. The applied electric field causes a lipid layer to peel off from the electrode surface and undergo self-assembly, forming giant vesicles in the buffer solution. It is believed that the electric field generates fluctuations in the lipid bilayers, which are responsible for the film detachment.

Kuribayashi et al. successfully implemented the electroformation technique in a microfluidic chip.[42] Here, channels fabricated between two glass layers patterned with indium tin oxide electrodes were used to produce liposomes encapsulating fluorescent polystyrene beads. When comparing to a gentle hydration-based method, the microfluidic device increased the number of giant liposomes and reduced the number of multilamellar vesicles. However, the technique did result in a polydisperse liposome population and requires further development to improve overall control.

LeBerre et al. were able to control vesicle size and size distribution by fragmenting the lipid film through pattering of the electrode surface with raised microstructures, as shown in Fig. 5.6.[43] The fragmentation of the lipid film allowed the formation of monodisperse vesicles, and it was found that the dimensions of the microstructures directly related to the size of the vesicles formed, thus allowing tunable production.

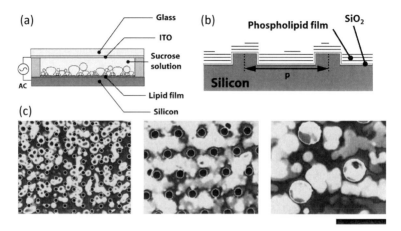

Figure 5.6   Liposome production by electroformation: (a) experimental setup for the electroformation on silicon, (b) phospholipid film on elevated microstructured, (c) reflection microscopy images in false colors of the film organization on microstructured Si with a pitch size of 7, 15, and 60 μm, respectively.[43] Reprinted with permission from Ref. [43], Copyright 2008, American Chemical Society, http://pubs.acs.org/doi/abs/10.1021/la703391q.

5.3.2   Hydration

Hydration techniques begin with a dried lipid film, similar to that used in electroformation; however, no electrical field is applied. Instead, a controlled flow of aqueous buffer solution is passed over the film, and the shear stress it produces causes the lipid layers to peel off, break, and self-assemble into liposomes. In bulk setups, this method notoriously produces polydisperse and multilamellar liposome populations.[44] Microfluidics, however, provides the ability to accurately control the buffer flow rate, allowing optimal conditions for obtaining different types of structures—a notable advantage in comparison to the macroscale hydration method. Lin et al. have described the use of hydration in a microfluidic device to form microtubes and connected vesicles under specific conditions.[45] Here, the dry lipid film was formed on a glass slide and later covered with a polydimethylsiloxane (PDMS) microchannel. Continuous flow of an aqueous buffer solution over the lipid film allows the formation of the microtubes and vesicles.

5.3.3 Extrusion

Unilamellar liposomes of a desired size can be achieved through extrusion. Essentially, a vesicle dispersion is forced through a membrane with pores of a specified size, causing lipid membranes to rupture and reseal. Often, multiple passes through the same membrane or membranes of decreasing pore size are required to achieve the desired product.[11]

Dittrich et al. implemented this technique in a microfluidic device.[46] In this work, the chip consisted of three layers, including a thin PDMS top layer and a thick PDMS bottom layer, sandwiching a silicon slide (Fig. 5.7). On the silicon slide, a 3 μm diameter aperture was created and later coated with a lipid film. Lipid vesicles and tubes with micrometer sizes were formed by applying a solution to either the top or the bottom channels causing

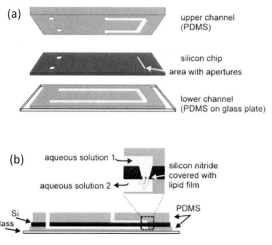

Figure 5.7 Schematic of a microfluidic device for on-chip extrusion of vesicles and microtubules, developed by Dittrich et al. (a) The three layers in the device are a thin PDMS layer, a silicon slide, and a thick PDMS layer. The white squares are the fluid reservoirs, and apertures are fabricated on the silicon substrate in a rectangular area of approximately 3 mm in length. (b) A cross section of the assembled device and one of its 3 μm diameter apertures. Lipids are coated over the aperture, from which vesicles and tubules are extruded.[46] Reproduced from Ref. [46] with permission of The Royal Society of Chemistry, http://dx.doi.org/10.1039/b517670K.

the lipid layer to protrude through the apertures and ultimately shear off. The size of apertures and the pressure difference between the top and bottom channels determined the dimensions of the vesicles and microtubes, with low-pressure differences yielding vesicles and higher differences producing lipid tubes. The authors state that this technique holds great promise for large-scale production as the vesicles could be produced with high speed by increasing the flow rate and the number of apertures. However, some limitations call for further investigation, such as polydispersity and encapsulation efficiency of the resulting liposomes. Additionally, similar to electroformation and hydration methods, lipid film coatings add significantly to the overall synthesis complexity and limit a continuous liposome generation.

5.3.4 Hydrodynamic Flow Focusing

Jahn et al. demonstrated an elegant technique to form sub-micrometer-sized liposome with monodisperse distribution by hydrodynamic flow focusing in a microfluidic chip.[47] In this strategy, lipids dissolved in isopropyl alcohol (IPA) flow through the center channel, while two streams of aqueous solution flow through the two side channels as depicted in Fig. 5.8a. The two aqueous streams hydrodynamically focus the stream of lipid solution at the cross junction of the channels, and as the IPA diffuses into the aqueous streams and dilutes at the interfacial region, the lipids self-assemble into liposomes. Based on this strategy, the size of the liposomes can be tuned by adjusting the relative flow rates of the solutions to control the width between the interfaces. In this regard, when the ratio of the flow rates in the side channels to the center inlet channel increases, the magnitude of the shear stress applied to the liposomes during self-assembly also increases, leading to a decrease in the average size and size distribution.

It was reported that sizes over the range of 100–300 nm could be achieved by tuning the flow rates of side channels in the range 2.4–59.8 mm/s, while that of the center channel was maintained at 2.4 mm/s. Furthermore, the authors demonstrated the ability of the technique to encapsulate fluorescent dye by adding it to the aqueous streams—here 1 mM carboxyfluorescein was used. The authors state that liposomes were able to encapsulate a high concentration of the dye as determined by confocal fluorescence microscopy, but no encapsulation efficiency and yield was provided.

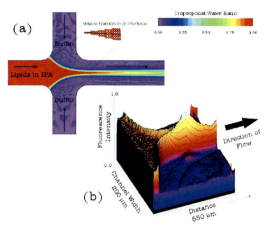

Figure 5.8   (a) Schematic of liposome formation process in the microfluidic channel. Color contours represent the concentration ratios of IPA to aqueous buffer. (b) Three-dimensional color contour map of DilC18 fluorescence intensity at focused region during liposome formation.[47] Copyright not subject to U.S. Copyright. Published 2004 American Chemical Society. http://pubs.acs.org/doi/abs/10.1021/ja0318030.

Since demonstrating the ability to control size over in the sub-micrometer range by simply manipulating the fluid flow rates, research in microfluidic hydrodynamic flow focusing for liposome synthesis has grown significantly.[48–57] For example, Zook et al. investigated the influence of temperature, hydrophobic chain length, and flow rate ratios on liposome size distribution.[49] The strategy was also employed to generate monodipserse liposome–hydrogel hybrid nanoparticles in which hydrogel precursors were mixed in aqueous buffer streams.[50] Jahn et al. suggested that microfluidic channel geometry in hydrodynamic flow focusing strongly affects vesicle size distributions and it can be used as a coarse control of liposome size followed by the total flow rate, which allows fine tuning.[51] Recently, Jin et al. successfully utilized hydrodynamic flow focusing to form liposomes entrapping SRB and conjugated to antibodies, as depicted in Fig. 5.9. A loading capacity of 10^5 dye molecules per liposome was reported, which is in the same order of magnitude obtained by conventional preparation techniques.[58]

(a)

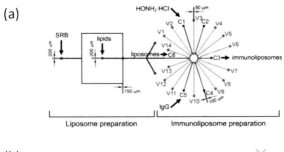

(b)

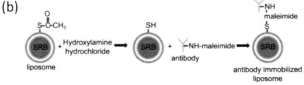

Figure 5.9   Immunoliposomes preparation using a microvalve-controlled microfluidic device. (a) Design of the microfluidic device, and (b) a schematic for antibody conjugation to liposomes.[54] Reproduced from Ref. [54] with permission from the Korean Chemical Society, Copyright 2013, http://dx.doi.org/10.5012/bkcs.2013.34.10.2921.

The authors have successfully demonstrated that the automation of liposome preparation and conjugation to reporter probes is feasible in this device as the loading and mixing steps simply require actuation of microvalves,[59] and scale-up can be realized through continuous operation over a long period.

Liposome synthesis-based microfluidic approaches, particularly by hydrodynamic flow focusing, can be very helpful for those applications in which the system requires a continuous supply of liposome, e.g., the study of cellular uptake mechanisms.[60] Synthesis of liposomes through hydration and extrusion realized in microfluidic systems might not be useful for analytical applications as microtubes are formed alongside the desired vesicles. Even though microfluidic chips offer a highly controllable manner for liposome production, the methods have still been inappropriate for large-scale production, which may be realized by massively parallelization, which in turn is easily realized with standard microfluidic designs.

5.4 Characterization and Study of Liposomes in Microfluidic Systems

Microfluidic systems also have a significant potential as highly efficient tools for the characterization and study of liposomes. Precise control and manipulation, as well as high-throughput capability, can be realized through microscale systems as will be discussed in this section.

Liposome characteristics that are of specific analytical interest include size and size distribution, lamellarity and lamellarity distribution, entrapment efficiency, formulation, and shelf-life stability. These are important factors in the successful translation of liposomes into analytical and other applications. The assessment of liposome quality leads to the comparison of liposome reproducibility in batch-to-batch preparations. Birnbaumer et al. successfully developed a microfluidic biochip capable of characterizing and identifying batch-to-batch variations of liposome formulations based on continuous monitoring of the dielectric properties of the lipid vesicles. The microfluidic chip consisted of contactless dielectric microsensors, which allowed the assessments of loading efficiency, variations in liposome formulations, and liposome stability.[61] In this work, the authors demonstrated the ability of the microfluidic chip to identify nine liposome formulations prepared by different methods. The combination of dielectric spectroscopy with microfluidics offers reproducible and well-defined measurement conditions because the contactless microsensors perceive the moving liposome suspension as bulk material. The presence of lipid vesicles contributes to the capacitive signal resulting in an impedance decrease, which mainly relates to intrinsic characteristics of liposomes, e.g., concentration, composition, and structure. Based on the demonstrated capabilities, this microfluidic analysis platform could be used as a high-throughput tool for quality assurance in liposome production.

Recently, Hoppe et al. demonstrated the use of microfluidic systems combined with transmission electron microscopy (TEM) to image liposome structures in aqueous solution.[62] The technique overcomes the limitation of the conventional method because contrast enhancement staining or cryogenic treatment are not required, allowing the study of native liposome structure. As shown in Fig. 5.10, liposome solution flowed between silicon nitride (SiN) windows separated by 150 nm spacers. Once liposomes stuck to one or both of the silicon nitride windows, the structures of liposome could be imaged by TEM.

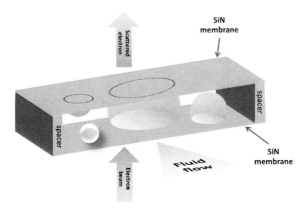

Figure 5.10 Schematic representation of a microfluidic cell during a liposome imaging by TEM. Transparent spheres with dash line exhibit the resultant liposome shapes that will present in TEM images (drawn as described in Ref. [62]).

Apart from being a tool for liposome characterization, microfluidic systems have been used to manipulate liposomes for further study. Liposomes are widely served as model biological membranes in which the mechanisms of fusion are of interest in various biotechnological applications, such as drug delivery. Microfluidic systems were utilized for investigating liposome fusion, particularly by employing electrofusion, as depicted in Fig. 5.11.[63–65] The technique relies mainly on applying AC voltage between two electrodes allowing liposome alignment. A subsequently applied DC pulse causes the breakdown of the membranes resulting in liposome fusion.

The microfluidic chip enabled accurate control of liposomes, realizing precise alignment, and a high-efficiency fusion process. Moreover, the short distance between the electrodes significantly reduces the required applied voltage, from thousands of volts to less than one hundred volts. The microdevice developed by Tresset and Takeuchi had a high aspect ratio channel, which is unfavorable for the observation of the liposome fusion process as low-density liposomes might float and form multiple layers hampering alignment and fusion.[65] Jiang et al., therefore, determined a suitable aspect ratio for liposome alignment and observation.[63] Moreover, they were able to manipulate a large number of liposomes at the same time with the aid of a high-density electrode array. This system allowed the authors to study the effects of cholesterol concentration on the flexibility of liposomes in the fusion process. This provides a great benefit to basic research applications in which liposomes are used as a cell model.

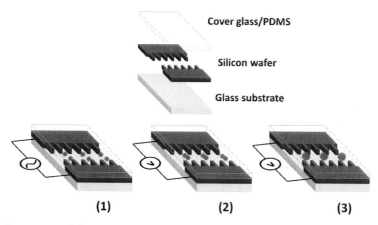

Cover glass/PDMS

Silicon wafer

Glass substrate

(1)   **(2)**   **(3)**

Figure 5.11 Schematic view exhibits the component of microfluidic device (top) and the process of electrofusion of liposomes inside the device (bottom). (1) An applied AC voltage for a few seconds results in liposome alignment, (2) DC pulses enable membrane disruption, and (3) adjacent vesicles are fused (drawn as described in Ref. [63]).

Trapping of liposomes for experimental studies has remained a challenge due to their small size and flexibility. Moreover, to perform statistical or combinatorial studies, processing vesicles simultaneously is required. Recently, Nuss et al. described a microfluidic device based on hydrodynamic trapping that allowed the study of many giant vesicles at the same time. This microfluidic platform provided a means to trap and manipulate liposomes with diameters in the range of 2–40 µm and could also efficiently narrow the size distribution of the vesicle population.[66] Figure 5.12a–c illustrates the working principle of the developed strategy.

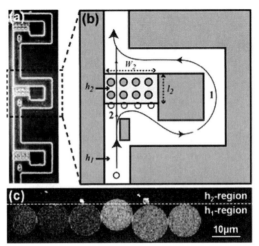

Figure 5.12 (a) Phase contrast microscopy picture of three traps in a row. (b) Schematic diagram of the microfluidic trap. The white channel (bypass) has a height h_1 = 40 μm and a typical width w_1 = 60 μm. The trap region (light grey area) has a height h_2 = 2 μm, a width w_2 = 130 μm, and a length l_2 = 70 μm. The detour length (path labeled as 1) has one of the following three values: l_1 = 800, 1300, or 2000 μm. The dark grey areas correspond to PDMS material, which forms the lateral walls of the microfluidic channel. The eight grey circles in the 2 μm high region correspond to supporting pillars. The rectangular PDMS block located in front of the trap forces the vesicles to reach the trap. (c) Micrograph, taken by laser scanning confocal microscopy (LSCM), of the trapped vesicles that contain the fluorophore Alexa Fluor1 488-dextran, 10,000 MW.[66] Reproduced from Ref. [66] with permission of The Royal Society of Chemistry. http://dx.doi.org/10.1039/C2LC40782E.

Here, liposomes were delivered through a channel with a height, h_1, of 40 μm. As the flow passed the trapping region (labeled as 2), some vesicles become trapped as the height, h_2, drops to 2 μm and the region contains eight micropillars. The decreased channel height of the trapping region increases the flow resistance leading to highly deformable objects such as vesicles to be trapped. By adjusting the flow rate, one can choose the size of trapped vesicles (Fig. 5.13a–d). Moreover, one can also change the size selection properties of the device by varying the trap height, h_2 (Fig. 5.13e).

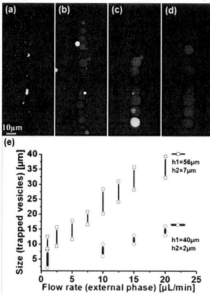

Figure 5.13 LSCM pictures (at $z = 2$ μm) of trapped vesicles ($h_2 = 2$ μm, $h_1 = 40$ μm, and $l_1 = 2000$ μm). By changing the flow rate, Q, of the external phase, one can choose the size interval of the trapped vesicles. (a) $Q = 1$ μL min^{-1}, $S = 2$–8 μm. (b) $Q = 10$ μL min^{-1}, $S = 6$–10 μm. (c) $Q = 15$ μL min^{-1}, $S = 10$–13 μm. (d) $Q = 20$ μL min^{-1}, $S = 13$–16 μm. The fact that some vesicles on the micrographs (a) to (c) appear darker or brighter than the vesicles on average originates from inhomogeneous encapsulation of the fluorophore during the electroformation process. On the left-hand side of each picture from (a) to (d), one can see a row of three black spots, which corresponds to the first row of PDMS pillars in the 2 μm region (the fourth pillar is missing). In (a) the pillars are surrounded by white circles to highlight their positions. (e) Graph of the trapped vesicle size S [μm] as a function of the external flow rate Q [μL min^{-1}] for two devices of different h_2 and h_1 values.[66] Reproduced from Ref. [66] with permission of The Royal Society of Chemistry. http://dx.doi.org/10.1039/C2LC40782E.

In their experiments, Nuss et al. found that the use of moderate flow rates enabled a substantial narrowing of the size distribution. Last, by inverting the flow in the device, the trapped vesicles could be released. The proposed platform is very well suited to the current research activity in the field of giant vesicles, e.g., physicochemical characterization of biological membranes (permeability, fusion, fission, pore opening), study of reconstituted membrane proteins, synthesis of artificial cells, or development of biosensors as well as design of biomimetic microreactors.

5.5 Liposomes in Microfluidic Separation Systems

Liposomes are able to assist separation processes in microfluidic systems, particularly those in which liposome surface properties play a major role. Alternatively, microstructures in microfluidic systems are capable of separating liposomes from unwanted species by size selection.

Utilizing surface properties of liposomes to aid liposome separation and removal in microfluidic channel has been recently demonstrated by our group.[67] Here, Matlock-Colangelo et al. successfully filtered negatively charged liposomes using positively charged nanofibers embedded in microfluidic channels. Moreover, we could selectively release the bound liposomes by increasing the pH of a 4-(2-hydroxyethyl)piperazine-1-ethanesulfonic acid (HEPES)-sucrose-saline (HSS) solution from pH 7 to pH 9. The pH change switched the zeta potential of the nanofibers from positive to negative, repelling the bound liposomes, releasing them from the nanofibers. In addition to electrostatic interaction, Kuhn et al. demonstrated a facile protocol to efficiently trap liposomes in microfluidic systems.[68] Here, biotinylated bovine serum albumin (bBSA) was initially adsorbed on the glass surface. Avidin was subsequently introduced and bound to the adhered bBSA. A cholesterol–polyethyleneglycol (PEG)–biotin linker was then bound to the immobilized avidin. Upon introduction to the microchannel and exposure to the modified surface, liposomes became trapped as the cholesterol tag of the linker inserted into the hydrophobic portion of the lipid bilayer membrane. The interaction is sufficient to withstand high flow rates in the microchannel, leaving the strategy very well suited for long-term studies of liposomes in which the fluid must be repeatedly changed.

In addition to using liposomes as a signal amplification reagent, our group also exploited their surface charge for a pre-concentration step in a microfluidic device for feline calicivirus

(FCV) detection.[69] In this work, an electric field was applied to drive a complex mixture of negatively charged liposome-tagged antibodies and bound and free analytes toward a nanoporous membrane creating a concentrated bolus. Switching the applied potential drove the bolus from the membrane sending it to a capture region of antibody-tagged magnetic beads enabling sandwich immunoassay-based detection. Upon releasing the encapsulated content with detergent, the strategy enabled an order of magnitude lower detection limit when compared to the measurement without the pre-concentration step.

Finally, the separation of liposomes from smaller molecules can be accomplished using microstructures in microfluidic systems. Recently, Wang et al. demonstrated a microfluidic device that consisted of ciliated micropillars to filter liposomes from smaller proteins and cellular debris.[70] The cilia on the micropillar sidewalls were porous silicon nanowires made by metal-assisted electroless nanowire etching. In addition, the trapped liposomes could be easily recovered by dissolving the porous silicon nanowires in PBS overnight. The technique provided high purity recovery of intact liposomes.

5.6 Conclusion and Future Perspective

In this chapter, we have described the major trends in the combination of microfluidics and liposomes as they relate to liposome use and synthesis. So what is next? Some questions, unknowns, challenges remain and provide future researchers with interesting scientific studies and valuable applications.

It can, for example, be concluded that liposomes have shown remarkable advantages when employed in microfluidic systems and vice versa. Signal enhancements in microfluidic analytical systems have been substantially realized through liposome labels. Further attempts should be focused on the integration of sample preparation modules enabling sample-to-answer devices, creating a powerful tool for point-of-care diagnostics.

We have also described many sensing strategies that have been shown to benefit from the use of liposomes. However, some have not been fully realized in microfluidic analytical systems, such as surface plasmon resonance and electrochemiluminescence. Furthermore, considering the vast application of liposomes in

LFAs, their use in paper-based microfluidic systems will surely follow.

A number of investigations have proven that microfluidic channels allow liposome synthesis in a highly controllable manner with the ability to adjust size and narrow the size distribution. However, scaling up of liposome production has remained a major challenge, which needs to be addressed so that these systems can move out of the research lab and find practical applications. Parallel multichannel designs might be a straightforward solution to overcoming the problem.

To date, there have not been many reports using the potential of microfluidic systems as a tool to characterize or study liposomes. Likewise, the use of liposomes as a tool for separations in microfluidic chips is also uncommon. Nonetheless, liposomes have been used as stationary phases in chromatography or as coating or carrier in capillary electrophoresis (Chapter 10). More studies should be exploiting the interesting phenomena afforded by liposomes for these purposes as conditions can be controlled well in microfluidic systems and enable single-particle studies that cannot be performed in bulk. The same holds true for the immense amplification power of liposomes, their cell-mimicking characteristics, and unique delivery properties.

References

1. Bangham AD, Standish MM, Watkins JC. Diffusion of univalent ions across the lamellae of swollen phospholipids. *J Mol Biol.* 1965; 13(1): 238–252.

2. Liu Q, Boyd BJ. Liposomes in biosensors. *The Analyst.* 2013; 138(2): 391–409.

3. Gómez-Hens A, Manuel Fernández-Romero J. The role of liposomes in analytical processes. *Trends Analyt Chem.* 2005; 24(1): 9–19.

4. Edwards KA, Baeumner AJ. Liposomes in analyses. *Talanta.* 2006; 68(5): 1421–1431.

5. Bally M, Voros J. Nanoscale labels: Nanoparticles and liposomes in the development of high-performance biosensors. *Nanomedicine.* 2009; 4(4): 447–467.

6. Whitesides GM. The origins and the future of microfluidics. *Nature.* 2006; 442(7101): 368–373.

7. Edwards KA, Bolduc OR, Baeumner AJ. Miniaturized bioanalytical systems: Enhanced performance through liposomes. *Curr Opin Chem Biol.* 2012; 16(3–4): 444–452.

8. Locascio LE, Hong JS, Gaitan M. Liposomes as signal amplification reagents for bioassays in microfluidic channels. *Electrophoresis.* 2002; 23(5): 799–804.

9. Baeumner AJ, Schlesinger NA, Slutzki NS, Romano J, Lee EM, Montagna RA. Biosensor for dengue virus detection: Sensitive, rapid, and serotype specific. *Anal Chem.* 2002; 74(6): 1442–1448.

10. Edwards KA, Baeumner AJ. Liposome-enhanced lateral-flow assays for the sandwich-hybridization detection of RNA. In: Rasooly A, Herold KE, eds. *Biosensors and Biodetection: Methods and Protocols.* Vol 2: Humana Press Books and Journals; 2009: 185–215.

11. Esch MB, Locascio LE, Tarlov MJ, Durst RA. Detection of viable *Cryptosporidium parvum* using DNA-modified liposomes in a microfluidic chip. *Anal Chem.* 2001; 73(13): 2952–2958.

12. Kwakye S, Baeumner A. A microfluidic biosensor based on nucleic acid sequence recognition. *Anal Bioanal Chem.* 2003; 376(7): 1062–1068.

13. Zaytseva NV, Goral VN, Montagna RA, Baeumner AJ. Development of a microfluidic biosensor module for pathogen detection. *Lab Chip.* 2005; 5(8): 805–811.

14. Zaytseva NV, Montagna RA, Baeumner AJ. Microfluidic biosensor for the serotype-specific detection of dengue virus RNA. *Anal Chem.* 2005; 77(23): 7520–7527.

15. Kuhn P, Eyer K, Allner S, Lombardi D, Dittrich PS. A microfluidic vesicle screening platform: Monitoring the lipid membrane permeability of tetracyclines. *Anal Chem.* 2011; 83(23): 8877–8885.

16. Wink T, van Zuilen SJ, Bult A, van Bennekom WP. Liposome-mediated enhancement of the sensitivity in immunoassays of proteins and peptides in surface plasmon resonance spectrometry. *Anal Chem.* 1998; 70(5): 827–832.

17. Alfonta L, Willner I, Throckmorton DJ, Singh AK. Electrochemical and quartz crystal microbalance detection of the cholera toxin employing horseradish peroxidase and GM1-functionalized liposomes. *Anal Chem.* 2001; 73(21): 5287–5295.

18. Patolsky F, Lichtenstein A, Willner I. Electronic transduction of DNA sensing processes on surfaces: Amplification of DNA detection and analysis of single-base mismatches by tagged liposomes. *J Am Chem Soc.* 2001; 123(22): 5194–5205.

19. Hyun S-J, Kim H-S, Kim Y-J, Jung H-I. Mechanical detection of liposomes using piezoresistive cantilever. *Sens Actuators, B.* 2006; 117(2): 415–419.

20. Genç R, Murphy D, Fragoso A, Ortiz M, O'Sullivan CK. Signal-enhancing thermosensitive liposomes for highly sensitive immunosensor development. *Anal Chem.* 2011; 83(2): 563–570.

21. Vreeland WN, Locascio LE. Using bioinspired thermally triggered liposomes for high-efficiency mixing and reagent delivery in microfluidic devices. *Anal Chem.* 2003; 75(24): 6906–6911.

22. Chong-Kook K, Kyung-Mi P. Liposome immunoassay (LIA) for gentamicin using phospholipase C. *J Immunol Methods.* 1994; 170(2): 225–231.

23. Liu D, Huang L. Trypsin-induced lysis of lipid vesicles: Effect of surface charge and lipid composition. *Anal Biochem.* 1992; 202(1): 1–5.

24. Hincha DK, Crowe JH. The lytic activity of the bee venom peptide melittin is strongly reduced by the presence of negatively charged phospholipids or chloroplast galactolipids in the membranes of phosphatidylcholine large unilamellar vesicles. *Biochim Biophys Acta.* 1996; 1284(2): 162–170.

25. Tanaka K, Takeda T, Nakamura M, Yamamura S, Miyajima K. Interactions of mixed surfactant solution with liposome membrane. *Colloid Polym Sci.* 1989; 267(6): 520–524.

26. Goral VN, Zaytseva NV, Baeumner AJ. Electrochemical microfluidic biosensor for the detection of nucleic acid sequences. *Lab Chip.* 2006; 6(3): 414–421.

27. Bunyakul N, Edwards KA, Promptmas C, Baeumner AJ. Cholera toxin subunit B detection in microfluidic devices. *Anal Bioanal Chem.* 2009; 393(1): 177–186.

28. Wongkaew N, He P, Kurth V, Surareungchai W, Baeumner AJ. Multi-channel PMMA microfluidic biosensor with integrated IDUAs for electrochemical detection. *Anal Bioanal Chem.* 2013; 405(18): 5965–5974.

29. Chaize B, Nguyen M, Ruysschaert T, et al. Microstructured liposome array. *Bioconjug Chem.* 2005; 17(1): 245–247.

30. Jiang X, Shao N, Jing W, Tao S, Liu S, Sui G. Microfluidic chip integrating high throughput continuous-flow PCR and DNA hybridization for bacteria analysis. *Talanta.* 2014; 122: 246–250.

31. Myers FB, Lee LP. Innovations in optical microfluidic technologies for point-of-care diagnostics. *Lab Chip.* 2008; 8(12): 2015–2031.

32. Qiagen. Fluo Sens Integrated. 2014; http://www.qiagen.com/about-us/contact/oem-services/ese-instruments/fluo-sens-integrated. Accessed 12 November 2014.

33. Wongkaew N, Kirschbaum SEK, Surareungchai W, Durst RA, Baeumner AJ. A novel three-electrode system fabricated on polymethyl methacrylate for on-chip electrochemical detection. *Electroanalysis.* 2012; 24(10): 1903–1908.

34. Connelly J, Skoupi M, Baeumner A. Optimization of microfluidic electrochemical detection channels for liposome nanovesicle-based signal amplification *Submitted.* 2014.

35. Mir M, Homs A, Samitier J. Integrated electrochemical DNA biosensors for lab-on-a-chip devices. *Electrophoresis.* 2009; 30(19): 3386–3397.

36. Damhorst G, Smith C, Salm E, et al. A liposome-based ion release impedance sensor for biological detection. *Biomed Microdevices.* 2013; 15(5): 895–905.

37. Nugen SR, Asiello PJ, Connelly JT, Baeumner AJ. PMMA biosensor for nucleic acids with integrated mixer and electrochemical detection. *Biosens Bioelectron.* 2009; 24(8): 2428–2433.

38. Bangham AD, De Gier J, Greville GD. Osmotic properties and water permeability of phospholipid liquid crystals. *Chem Phys Lipids.* 1967; 1(3): 225–246.

39. Zumbuehl O, Weder HG. Liposomes of controllable size in the range of 40 to 180 nm by defined dialysis of lipid/detergent mixed micelles. *Biochim Biophys Acta.* 1981; 640(1): 252–262.

40. Pons M, Foradada M, Estelrich J. Liposomes obtained by the ethanol injection method. *Int J Pharm.* 1993; 95(1–3): 51–56.

41. Angelova MI, Dimitrov DS. Liposome electroformation. *Faraday Discuss Chem Soc.* 1986; 81(0): 303–311.

42. Kuribayashi K, Tresset G, Ph C, Fujita H, Takeuchi S. Electroformation of giant liposomes in microfluidic channels. *Meas Sci Technol.* 2006; 17(12): 3121.

43. Le Berre M, Yamada A, Reck L, Chen Y, Baigl D. Electroformation of giant phospholipid vesicles on a silicon substrate: Advantages of controllable surface properties. *Langmuir.* 2008; 24(6): 2643–2649.

44. van Swaay D, deMello A. Microfluidic methods for forming liposomes. *Lab Chip.* 2013; 13(5): 752–767.

45. Lin Y-C, Huang K-S, Chiang J-T, Yang C-H, Lai T-H. Manipulating self-assembled phospholipid microtubes using microfluidic technology. *Sens Actuators, B.* 2006; 117(2): 464–471.

46. Dittrich PS, Heule M, Renaud P, Manz A. On-chip extrusion of lipid vesicles and tubes through microsized apertures. *Lab Chip.* 2006; 6(4): 488–493.

47. Jahn A, Vreeland WN, Gaitan M, Locascio LE. Controlled vesicle self-assembly in microfluidic channels with hydrodynamic focusing. *J Am Chem Soc.* 2004; 126(9): 2674–2675.

48. Jahn A, Vreeland WN, DeVoe DL, Locascio LE, Gaitan M. Microfluidic directed formation of liposomes of controlled size. *Langmuir.* 2007; 23(11): 6289–6293.

49. Zook JM, Vreeland WN. Effects of temperature, acyl chain length, and flow-rate ratio on liposome formation and size in a microfluidic hydrodynamic focusing device. *Soft Matter.* 2010; 6(6): 1352–1360.

50. Hong JS, Stavis SM, DePaoli Lacerda SH, Locascio LE, Raghavan SR, Gaitan M. Microfluidic directed self-assembly of liposome-hydrogel hybrid nanoparticles. *Langmuir.* 2010; 26(13): 11581–11588.

51. Jahn A, Stavis SM, Hong JS, Vreeland WN, DeVoe DL, Gaitan M. Microfluidic mixing and the formation of nanoscale lipid vesicles. *ACS Nano.* 2010; 4(4): 2077–2087.

52. Wi R, Oh Y, Chae C, Kim D. Formation of liposome by microfluidic flow focusing and its application in gene delivery. *Korea-Aust Rheol J.* 2012; 24(2): 129–135.

53. Balbino TA, Aoki NT, Gasperini AAM, et al. Continuous flow production of cationic liposomes at high lipid concentration in microfluidic devices for gene delivery applications. *Chem Eng J.* 2013; 226: 423–433.

54. Jin Y, Kim SH, Kim M, Park S. Continuous Production of Immunoliposomes using a microvalve-controlled microfluidic device (μFD). *Bull Korean Chem Soc.* 2013; 24: 2921–2924.

55. Balbino TA, Azzoni AR, de la Torre LG. Microfluidic devices for continuous production of pDNA/cationic liposome complexes for gene delivery and vaccine therapy. *Colloids Surf B Biointerfaces.* 2013; 111: 203–210.

56. Mijajlovic M, Wright D, Zivkovic V, Bi JX, Biggs MJ. Microfluidic hydrodynamic focusing based synthesis of POPC liposomes for model biological systems. *Colloids Surf B Biointerfaces.* 2013; 104(0): 276–281.

57. Hood R, Shao C, Omiatek D, Vreeland W, DeVoe D. Microfluidic synthesis of PEG- and folate-conjugated liposomes for one-step formation of targeted stealth nanocarriers. *Pharm Res.* 2013; 30(6): 1597–1607.

58. Lee M, Durst RA, Wong RB. Comparison of liposome amplification and fluorophor detection in flow-injection immunoanalyses. *Anal Chim Acta* 1997; 354(1–3): 23–28.

59. Kou S, Lee HN, van Noort D, et al. Fluorescent molecular logic gates using microfluidic devices. *Angew Chem Int Ed.* 2008; 47(5): 872–876.

60. Andar A, Hood R, Vreeland W, DeVoe D, Swaan P. Microfluidic preparation of liposomes to determine particle size influence on cellular uptake mechanisms. *Pharm Res.* 2014; 31(2): 401–413.

61. Birnbaumer G, Kupcu S, Jungreuthmayer C, et al. Rapid liposome quality assessment using a lab-on-a-chip. *Lab Chip.* 2011; 11(16): 2753–2762.

62. Hoppe SM, Sasaki DY, Kinghorn AN, Hattar K. In-situ transmission electron microscopy of liposomes in an aqueous environment. *Langmuir.* 2013; 29(32): 9958–9961.

63. Jiang F, Yang J, Wang Z-Y, et al. Study of liposome electrofusion on microelectrode array chip. *Chin J Anal Chem.* 2012; 40(4): 551–555.

64. Tresset G, Takeuchi S. Utilization of cell-sized lipid containers for nanostructure and macromolecule handling in microfabricated devices. *Anal Chem.* 2005; 77(9): 2795–2801.

65. Tresset G, Takeuchi S. A microfluidic device for electrofusion of biological vesicles. *Biomed Microdevices.* 2004; 6(3): 213–218.

66. Nuss H, Chevallard C, Guenoun P, Malloggi F. Microfluidic trap- and-release system for lab-on-a-chip-based studies on giant vesicles. *Lab Chip.* 2012; 12(24): 5257–5261.

67. Matlock-Colangelo L, Cho D, Pitner CL, Frey MW, Baeumner AJ. Functionalized electrospun nanofibers as bioseparators in microfluidic systems. *Lab Chip.* 2012; 12(9): 1696–1701.

68. Kuhn P, Eyer K, Robinson T, Schmidt FI, Mercer J, Dittrich PS. A facile protocol for the immobilisation of vesicles, virus particles, bacteria, and yeast cells. *Integr Biol.* 2012; 4(12): 1550–1555.

69. Connelly JT, Kondapalli S, Skoupi M, Parker JL, Kirby BJ, Baeumner AJ. Micro-total analysis system for virus detection: Microfluidic pre-concentration coupled to liposome-based detection. *Anal Bioanal Chem.* 2012; 402(1): 315–323.

70. Wang Z, Wu H-J, Fine D, et al. Ciliated micropillars for the microfluidic-based isolation of nanoscale lipid vesicles. *Lab Chip.* 2013; 13(15): 2879–2882.

Chapter 6

Redox Liposomes in the Development of Electrochemical Sensors

Wei-Ching Liao,[a,b,†] Amily Fang-ju Jou,[a,†] Cheng-Huang Lin,[b]
and Ja-An Annie Ho[a]

[a]*BioAnalytical Chemistry and Nanobiomedicine Laboratory,*
Department of Biochemical Science and Technology,
National Taiwan University, Taipei, Taiwan
[b]*Department of Chemistry, National Taiwan Normal University, Taipei, Taiwan*

jaho@ntu.edu.tw, chenglin@ntnu.edu.tw

6.1 Introduction

Liposomes, first described by British hematologist A.D. Bangham[1-3] at the Babraham Institute, UK, in 1961, are artificially prepared spherical vesicles composed of phosphatidylcholine-enriched phospholipid bilayers. They can be categorized into multilamellar vesicles, small unilamellar vehicles, large unilamellar vesicles, and cochleate vesicles.[4] Liposomes are formed spontaneously when amphipathic lipids are dispersed in an aqueous environment, and during the formation, they encapsulate a portion of the solution containing marker molecules (intended to be entrapped inside of liposome cavity) in which they were dispersed. Thereafter, liposomes have been regarded as models for artificial cells or

---

[†]Authors contributed equally.

Liposomes in Analytical Methodologies
Edited by Katie A. Edwards
Copyright © 2016 Pan Stanford Publishing Pte. Ltd.
ISBN 978-981-4669-26-9 (Hardcover), 978-981-4669-27-6 (eBook)
www.panstanford.com

used as a vehicle for the delivery of pharmaceutical drugs and administration of nutrients.

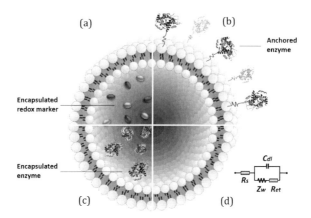

Figure 6.1   A schematic overview of liposomal structure implemented in electrochemical detection: (a) redox bench marker encapsulated in liposomal vesicle; (b) liposomal vesicle with surface-anchored enzyme; (c) enzyme encapsulation in liposomal vesicles; (d) electroanalytical methods that can be used to characterize liposomes, or electroanalytical methods involving the participation of liposomes.

The utilization of liposomes in the development of immunoanalytical tools has been intensively described in the last two–three decades.[5-18] Several previous studies have demonstrated the use of liposomes in solid-phase immunoassays, such as the immunomigration strip format (Chapter 2),[19,20] or in continuous-flow competitive liposome immunoassay.[3,7-9] Liposomes, encapsulating detectable molecules (e.g., electroactive molecules or other signal-producing markers), play a pivotal role in signal amplification. Such liposomal signal amplifiers are capable of providing instantaneous enhancement rather than time-dependent enhancement as in enzyme immunoassays. The advantages of applying liposome-encapsulated electroactive markers to enhance the signal obtained in the competitive reaction have been long established.[10-16] Electroactive markers such as potassium ferrocyanide, ruthenium(III) hexamine chloride, and methylene blue were previously used in liposome immunoassays (LIA), which can be conveniently measured by an amperometric technique.[21] The current chapter aims to present an extensive review on the preparation of electroactive liposomes and their application in analytical science in accordance with the four different constructions indicated in Fig. 6.1. Additionally, electroanalytical methods developed for the characterization of liposomes are briefly discussed. Appendix A summarizes the various electrochemical applications of the liposomes for the development of the analytical platforms, in terms of signal-labeling agent, electrochemical technique, electrode, lipid composition, analyte, assay format, and detection range, respectively, as described by the selected works.

6.2   Redox Bench Marker-Encapsulating Liposomes

Various sensing platforms, combined with liposomal signal-amplification schemes as selected in this section, promise a sensitive and inexpensive solution to the heightened need for a technology that can rapidly and accurately detect biologically or environmentally important targets in the wake of recent threats of bioterrorism. Liposome technology has been used in membrane strip detection systems,[20,22,23] flow injection systems,[24,25] and microfluidic systems[26,27] with great success. We herein focus on the development of the electrochemical sensing platforms in conjunction with liposomal amplification.

One key point of utilization of liposomes in electrochemical sensing platforms is to entrap electroactive markers within lipid bilayers without nonspecific leakage of the markers. The maintenance of the entrapped marker within the aqueous cavity of a liposome largely depends on the solubility and charge of the marker. If molecules contain large hydrophobic regions, they can easily partition into the lipid bilayer and leak out of the liposome over a relatively short period of time. The use of molecules with low oxidation potential minimizes interferences by other oxidizable species and eliminates the need of solution deaeration. Also, the stability of the lipid bilayer is important, which depends on the lipid components used in the liposome preparation. Commonly, saturated lipids are used because of their resistance to oxidation. Cholesterol has been found to associate in the hydrophobic bilayer region thereby reducing the leakage of the contents across the bilayer structure as well as reducing the effects of temperature on the lipid physical state. Finally, anionic lipid doping provides the membrane with a net negative charge to reduce aggregation and fusion.

In 1988, Durst et al. demonstrated a way to characterize ferrocyanide-loaded liposomes and also the feasibility of using liposomes reliably for the selective and sensitive determination of immuno-agents in serum matrices.[28] According to their characterization method, it was revealed that approximately 10^4 molecules of potassium ferrocyanide ($K_4[Fe(CN)_6]$) are encapsulated in the aqueous cavity of a liposome, which led to a sensitive assay for dinitrophenol with a detection limit of 10 nM (10^{-8} mol/L). This study provided a pioneering insight into both homogeneous and heterogeneous immunoassays based on the ferrocyanide/liposome system and facilitated the application of an electrochemical detector for this type of immunoassay.

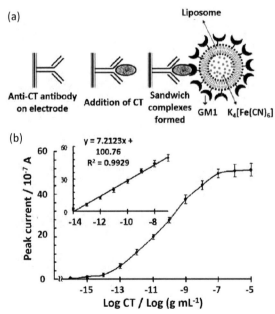

Figure 6.2   (a) Schematic outlines of immunosensor for cholera toxin. (b) Calibration plot for different concentration of cholera toxin. The inset shows a linear part of the main curve. (Reprinted with permission from Ref. [10], Copyright 2006, American Chemical Society. http://pubs.acs.org/doi/abs/10.1021/ac051435d)

Inspired by the design of an assay described by Durst et al.,[28,29] a sensitive electrochemical "sandwich-type" immunosensor for the detection of cholera toxin (CT) with liposomal magnification, followed by adsorptive square-wave stripping voltammetry, was designed and developed by our group in 2006 (Fig. 6.2a).[10] CT is toxic in very small quantities; therefore, sensitive detection methods for ultra-trace levels of CT are in urgent need. Potassium-ferrocyanide-encapsulating and ganglioside (GM1)-functionalized liposomes were fabricated and functioned as specific recognition labels for the amplified detection of CT. The combination of the multiwalled carbon nanotube (MWCNT)-poly(3,4-ethylenediox ythiophene)(PEDOT)-modified sensing interface, consisting of monoclonal antibodies against the B subunit of CT that is linked with PEDOT coated on Nafion-supported MWCNT caste film on a glassy carbon electrode, and the aforementioned liposomal biolabels were confirmed to yield an analytically attractive performance. The CT is detected on the electronic transducers, where the toxin is first bound to the anti-CT antibody and then to the GM1-functionalized liposome. The potassium ferrocyanide molecules are released from liposomes bound to the electrode by lysis with methanolic Triton X-100. The sandwich assay allows an ultrasensitive detection limit of 10^{-16} g of CT (equivalent to 100 µL of 10^{-15} g mL^{-1}), shown in Fig. 6.2b.

In a similar manner, later in 2012 we developed a simple, yet novel and sensitive electrochemical sandwich immunosensor for the detection of P-selectin, which operates through covalent linkage of anti-P-selectin antibodies on CNT@GNB nanocomposite-modified disposable screen-printed electrodes (SPEs) as the detection platform, with $K_4[Fe(CN)_6]$-encapsulating, anti-P-selectin-tagged liposomal biolabels as electrochemical signal amplifiers.[15] The CNT@GNB is a nanoassembly of carbon nanotube and gold nonobone that serves as the electrode modifier and promotes signal transduction due to its excellent conductivity. On the sensing surface, the immunorecognition of the antibody-captured sample P-selectin by the liposomal biolabels occurred; the release of $K_4[Fe(CN)_6]$ from the bound liposomal biolabels extensively contributed to the increase in electrochemical signal, which could be acquired in HCl solution at +0.32 V by the square-wave voltammetric (SWV) technique. A detection limit as low as 4.3 fg (equivalent to 5 µL of 0.85 pg/mL solution) was achieved for detecting P-selectin at trace levels attributed to the unique amplification route offered by this liposome-based electrochemical immunoassay. The performance of this new liposomal assay was validated by a commercial enzyme-linked immunosorbent assay (ELISA) kit as a reference method through the analysis of mouse serum samples. A strong correlation was observed between the two datasets as the R-squared value of 0.997 from the linear regression line, meaning that this electrochemical immunosensor will be useful for the detection of P-selectin in biological fluids and tissue extracts (as indicated in Fig. 6.3a,b).

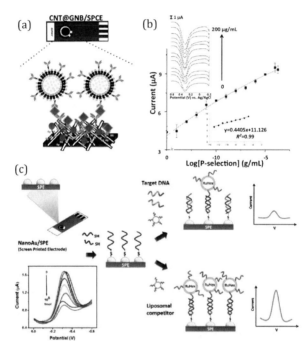

Figure 6.3   (a) Schematic diagrams of CNT@GNB/SPCE for the immunosensing of P-selectin using electroactive liposomal biolabels and (b) the corresponding dose-response curve (Inset: square-wave voltammograms for different concentrations of P-selectin) (Reprinted with permission from Ref. [15], Copyright 2012, Elsevier. http://dx.doi.org/10.1016/j.ymeth.2011.10.014.) (c) Flow diagram illustrating the design concept for the competitive assay- type genosensor (Inset: SWV traces for various amounts of the target rfbE gene). (Reprinted with permission from Ref. [12], Copyright 2009, American Chemical Society. http://pubs.acs.org/doi/abs/10.1021/ac8020517)

As we have introduced several examples in which liposomal amplifiers were used in the sandwich-type assay format, the following example demonstrated the feasibility of liposomal amplifiers to be used in competitive assay. The development of a cost-effective, user-friendly immunoanalytical sensing platform with acceptable sensitivity for use in the detection of biotin, known as vitamin H, was described by our group in 2009.[13] The detection system consisted of biotin-tagged, $K_4[Fe(CN)_6]$-encapsulating liposomes as the signal amplifier, and polyallylamine hydrochloride (PAH)-modified, nanosized-Au (nanoAu) particles assembled on an SPE as the sensing transducer. The determination of biotin was based on a "competitive-type" immunoassay where competition occurs between the analyte biotin and $K_4[Fe(CN)_6]$-encapsulating, biotin-tagged liposomes for a limited number of anti-biotin antibody-binding sites immobilized on the PAH/nanoAu/SPE surface. The SWV technique was used to measure the current signal produced by the ferrocyanide released after the lysis of bound liposomes. The detection limit of this sensor is as little as 9.1 pg of biotin (equivalent to 4.5 μL of 8.3×10^{-9} M).

Further, in 2009 our group also developed a novel electrochemical competitive genosensor (schematic diagram shown in Fig. 6.3c),[12] operated on gold-electrodeposited SPE for the detection of the *rfb*E gene, which is specific to a verocytotoxin (VT1/2)-producing pathogen *Escherichia coli* O157. The fabrication of nanoAu/SPE-sensing surface was initiated by the modification of a self-assembled monolayer of thiol-capped single- stranded DNA (capture probe), and this sensor functioned based on competition between the target gene (complementary to the capture probe DNA) and reporter DNA-tagged, hexaammineruthenium(III) chloride-encapsulating liposomes. SWV was then used to acquire the current signal generated by the released liposomal $Ru(NH_3)_6$. This liposomal competitive assay was able to detect as little as 0.75 amol of the target *rfb*E DNA (equivalent to the amount present in 5 μL of a 0.15 pM solution).

Moreover, in 2013 our group also presented the successful synthesis of methylene blue-encapsulating liposomes and their further functionalization with progesterone.[16] This methylene blue-encapsulating liposomal preparation tagged with progesterone (LP) through carboxyl-to-amine crosslinkage endorsed an amplification merit beneficial for electroanalytical applications. A new disposable electrochemical immunosensing strip assay for the leveling of progesterone, a hormone that helps to regulate the menstrual cycle of women, was designed and developed. This competitive immune-recognition assay utilizing anti-progesterone antibodies conjugated to a screen-printed electrode for the simultaneous detection of target progesterone and liposomal progesterone enabled the reliable quantification of progesterone with limit of detection as low as 0.83 pg/mL. By virtue of the robustness of electrochemical strips and liposomal biolabels, it was anticipated that the present sensor is useful in facilitating the analysis of progesterone with versatile applications.

Different from the conventional format operated on the disposable single-use electronic transducer, the Baeumner group demonstrated the application of DNA-probe-coated paramagnetic beads and DNA-probe-tagged, ferri/ferrohexacyanide-encapsulating liposomes (as the redox marker) in developing a multichannel poly(methyl methacrylate) (PMMA) microfluidic biosensor with interdigitated ultramicroelectrode arrays (IDUAs) for electrochemical nucleic acid detection.[30] The simple fabrication strategy described in this study enabled a strong sealing for all channels of the microfluidic chip. In addition, the chip shows desirable electrochemical performance in terms of analytical sensitivity (limit of detection: 12.5 µM), linearity, and reproducibility. The as-obtained results suggest that the multichannel device was capable of offering an excellent opportunity for multi-analyte and high-throughput bioanalytical detection.

In addition, the Bard group in 2006 revealed the use of scanning electrochemical microscopy (SECM) to probe outside and inside single giant liposomes containing $Ru(bpy)_3^{2+}$.[31] The authors discovered the practicality of SECM in studying liposomes, with potential applications to investigate biomembranes and redox regulation of cellular processes. It was found that the individual redox-marker-encapsulating giant liposomes could be probed by microelectrode tips to obtain meaningful evidence about molecular transport through a biomembrane. Based on what has been discussed in this work, it can be concluded that an alternative probe to those based on fluorescence and radioactivity was offered to study biomembranes. In comparison to a bilayer lipid membrane setup that Bard's group previously demonstrated to study charge and ion transfer through the bilayer lipid, this present system based on giant liposomes allows one to perform measurements over a more extended period of time. With a stable biomembrane system in hand, it becomes more feasible to conduct more detailed studies on the liposome membrane modified by natural or synthetic proteins (as pores and ion channels) at higher resolution.

6.3   Enzyme-Encapsulating Liposomes

Enzymes are commonly used as signal amplifiers in the development of electrochemical sensors. Unlike in ELISAs, the signal generation is due to the oxidation/reduction of an electroactive product converted by the enzyme labeled on the surface of transducer, or the recycling of signal molecules to their reduced/oxidized state by the enzyme, so that multiple signal generation processes can proceed. However, the analytical sensitivity and detection limit of enzyme-based assays are exclusively limited by the number of enzyme labels existing on the reporting molecules (antibody or DNA probe), typically in a 1:1 ratio. Liposomes, serving as promising signal enhancers, can be the solution to circumvent the suboptimal property of enzyme labels, owing to liposomes' superior capability to entrap hydrophilic agents in their internal aqueous compartment or lipophilic molecules within the lipid membrane. The liposomal signal amplification is due to the large number of enzymes that can be encapsulated inside the liposomal cavity. Accordingly, the more the enzymes encapsulated in the liposomes, the higher the sensitivity of the enzyme-based liposomal electrochemical sensors. In addition, the biocompatible microenvironments of the liposomes, along with the careful tuning and maintenance of their physicochemical properties, enable the stabilization of enzyme labels, preventing them from denaturation. Therefore, in this section, an overview and essential information are provided to allow the design of liposomal signal enhancers and employment of enzyme-encapsulating liposomes in the development of electrochemical sensing platforms.

In 1980, the first enzyme-encapsulating liposome immunosensor was demonstrated by Haga et al.[32,33] The authors revealed the detection capability of enzyme-encapsulating liposomes for theophylline, which is widely used in treating acute and chronic respiratory diseases. The liposome immunosensing system is composed of a Clark-type oxygen electrode and theophylline-tagged liposomes, as shown in Fig. 6.4a.

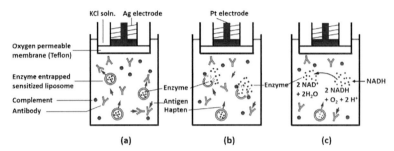

(a)   (b)   (c)

Figure 6.4 Schematic diagram of liposome immunosensor based on activation of complement system and enzymatic reaction. (Adapted with permission from Ref. [33], Copyright 1981, Elsevier. http://dx.doi.org/10.1016/0003-2697(81)90584-4)

The detection is based on monitoring the release of entrapped enzymes from ruptured liposomes induced by specific anti-theophylline antibody and complement. As an unknown concentration of theophylline, a known amount of theophylline-tagged liposomes and complement were mixed together and then incubated with the limited number of antibodies, competitive binding occurred between theophylline presented in the tested solution and theophylline-bound liposomes. The complement system was acted upon by the antigen–antibody reaction, resulting in the lysis of liposomes and subsequent release of entrapped enzyme (e.g., horseradish peroxidase, HRP). It was reported by the authors that the enzymatic activity was directly proportional to the immuno-lysis of liposomes and related inversely to the concentration of free theophylline. Further, a known concentration of NADH substrates was introduced into the system. The more NADH molecules were oxidized, the more oxygen in the solution was consumed. The signal collection was achieved by amperometric monitoring of oxygen depletion using Clark oxygen electrode.

By virtue of enzyme-loaded liposomes that have been successfully adopted in homogeneous immunoassays, Wu and Durst introduced enzyme-encapsulating liposomes into a flow injection analysis system.[34] The sensing principle was based on the competition between the analyte molecules (theophylline) and theophylline-derivatized liposomes for a fixed number of antibodies immobilized in a flow-through immunoreactor column. In this system, unbound enzyme-encapsulating liposomes were carried downstream and ruptured by free radicals in the presence of hydrogen peroxide and p-fluorophenol. The released peroxidases from liposomes enzymatically cleave organofluorine substrates to produce fluoride ions, which could then be potentiometrically measured with an ion-selective electrode. The acquired signal was directly proportional to the theophylline concentration presented in the sample. This flow injection operation allows repetitive column regeneration, reduction in reaction time, improved precision over manual procedures, and most importantly the double signal-amplification strategy (enzymatic amplification and liposomal amplification).

Moreover, in 2010 Chu's group described the design of a novel electrochemical immunosensor that integrated double signal amplification of enzyme-encapsulating liposomes with biocatalytic metal deposition for the detection of human prostate-specific antigen (PSA).[35] Alkaline phosphatase (ALP)-encapsulating, antibody-functionalized liposomes were prepared and used as the detection reagent. As illustrated in Fig. 6.5, the sensing method was based on a sandwich immunoassay, where the PSA was first captured by anti-PSA antibody immobilized on the electrode and subsequently sandwiched with the functionalized liposomes. Finally, the encapsulated ALPs were released from bound liposomes with the addition of surfactants, serving as secondary signal amplifier. In the presence of substrates, ALP initiated the hydrolysis of ascorbic acid 2-phosphate (AA-p) to produce ascorbic acid, which was able to reduce silver ions on the electrode surface, resulting in the deposition of metal silver on the electrode surface.

Finally, linear sweep voltammetry (LSV) was employed to measure the amount of the deposited silver. The detection limit of PSA, as low as 0.007 ng/mL, was obtained. Since the cut-off value of human PSA is 4 ng/mL, the authors claimed that their electrochemical immunosensor holds great potential for the detection of PSA in clinical samples, due to sensitive LOD.

In 2011, Genc et al. reported the development of an amperometric immunosensor, which utilizes enzyme-encapsulating, thermosensitive liposomes for the detection of carcinoembryonic antigens (CEA) with high sensitivity (Fig. 6.6).[36]

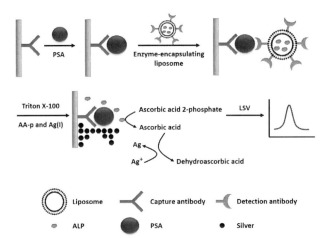

Figure 6.5 An electrochemical immunosensor based on double signal amplification of enzyme-encapsulated liposomes and biocatalytic metal deposition. (Adapted with permission from Ref. [35], Copyright 2010, Elsevier. http://dx.doi.org/10.1016/j.aca.2010.01.050)

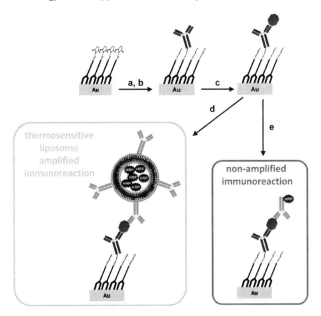

Figure 6.6 Liposome-based sandwich immunosensor for the detection of carcinoembryonic antigen. (Reprinted with permission from Ref. [36], Copyright 2011, American Chemical Society. http://pubs.acs.org/doi/abs/10.1021/ac1023765)

This group demonstrated a standard sandwich immunoassay and studied five different bioconjugation approaches to couple anti-CEA antibodies to HRP-encapsulating liposomes and comparing them to conventional HRP-conjugated antibodies. Five bioconjugation strategies were depicted in Fig. 6.7, including (I) biotin-streptavidin, (II) SATA/sulfo-SMCC, (III) EDC/NHS, (IV) sodium periodate, and (V) glutaraldehyde methods.

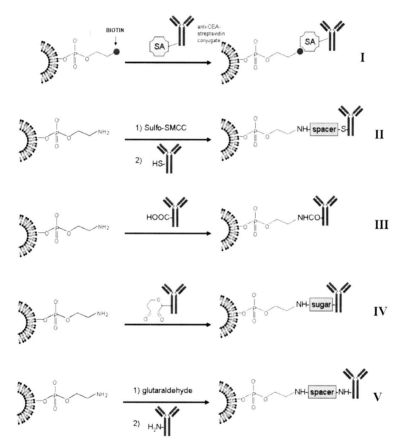

Figure 6.7   Various antibody–liposome conjugation methods. (Reprinted with permission from Ref. [36], Copyright 2011, American Chemical Society. http://pubs.acs.org/doi/abs/10.1021/ac1023765)

The concept of using liposomes to serve as signaling labels in developing sensing platforms has been described and demonstrated through Chi's group, which differs from others by employing liposomes as a sensing bioreactor,[37,38] as shown in Fig. 6.8a. The liposome-based bioreactors were constructed by encapsulating acetylcholinesterase (AChE) in liposomes, consisting of L-α-phosphatidylcholine. Porins were subsequently embedded into the lipid membrane, facilitating the transport of free and small-size substrates. AChE is capable of stabilizing the levels of the neurotransmitter acetylcholine by catalyzing the hydrolysis of acetylcholine to thiocholine, but its catalytic activity can be inhibited by trace amounts of organophosphate pesticides. Dichlorvos, an organophosphate pesticide, was chosen herein as a target compound. Based on the inhibitory effect exerted by organophosphate pesticides on the AChE activity, the inhibition induced by dichlorvos was proportional to its concentration. The schematic diagram of the AChE-based inhibitor liposomal bioreactor is shown in Fig. 6.8b, which is based on the multilayer films composed of [chitosan (CS)/AChE liposomal bioreactors (ALB)]$_5$ or [(MWCNTs)/ALB]$_6$, respectively, on the surface of glassy

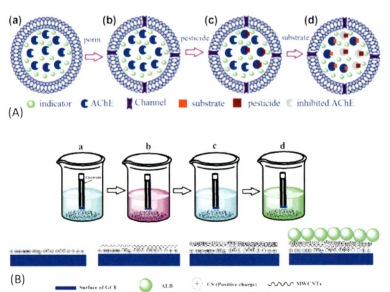

Figure 6.8   (a) Schematic diagram of the AChE-based inhibitor liposome bioreactor. (b) The schematic diagram of the MWCNTs/ALB multilayer films. (Reprinted with permission from Ref. [38], Copyright 2013, Elsevier. http://dx.doi.org/10.1016/j.pestbp.2013.02.003)

carbon electrodes. The resulting AChE biosensor exhibited high sensitivity, good reproducibility, long-term stability, and low-cost operation for the analysis of pesticides and characterization of enzyme inhibitors.

6.4 Liposomes with Surface-Anchored Enzymes

Owing to the large surface area of liposomes, rather than limited to being a versatile carrier to entrap a large number of cargo molecules, it is also feasible to anchor a number of functioning enzymes onto the surface of liposomes. The surface-anchored enzymes can be directly in contact with substrates, leading to the direct utilization of enzyme-anchored liposomes, and omitting the need for liposomal lysis.

Willner's group first demonstrated the application of enzyme-anchored liposomes for the detection of CT, anti-dinitrophenyl antibody (DNP–Ab), and oligonucleotide (DNA), respectively.[39,40] In one of their studies (depicted in Fig. 6.9), HRP and ganglioside GM1-functionalized liposomes were fabricated as catalytic recognition labels for the amplified detection of the CT. The sensing interface consisted of the monoclonal antibody against the B subunit of CT that was linked to protein G and assembled as a monolayer on an Au electrode or an Au/quartz crystal. The CT was detected by a sandwich assay on the electrodes, where the toxin was first bound to the anti-CT antibody and then to the HRP-GM1-ganglioside-functionalized liposome. The enzyme-labeled liposome mediated the oxidation of 4-chloronaphthol (**1**) in the presence of H_2O_2 to form the insoluble product benzo-4-chlorohexadienone (**2**) on transducer surfaces. The precipitation of the insoluble product on the transducer was anticipated to alter the interfacial properties. Thus, constant-current chronopotentiometry and microgravimetric quartz crystal microbalance (QCM) measurements were used as characterization methods, and Faradaic impedance spectroscopy was then employed as an electronic transduction approach for the detection of CT with detection limits of 0.1 pM.

For a wider range of applications, instead of conjugating affinity probes directly on liposomes, liposomes labeled with biotin and HRP were used as an amplification probe in the sensing of antigen–antibody interactions or oligonucleotide bindings.[39]

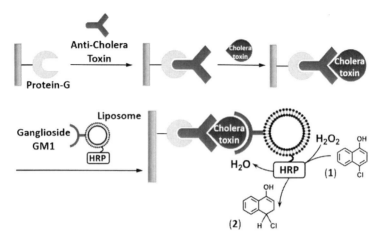

Figure 6.9   Amplified sensing of cholera toxin using a GM1-tagged HRP-functionalized liposome. (Adapted with permission from Ref. [40], Copyright 2001, American Chemical Society. http://pubs.acs.org/doi/abs/10.1021/ac010542e)

Figure 6.10a,b outlines the concept for the amplified electronic transduction of the biotin-labeled HRP liposome. The DNP–Ab was sensed by a dinitrophenyl-L-cysteine antigen monolayer functionalized on an Au electrode (Fig. 6.10a). A biotinylated anti-IgG-antibody (Fc-specific) was subsequently applied to the antigen-DNP–Ab complex, followed by an addition of avidin. The formation of immunocomplexes, consisting of biotin-labeled HRP-liposomes and the assembly, was achieved through an avidin bridge. In a similar manner, DNA-based targets were partially recognized by capture probes immobilized on Au electrode (Fig. 6.10b). The biotin-labeled oligonucleotide was complementary to the exposed part of an analyte DNA associated with double-stranded complexes presented on the electrode by a sandwich-type DNA hybridization. After treating with avidin, the final configuration subsequently interacted with the biotinylated HRP-modified liposomes.

To be brief, the principle underlying the utilization of enzyme-anchored liposomes in biosensor technology relies on two strategies. The primary binding of the analyte assembly with the liposome results in the generation of a micromembrane environment that alters the interfacial properties of the sensing transducer, e.g., electron-transfer resistance or mass density.

The secondary biocatalyzed precipitation (via enzyme, such as HRP) of an insoluble product intensifies further the primary recognition of the corresponding antibody, protein, or target DNA by insulating the sensing transducer to enable the amplification of the sensing event. In addition, Willner et al. also provided an important take-home message: the functionalized liposomes were able to serve as cleaning agents to remove nonspecific protein (antibody or avidin) or DNA adsorbents, enabling the selective sensing of the target analyte.

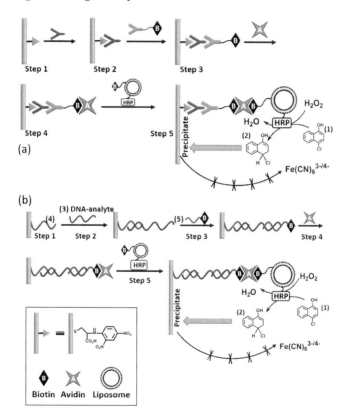

Figure 6.10 (a) Sensing of the anti-DNP antibody and (b) a target DNA with an aid of biotin-tagged HRP-functionalized liposomes and the electronic transduction of the sensing event by following the interfacial electron-transfer resistance as a result of the biocatalyzed precipitation of an insoluble product. (Adapted with permission from Ref. [39], Copyright 2001, American Chemical Society. http://pubs.acs.org/doi/abs/10.1021/ac000819v)

6.5 Electroanalytical Methods Based on the Unique Characteristics of Liposomes

Functionalized liposomes are commonly regarded as a simple model system of cells and widely used as a carrier for drug delivery. The first challenge encountered is their possible interaction with cells before executing their function. Therefore, it is of great importance to realize how the interaction takes place between the functionalized liposome and the cell membrane before the functionalization strategies designed for liposomes can be further improved. To address the issue, electrochemical techniques were confirmed as simple tools to analyze functionalized liposomes. In 2006, Janshoff and Wegener described a novel approach for studying the adsorption of giant liposomes on protein-coated solid surfaces with a time resolution in the order of seconds using electrochemical impedance measurement (Fig. 6.11a,b).[41] In addition to monitoring the adsorption of liposomes on protein-coated surfaces, such a technique can also be extended to study the shape fluctuations of the adsorbed vesicles, distinguishing between the adsorption of intact liposomes and planar lipid bilayers. It enables the comparison of the corresponding power spectra with those acquired for hard particles and living animal cells. The device fabricated based on the aforementioned principle can be further miniaturized to provide the technical basis for screening arrays on the micrometer scale.

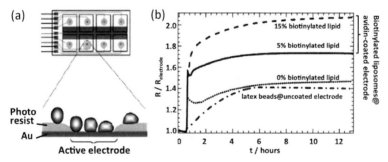

Figure 6.11 (a) Schematic diagram of the electrode that is able to monitor adsorption and shape fluctuations of liposomes and (b) the corresponding time course responses of the resistance measured during the adsorption of liposomes. (Reprinted with permission from Ref. [41], Copyright 2006, American Chemical Society. http://pubs.acs.org/doi/abs/10.1021/la051344b)

Gene therapy is an emerging treatment for clinical therapeutic procedures achieved by introducing the corrected copies of the malfunctioning genes into cells to cure or eventually prevent diseases. The design of a vector to function as a safe and efficient gene-delivery vehicle becomes the key to success for gene therapy strategy. The liposomal DNA-delivery system has been extensively studied as a gene therapy vector; therefore, it is central to unravel the effect of different lipid constituent on the self-assembly process that subsequently leads to the formation of a DNA–liposome complex.

In 2004, Oliveira-Brett et al. demonstrated the use of differential pulse voltammetry (DPV) to explore the complex (ODN lipoplexes) formation between short oligodeoxynucleotides (ODN) with a variable dGxdCy base composition, and liposomes composed of the cationic lipid DOTAP at the electrode surface/ solution interface.[42] It was verified that the oxidation of guanosine resulted in the production of peak current in the voltammograms for ODN lipoplexes (Fig. 6.12a), which was found to be influenced by the (±) charge ratio of lipoplex and the applied adsorption potential. Moreover, a model that explains the organization of ODN lipoplexes at the electrode surface/ solution interface was proposed in this study (Fig. 6.12b). The electrochemical results presented by the authors provided details on not only the physicochemical characterization of lipoplexes at charged interfaces, but also the quantification of the amount of genetic material protected or released by the lipoplex formulation when in contact with a charged interface. Such information is vital for the understanding and development of gene therapy vectors based on ODN lipoplexes.

Liposomes, consisting of phospholipids with various functional groups, can be regarded as a multivalent ligand system, which enables scientists to design them as either capture probes or signaling labels based on a sandwich-format assay. It was reported previously that DNA or protein-functionalized liposomes are able to serve as multivalent capture probes, situated at the first layer of a sandwich complex for the biorecognition with its counterparts. Such functionalized liposomes, on the other hand, are capable of functioning as signaling labels with multiple binding sites, positioned at the third layer of a sandwich complex for not only the biorecognition with targets captured by the first probes bound on surfaces, but also for the generation of signal outputs. Therefore, the fabrication of electrodes using functionalized liposomes combined with Faradaic impedance spectroscopy (EIS) provides a novel amplification strategy for the analyses of target DNAs, and especially the detection of single-base mismatch. The principle of such a sensing platform is based on the signal differences in which the formation of the liposomal sandwich complexes on the electrode often leads to a higher electron-transfer resistance attributed to the presence of bulky liposomes.

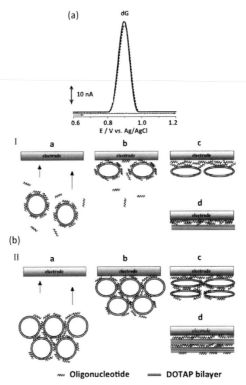

Figure 6.12 (a) Differential pulse voltammograms for oligonucleotide-I (full line), DOTAP liposome suspension (dashed line), and ODN-I lipoplex after base line correction; (b) a proposed model for layer organization of the low (I) and high (II) molar charge ratio of ODN lipoplexes at the electrode/solution charged interface. (Reprinted with permission from Ref. [42], Copyright 2004, Elsevier. http://dx.doi.org/10.1016/j.bios.2004.06.014)

In addition, the formation of DNA duplex onto liposomes sheltered the negatively charged redox markers from approaching the surface of the electrode.

In 2013, Dharumana et al. demonstrated for the first time a covalent immobilization of 1,2-dioleoyl-*sn*-glycero-3-phosphoethanolamine (DOPE) liposome–gold nanoparticle (DOPE-AuNP) nanocomposite on a 3-mercaptopropionic acid (MPA)-derivatized gold surface for electrochemical label-free DNA sensing (Fig. 6.13a).[43] The appearance of the sigmoidal voltammetric profile, which is the representative behavior of linear diffusion for the MPA–DOPE in the presence of $[Fe(CN)_6]^{3-/4-}$ and $[Ru(NH_3)_6]^{3+}$, provided the evidence for the successful coating of spherical DOPE vesicles on the MPA monolayer. It was followed by the electroless deposition of AuNP on the hydrophilic amine headgroups of the DOPE. Finally, DNA hybridization sensing platform was established by the fixation of single-stranded DNA (ssDNA) probe onto AuNP via simple gold–thiol linkage. The authors claimed their sensor was able to discriminate the complementary target, noncomplementary target, and single-base mismatch target sensitively and selectively without further signal amplification, and its detection limit was calculated as low as 1×10^{-13} M (Fig. 6.13b). The principle of such sensors is based on the electrostatic repulsion between negatively charged $Fe(CN)_6]^{3-/4-}$ and the hybridized DNA duplex formed on liposome–AuNP nanocomposite. Cyclic voltammetric (CV), electrochemical impedance (EIS), DPV, and QCM techniques were used in this study for DNA sensing in the presence of $Fe(CN)_6]^{3-/4-}$. This method holds great potential to be extended to cell transfection studies at relatively low costs.

In fact, the utilization of negatively charged liposomes as signaling labels was demonstrated by Willner's group back in 2000 (schematic diagram is shown in Fig. 6.14a).[44] The analyses of the target DNA were transduced electrochemically using either Faradaic impedance spectroscopy or microgravimetric measurements with Au–quartz crystals, in which a single-strand probe oligonucleotide (1) was first assembled on Au electrodes. The formation of the double-stranded duplex with the analyte DNA (2) was amplified by the association of the oligonucleotide (3)-functionalized liposomes to the sensing interface. The target DNA is analyzed by this method with a sensitivity limit that corresponds to 1.2×10^{-12} M (Fig. 6.14b). Willner et al. successfully demonstrated highly sensitive sensing processes that were transduced by Faradaic impedance measurements, and the sensing interfaces revealed superior selectivity in the analysis of the target DNA based on a sandwich DNA hybridization format.

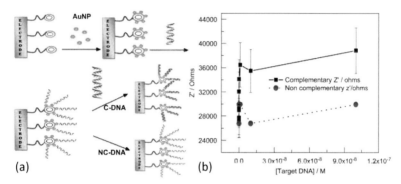

Figure 6.13 (a) Formation of spherical DOPE-AuNP nanocomposite and DNA detection. (b) Electrical impedance of different concentrations of the complementary (filled square, solid line) or noncomplementary (filled circle, dotted line) target DNA. (Adapted from with permission from Ref. [43], Copyright 2013, Elsevier. http://dx.doi.org/10.1016/j.bios. 2012.10.017)

Different from the scheme depicted in Fig. 6.14a, another sensing mechanism shown in Fig. 6.15a was described by the same group, highlighting the use of avidin/biotin-tagged liposomes as a particulate building unit for the dendritic amplification of DNA sensing through a two-step amplification, leading to unprecedented sensitive and specific detection of DNA with a detection limit of 0.5 fM (Fig. 6.15b). It involves the interaction of the (1)-functionalized electrode with the target DNA sample (2) that is pretreated with the biotinylated oligonucleotide (4). The formation of the three-component double-stranded complex among DNAs (1), (2), and (4) could be further intensified by interacting with avidin and biotin-labeled liposomes to the sensing interfaces, resulting in dendritic-type amplification for DNA analysis. The authors also described the possibility of adopting this design to the organization of microelectrode arrays on transducers, enabling the development of electrochemical DNA chips for the multicomponent DNA analyses.

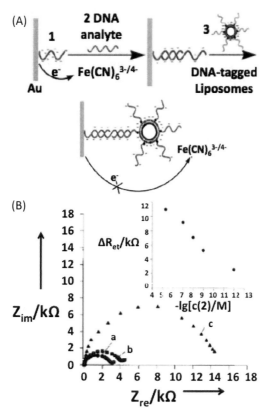

Figure 6.14 (A) Schematic illustration of the amplified sensing for the target DNA utilizing oligonucleotide-functionalized liposomes, and (B) the Faradaic impedance spectra of (a) 1-functionalized Au electrode, (b) after interaction of the sensing electrode with 2, and (c) finally interacting with the 3-functionalized liposome. (Adapted from with permission from Ref. [44], Copyright 2000, Wiley-VCH Verlag GmbH & Co. KGaA. http://onlinelibrary.wiley.com/doi/10.1002/(SICI)1521-3773(20000303)39:5<940::AID-ANIE940>3.0.CO;2-Y/abstract)

In addition, Willner's group in 2001 also confirmed the feasibility of using the biotin-tagged liposomes in probing and amplifying single-base mismatches in an analyte DNA (Fig. 6.16a), in which the (6)-oligonucleotide-functionalized Au–quartz crystal or Au electrode (Fig. 6.16b) was used to distinguish the single-base mismatch (G) in the mutant (5) from the normal A-containing gene (5a).[45] The sensing principle to probe the single-base mismatch relies on the polymerase-induced coupling of the biotinylated-C-base to the double-stranded duplex generated between (6) and (5), followed by the recognition between avidin and biotin-tagged liposomes. The functionalized liposomes functioned as a particulate building unit, featuring the dendritic amplification that enabled the discrimination between the mutant gene (1×10^{-13} M) and the normal gene (1×10^{-9} M). Moreover, the authors also mentioned an important advantage of liposomes as "nanocontainers" for additional components that may stimulate secondary amplification processes in the amplified DNA sensing.

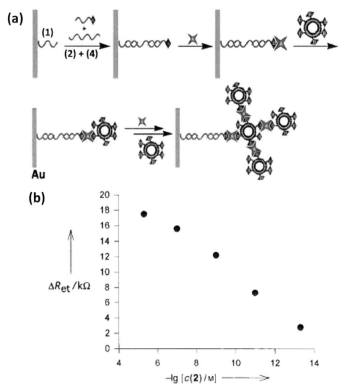

Figure 6.15 (a) Schematic diagram of amplified sensing of a target DNA with a biotinylated oligonucleotide, avidin, and liposomes labeled with biotin as an amplification conjugate, and (b) the corresponding calibration curve. (Reprinted with permission from Ref. [44], Copyright 2000, Wiley-VCH Verlag GmbH & Co. KGaA. http://onlinelibrary.wiley.com/doi/10.1002/(SICI)1521-3773(20000303)39:5<940::AID-ANIE940>3.0.CO;2-Y/abstract)

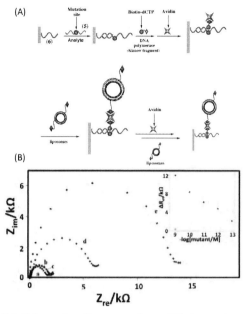

Figure 6.16 (A) Schematic diagram of amplified sensing of a single-base mutation based on polymerase-induced coupling of a biotinylated-base and biotin-labeled liposomes, and (B) the Faradaic impedance spectra of (a) (6)-functionalized electrodes before and (b) after hybridization with (5), followed by stepwise interaction with (c) biotinylated-dCTP, (d) avidin, and (e) biotinylated liposomes (Inset: the corresponding calibration curve). (Adapted and reprinted with permission from Ref. [45], Copyright 2001, American Chemical Society. http://pubs.acs.org/doi/abs/10.1021/ja0036256)

6.6 Future Perspectives

Liposome technologies have been applied to design novel electrochemical sensing devices for years. By combining with modern components, such as advanced nanomaterials, or electronic elements, the technology further highlights the utility of liposome-based sensing platforms, ensuring a mobile, low-cost, user-friendly, and highly sensitive diagnostics. Multiplex sensing configurations used toward the detection of small molecules, proteins, or oligonucleotides involving liposomal amplification with single or multiple selective reagents can potentially contribute to the monitoring or surveillance of environmentally, clinically, and biologically important targets.

Appendix A Summary of electrochemical applications of liposomes for analyte detection

Labeling agent	Technique	Electrode	Liposome composition (diameter)	Analyte[Ref]	Assay format	Detection range (detection limit, signal output)
			Redox bench marker-encapsulating liposomal vesicles			
$K_4Fe(CN)_6$	SWV	GCE	DPPC/Chol/DPPG/GM1 (238 nm)	Cholera toxin[10]	Sandwich	10^{-14}–10^{-7} g/mL (0.1 fg)
Fc	SWV	SPCE	DPPC/Chol/DPPG/DPPE–acetylthioacetate (250 ± 30 nm)	CEA[11]	Sandwich	5×10^{-12}–5×10^{-7} g/mL (1×10^{-12} g/mL)
$Ru(NH_3)_6Cl_3$	CV, SWV	Au/SPCE	DPPC/Chol/DPPG/PE-MCC (212.4 nm)	DNA[12]	Sandwich	1–10^6 fmol (0.75 amol, SWV)
$K_4Fe(CN)_6$	CV, SWV	SPCE	DPPC/Chol/DPPG/DHPE–X–biotin (213 nm)	Biotin[13]	Competitive	10^{-11}–10^{-2} M (9.1 pg, SWV)
$K_4Fe(CN)_6$	CV, SWV	Au/SPCE	DPPC/Chol/DPPG/DHPE–X–biotin (185 nm)	Biotin[14]	Sandwich	10^{-3}–10^{-10} M (0.19 pg, SWV)
$K_4Fe(CN)_6$	CV, SWV	CNT@GNB/SPCE	DPPC/Chol/DPPG/DSPE–PEG_{2000}–amine (158 nm)	P-selectin[15]	Sandwich	10^{-13}–10^{-5} g/mL (0.85 pg/mL, SWV)
MB	SWV	SPCE	DPPC/Chol/DPPG/DSPE–PEG_{2000}–amine (220 ± 30 nm)	Progesterone[16]	Sandwich	10^{-6}–10^{-11} g/mL (0.83 pg/mL)
$K_4Fe(CN)_6$	DPV	Pt	DMPC/chol/dicetyl-phosphate	liposome[28]	—	—

Labeling agent	Technique	Electrode	Liposome composition (diameter)	Analyte[Ref]	Assay format	Detection range (detection limit, signal output)
$K_4Fe(CN)_6$/ $K_3Fe(CN)_6$	Amperometry	IUDA	DPPC/DPPG/Chol	DNA[30]	—	0–38 μM (3.48 μM)
$Ru(bpy)_6Cl_2$	SECM	Glass	(1) DSPC/(PSPG or SOPG) (2 μm) (2) DHPE-X-biotin/DSPC/(PSPG or SOPG) (2 μm)	Liposome[31]	—	—
Enzymes encapsulated in liposomal vesicles						
HRP	Amperometry	ISE (Oxygen)	Theophylline–PE/PC/Chol/DCP	Theophylline[32,33]	Competitive	4×10^{-9}–2×10^{-8} M (4 nM)
HRP	Potentiometry	ISE (Fl⁻)	Theophylline–PE/PC/ hol/DCP	Theophylline[34]	Competitive	0–43 μg/mL (0.2 ng/mL)
ALP	LSV	Au	PC/Chol/PE (352 nm)	PSA[35]	Sandwich	0.01–100 ng/mL (0.007 ng/mL)
HRP	Amperometry	Au	DPPC/DPPE/lyso-PPC	CEA[36]	Sandwich	0.59–37.5 ng/mL (0.08 ng/ mL) 1.17–37.5 ng/mL (0.113 ng/mL)
AChE	Amperometry	GCE	LPC/Chol (7.3 μm)	Dichlorvos[37]	Inhibition	0.25–1.50 μM 1.75–10 μM (0.86 ± 0.098 μg/L)
AChE	Amperometry	GCE	LPC/Chol (7.3 μm)	Dichlorvos[38]	Inhibition	0.25–1.75 μM 2–10 μM (0.68 ± 0.076 μg/L)

(Continued)

Appendix A *(Continued)*

Labeling agent	Technique	Electrode	Liposome composition (diameter)	Analyte[Ref]	Assay format	Detection range (detection limit, signal output)
			Liposomal vesicles with surface-anchored enzymes			
HRP	EIS, CCCP	Au	DSPC/Chol/DMPE/DHPE-X-biotin (148 nm)	(1) DNP–Ab (2) DNA[39]	Sandwich	(1) DNP-Ab 0.01–10 ng mL^{-1} (1 × 10^{-11} g/mL, CCCP) (2) DNA 6.5 × 10^{-13} – 6.5 × 10^{-10} M (6.5 × 10^{-13} M)
HRP	EIS, CCCP	Au	GM1/PA/DMPE/ DSPC/Chol (130.5 nm)	Cholera toxin[40]	Sandwich	1 × 10^{-13}–1 × 10^{-7} M (1 × 10^{-13} M, CCCP)
			Redox bench marker-encapsulated liposomes based on their unique characteristics			
—	EIS	Au	Asolectin/POPG/chol/ N-biotinyl Cap–PE	—[41]	Sandwich	—
—	DPV	GCE	DOTAP	—[42]	—	—
K$_4$Fe(CN)$_6$/ K$_3$Fe(CN)$_6$ Ru(NH$_3$)$_6$Cl$_3$	EIS, CV, DPV	Au	DOPE (700 nm)	DNA[43]	Sandwich	10^{-6}–10^{-11} M (1 × 10^{-13} M, EIS)
K$_4$Fe(CN)$_6$/ K$_3$Fe(CN)$_6$	EIS, amperometry	Au	PA/PC/maleimide-PE/chol (220 ± 20 nm)	DNA[45]	Sandwich	10^{-5}–10^{-12} M (1 × 10^{-12} M, EIS) 10^{-9}–10^{-13} M (1 × 10^{-13} M, EIS)

Appendix A: Abbreviations

SWV: square-wave voltammetry

CV: cyclic voltammetry

DPV: differential pulse voltammetry

SECM: scanning electrochemical microscopy

LSV: linear sweep voltammetry

EIS: electrochemical impedance spectroscopy

CCCP: constant-current chronopotentiometry

GCE: glass carbon electrode

SPCE: screen-printed carbon electrode

Au: gold disc electrode

Pt: platinum disk electrode

IUDA: interdigitated ultramicroelectrode array

ISE: ion-selective electrode

DPPC: dipalmitoylphosphatidylcholine

Chol: cholesterol

DPPG: dipalmitoylphosphatidylglycerol

GM1: monosialoganglioside

PE–MCC: 1,2-dihexadecanoyl-*sn*-glycero-3-phosphoethanolamine-N-[4-(p-maleimidomethyl)cyclohexanecarboxamide]

DHPE–X–biotin: N-(Biotinoyl)-1,2-dihexadecanoyl-*sn*-glycero-3-phosphoethanolamine, triethylammonium salt

DSPE–PEG2000–amine: 1,2-distearoyl-*sn*-glycero-3-phosphoethanolamine-N-[amino(polyethyleneglycol)-2000] (ammonia salt)

DMPC: dimyristoylphosphatidylcholine

DSPC: distearoylphosphatidylcholine

PSPG: palmitoylstearolphosphatidylglycerol

SOPG: 1-stearoyl-2-oleoyl-*sn*-glycero-3-[phospho-rac-(1-glycerol)] (sodium salt)

Theophylline–PE: theophylline-cap-phosphatidylethanolamine

Theophylline–DPPE: theophylline-cap-dipalmitoylphosphatidylethanolamine

PC: phosphatidylcholine

DCP: dicetylphosphate

PE: phosphatidylethanolamie

DPPE: 1,2-dipalmitoylphosphoethanolamine

lyso–PPC: lyso-palmitoylphosphatidylcholine

LPC: L-α-phosphatidylcholine

DMPE: dimyristoylphosphatidylethanolamine

DHPE–X–biotin: N-(Biotinoyl)-1,2-dihexadecanoyl-*sn*-glycero-3-phosphoethanolamine, triethylammonium salt

PA: phosphatidic acid

POPG: 1-palmitoyl-2-oleoyl-*sn*-glycero-3-[phospho-rac-(1-glycerol)]

N–biotinyl Cap–PE: 1,2-dipalmitoyl-*sn*-glycero-3-phosphoethanolamine-N-(CapBiotinyl)

DOTAP: 1,2-dioleoyl-3-trimethylammoniumpropane

Maleimide-PE: maleimide-phosphatidylethanolamie

DOPE: 1,2-dio-leoyl-*sn*-glycero-3-phosphoethanolamine

CEA: carcinoembriyonic antigen

PSA: prostate specific antigen

References

1. Bangham A, Horne R. Negative staining of phospholipids and their structural modification by surface-active agents as observed in the electron microscope. *J Mol Biol.* 1964; 8(5): 660-IN610.

2. Finean J, Rumsby M. Negatively stained lipoprotein membranes. *Nature.* 1963; 200(4913): 1340–1340.

3. Bangham A, Horne R. Action of saponin on biological cell membranes. *Nature.* 1962; 196: 952–953.

4. New RR. *Liposomes: A Practical Approach.* Vol 58. Oxford University Press, USA; 1990.

5. Ullman EF, Tarnowski T, Felgner P, Gibbons I. Use of liposome encapsulation in a combined single-liquid reagent for homogeneous enzyme immunoassay. *Clin Chem.* 1987; 33(9): 1579–1584.

6. Reeves SG, Rule GS, Roberts MA, Edwards AJ, Durst RA. Flow-injection liposome immunoanalysis (FILIA) for alachlor. *Talanta.* 1994; 41(10): 1747–1753.

7. Rule GS, Palmer DA, Reeves SG, Durst RA. Use of protein A in a liposome-enhanced flow-injection immunoassay. Paper presented at: *Anal. Proc.* 1994.

8. Edwards AJ, Durst RA. Flow-injection liposome immunoanalysis (FILIA) with electrochemical detection. *Electroanalysis.* 1995; 7(9): 838–845.

9. Lee M, Durst RA. Determination of imazethapyr using capillary column flow injection liposome immunoanalysis. *J Agric Food Chem.* 1996; 44(12): 4032–4036.

10. Viswanathan S, Wu L-C, Huang M-R, Ho J-A. Electrochemical immunosensor for cholera toxin using liposomes and poly(3, 4-ethylenedioxythiophene)-coated carbon nanotubes. *Anal Chem.* 2006; 78(4): 1115–1121.

11. Viswanathan S, Rani C, Vijay Anand A, Ho J-A. Disposable electrochemical immunosensor for carcinoembryonic antigen using ferrocene liposomes and MWCNT screen-printed electrode. *Biosensors Bioelectron.* 2009; 24(7): 1984–1989.

12. Liao W-C, Ho J-A. Attomole DNA electrochemical sensor for the detection of *Escherichia coli* O157. *Anal Chem.* 2009; 81(7): 2470–2476.

13. Ho J-A, Chiu J-K, Hong J-C, Lin C-C, Hwang K-C, Hwu J-RR. Gold-nanostructured immunosensor for the electrochemical sensing of biotin based on liposomal competitive assay. *J Nanosci Nanotechnol.* 2009; 9(4): 2324–2329.

14. Ho J-A, Hsu W-L, Liao W-C, et al. Ultrasensitive electrochemical detection of biotin using electrically addressable site-oriented antibody immobilization approach via aminophenyl boronic acid. *Biosensors Bioelectron.* 2010; 26(3): 1021–1027.

15. Ho J-A, Jou AF-J, Wu L-C, Hsu S-L. Development of an immunopredictor for the evaluation of the risk of cardiovascular diseases based on the level of soluble P-selectin. *Methods.* 2012; 56(2): 223–229.

16. Tien CY, Jou AF-J, Fan NC, Chuang MC, Ho J-A. Preparation of liposomal progesterone and its application on the measurement of progesterone interpreted via electrochemical and colorimetric sensing platforms. *Electroanalysis.* 2013; 25(4): 1017–1022.

17. Mercadal M, Domingo JC, Bermudez M, Mora M, de Madariaga MA. N-Palmitoylphosphatidylethanolamine stabilizes liposomes in the presence of human serum: Effect of lipidic composition and system characterization. *Biochimica et Biophysica Acta (BBA): Biomembranes.* 1995; 1235(2): 281–288.

18. Ueno T, Tanaka S, Umeda M. Liposome turbidimetric assay (LTA). *Adv Drug Del Rev.* 1997; 24(2): 293–299.

19. Siebert TA, Reeves SG, Roberts MA, Durst RA. Improved liposome immunomigration strip assay for alachlor determination. *Anal Chim Acta.* 1995; 311(3): 309–318.

20. Roberts MA, Durst RA. Investigation of liposome-based immunomigration sensors for the detection of polychlorinated biphenyls. *Anal Chem.* 1995; 67(3): 482–491.

21. Axelsson B, Eriksson H, Borrebaeck C, Mattiasson B, Sjögren H. Liposome immune assay (LIA). Use of membrane antigens inserted into labelled lipid vesicles as targets in immune assays. *J Immunol Methods.* 1981; 41(3): 351–363.

22. Ho J-A, Wauchope R. A strip liposome immunoassay for aflatoxin B1. *Anal Chem.* 2002; 74(7): 1493–1496.

23. Esch MB, Baeumner AJ, Durst RA. Detection of cryptosporidium parvum using oligonucleotide-tagged liposomes in a competitive assay format. *Anal Chem.* 2001; 73(13): 3162–3167.

24. Locascio-Brown L, Plant AL, Horvath V, Durst RA. Liposome flow injection immunoassay: Implications for sensitivity, dynamic range, and antibody regeneration. *Anal Chem.* 1990; 62(23): 2587–2593.

25. Locascio-Brown L, Plant A, Chesler R, Kroll M, Ruddel M, Durst R. Liposome-based flow-injection immunoassay for determining theophylline in serum. *Clin Chem.* 1993; 39(3): 386–391.

26. Esch MB, Locascio LE, Tarlov MJ, Durst RA. Detection of viable cryptosporidium parvum using DNA-modified liposomes in a microfluidic chip. *Anal Chem.* 2001; 73(13): 2952–2958.

27. Kwakye S, Baeumner A. A microfluidic biosensor based on nucleic acid sequence recognition. *Anal Bioanal Chem.* 2003; 376(7): 1062–1068.

28. Kannuck RM, Bellama JM, Durst RA. Measurement of liposome-released ferrocyanide by a dual-function polymer modified electrode. *Anal Chem.* 1988; 60(2): 142–147.

29. Ahn-Yoon S, DeCory TR, Baeumner AJ, Durst RA. Ganglioside-liposome immunoassay for the ultrasensitive detection of cholera toxin. *Anal Chem.* 2003; 75(10): 2256–2261.

30. Wongkaew N, He P, Kurth V, Surareungchai W, Baeumner AJ. Multi-channel PMMA microfluidic biosensor with integrated IDUAs for electrochemical detection. *Anal Bioanal Chem.* 2013; 405(18): 5965–5974.

31. Zhan W, Bard AJ. Scanning electrochemical microscopy. 56. Probing outside and inside single giant liposomes containing Ru(bpy)32+. *Anal Chem.* 2006; 78(3): 726–733.

32. Haga M, Itagaki H, Sugawara S, Okano T. Liposome immunosensor for theophylline. *Biochem Biophys Res Commun.* 1980; 95(1): 187–192.

33. Haga M, Sugawara S, Itagaki H. Drug sensor: Liposome immunosensor for theophylline. *Anal Biochem.* 1981; 118(2): 286–293.

34. Wu T-G, Durst RA. Liposome-based flow injection enzyme immuno-assay for Theophylline. *Microchim Acta.* 1990; 100(3–4): 187–195.

35. Qu B, Guo L, Chu X, Wu D-H, Shen G-L, Yu R-Q. An electrochemical immunosensor based on enzyme-encapsulated liposomes and biocatalytic metal deposition. *Anal Chim Acta.* 2010; 663(2): 147–152.

36. Genç R, Murphy D, Fragoso A, Ortiz M, O'Sullivan CK. Signal-enhancing thermosensitive liposomes for highly sensitive immunosensor development. *Anal Chem.* 2010; 83(2): 563–570.

37. Guan H, Zhang F, Yu J, Chi D. The novel acetylcholinesterase biosensors based on liposome bioreactors–chitosan nanocomposite film for detection of organophosphates pesticides. *Food Res Int.* 2012; 49(1): 15–21.

38. Yan J, Guan H, Yu J, Chi D. Acetylcholinesterase biosensor based on assembly of multiwall carbon nanotubes on to liposome bioreactors for detection of organophosphates pesticides. *Pestic Biochem Physiol.* 2013; 105(3): 197–202.

39. Alfonta L, Singh AK, Willner I. Liposomes labeled with biotin and horseradish peroxidase: A probe for the enhanced amplification of antigen–antibody or oligonucleotide–DNA sensing processes by the precipitation of an insoluble product on electrodes. *Anal Chem.* 2001; 73(1): 91–102.

40. Alfonta L, Willner I, Throckmorton DJ, Singh AK. Electrochemical and quartz crystal microbalance detection of the cholera toxin employing horseradish peroxidase and GM1-functionalized liposomes. *Anal Chem.* 2001; 73(21): 5287–5295.

41. Sapper A, Reiss B, Janshoff A, Wegener J. Adsorption and fluctuations of giant liposomes studied by electrochemical impedance measurements. *Langmuir.* 2006; 22(2): 676–680.

42. Piedade J, Mano M, Pedroso de Lima M, Oretskaya T, Oliveira-Brett A. Electrochemical sensing of the behaviour of oligonucleotide

lipoplexes at charged interfaces. *Biosensors Bioelectron.* 2004; 20(5): 975–984.

43. Bhuvana M, Narayanan JS, Dharuman V, Teng W, Hahn JH, Jayakumar K. Gold surface supported spherical liposome–gold nano-particle nano-composite for label free DNA sensing. *Biosensors Bioelectron.* 2013; 41(0): 802–808.

44. Patolsky F, Lichtenstein A, Willner I. Electrochemical transduction of liposome-amplified DNA sensing. *Angew Chem, Int Ed.* 2000; 39(5): 940–943.

45. Patolsky F, Lichtenstein A, Willner I. Electronic transduction of DNA sensing processes on surfaces: Amplification of DNA detection and analysis of single-base mismatches by tagged liposomes. *J Am Chem Soc.* 2001; 123(22): 5194–5205.

Chapter 7

Coupling Liposome-Encapsulated Nucleic Acids with the Polymerase Chain Reaction: A Generic Assay Platform for High-Sensitivity Analyte Detection

David L. Evers,[a] Carol B. Fowler,[a] Timothy J. O'Leary,[b] and Jeffrey T. Mason[a]

[a]Research Service, VA Maryland Healthcare System, Baltimore, Maryland 21201, USA
[b]Office of Research and Development, Veterans Health Affairs, Washington DC 20002, USA

jeffrey.mason2@va.gov

The accurate quantification of proteins at low concentrations over a wide dynamic range is needed to identify biological toxins and biomarkers associated with diseases and proteins captured by high-throughput microarrays used in proteomics. In this chapter, we describe an ultrasensitive and quantitative generic assay format called liposome-polymerase chain reaction (LPCR). LPCR uses liposomes with ganglioside or antibody (Ab)-binding receptors on their outer surface that bind biological toxins and antigens (Ags), respectively. These liposomes encapsulate DNA templates to serve as analyte surrogates that can be quantified by real-time polymerase chain reaction (PCR). Ganglioside-based

Liposomes in Analytical Methodologies
Edited by Katie A. Edwards
Copyright © 2016 Pan Stanford Publishing Pte. Ltd.
ISBN 978-981-4669-26-9 (Hardcover), 978-981-4669-27-6 (eBook)
www.panstanford.com

LPCR (gLPCR) assays for cholera and botulinum toxins were several orders of magnitude more sensitive than current detection methods. Likewise, Ab-based LPCR (immunoliposome-PCR or ILPCR) detected carcinoembryonic antigen (CEA), HIV-1 p24 core protein, and plasminogen activator inhibitor type-1 (PAI-1) with greatly improved sensitivities and dynamic ranges compared to current assays for these analytes.

7.1 Introduction

The ability to accurately quantify proteins such as biological toxins and disease biomarkers at low concentrations over a wide dynamic range is important in clinical medicine and many fields within the life sciences.[1-4] For example, botulinum neurotoxin type A (BoNT/A) protein is the most lethal human toxin known, with a 50% lethal human dose of approximately 1 ng/kg. This is approximately 100 billion times more toxic than cyanide.[5] Thus, assays for biological toxins must be not only highly specific but also highly sensitive, with the ability, in some applications, to detect toxins down to the level of a few hundred molecules. Other examples include the detection of proteins in microgram tissue specimens isolated by laser capture microdissection[6] and the detection of proteins in nanoliter sample volumes used in high-throughput proteomic microarrays.[7] Disease biomarkers such as HIV-1 p24 core protein, interleukins, Abs to Lyme disease, and troponins released due to cardiovascular disease are present at very low levels in circulation. Conventional enzyme-linked immunosorbent assay (ELISA)[8,9] methods are inadequate to accurately quantify these proteins over a wide dynamic range at this level of sensitivity.[10] New and improved bioanalytical methods are needed to rise to the challenge of miniaturization. To this end, we present methods for high-sensitivity detection assays[11-13] with particular emphasis on gLPCR and ILPCR.

7.2 Methods for High-Sensitivity Detection Assays

High-sensitivity analyte detection assays currently available follow one of two general formats: signal-based amplification or target-based amplification.[14] Signal-based amplification increases the measurable output that results from fixed binding events. Sandwich ELISA is the standard for signal-based amplification. The generic sandwich ELISA has four steps. First, a capture Ab is adsorbed to a microwell plate. Second, samples are added and the nonspecifically bound material is washed away. Third, a second Ab, which is tagged with an enzyme reporter moiety, is added. Fourth, the enzyme amplifies the binding signal by catalysis. Target-based amplification produces many copies of the analyte prior to detection by conventional unamplified means. PCR[15] is the standard for target-based amplification.

Emerging biodiagnostic assays frequently employ advances in biomaterials and microfabrication techniques. For example, carbon nanotubes and silicon nanowires produce electrical signals and show limits of detection (LOD) of low femtomolar (fM) to high picomolar (pM) concentrations.[14,16] The most common electrochemical biosensors employ amperometric detection coupled to binding events, such as Ab–Ag interactions.[17] Electrochemical detection continues to develop with nanomaterials, such as gold nanoparticles, magnetic particles, and quantum dots for detection.[18] Detection limits at the fM range are possible with immunoassays that are coupled to mass spectrometry. However, the equipment is expensive and throughput is typically low. The same drawbacks apply to the highly sensitive surface plasmon resonance and surface-enhanced Raman scattering methods. Gains in sensitivity, specificity, multiplexing, and throughput suggest that some of these technologies will eventually replace the ELISA and PCR standards for target- and signal-based amplification bioanalytical detection.[14] Two detection methods that obtain their specificity from Ab–Ag binding and produce their signal with PCR are immuno-PCR (iPCR) and LPCR. The following sections describe both methods, focusing on our own work with gLPCR and ILPCR.

7.2.1 Immuno-PCR Method

PCR is highly sensitive, capable of detecting the equivalent of a needle in a haystack and amplifying it into quantities that can be productively manipulated by those with minimal laboratory skills.[15] The method of iPCR[19-21] combines the specificity of Ab–Ag binding with PCR amplification for Ag quantification. Specifically, iPCR follows a direct sandwich ELISA immunoassay format where a capture Ab and blocking reagent are added to an assay plate well followed by the sample solution containing the Ag of interest. After rinsing to remove the sample solution, a second Ab specific to the target Ag is added. In colorimetric ELISA, an enzyme, such as alkaline phosphatase, is covalently coupled to the second Ab and detection is achieved by enzymatic generation of a chromogenic reagent. In iPCR, the enzyme is replaced by a nucleic acid segment (typically 70–120 base pairs in length) and detection is achieved by quantitative PCR amplification of the Ab-coupled nucleic acid segment. Two methods are used to couple nucleic acids to the second Ab. The first is a covalent attachment in which a free amine on the 5′-end of the nucleic acid is coupled to a free thiol on the Ab by a bifunctional coupling agent such as succinimidyl-4-(N-maleimidomethyl)cyclohexyl-1-carboxylate.[20] In the second method, a 5′-biotinylated nucleic acid segment is coupled to a biotinylated second Ab through a streptavidin bridge. This method is referred to as universal iPCR.[22] Coupling can occur prior to the addition of the second Ab to the assay solution, or the coupling step can take place as part of the assay following the addition of the second Ab to the assay plate well. The detection limits of an ELISA converted to an iPCR assay often improve 100- to 10,000-fold.[20]

Yet there are limitations to iPCR. First, the most sensitive iPCR assays use covalently coupled reporter DNA–Ab conjugates.[23,24] The preparation and purification of these conjugates require expertize in protein conjugation chemistry, is time consuming, and can result in low yields of the conjugate.[25] Second, in most iPCR assay formats, there are no more than a few nucleic acid reporters coupled to each Ab, which makes detection of low copy number targets difficult in many specimens due to matrix effects, including the presence of polymerase inhibitors. Third, even when amplification is successful, a large and time-consuming number of amplification cycles are necessary to produce enough DNA to allow for reliable detection of the amplified product. Fourth, in all current iPCR methods, the nucleic acid reporter of the conjugate is exposed to the assay solution, rendering it indistinguishable from nonspecific reporters that can arise from incomplete purification of the conjugates and inadvertent contamination during the iPCR assay procedure. Contamination of samples with extraneous DNA is a critical concern for samples with low DNA copy number, particularly outside a controlled laboratory environment. This nonspecific reporter contamination is likely to be the source of the high and variable background signals that are common in the negative controls of iPCR assays.[23,26-28] Recent advances in iPCR technology, such as commercial coupling reagents and nanoparticle conjugation strategies, show great promise.[20] However, iPCR remains elegant in design but difficult in implementation.

7.3 Liposome-PCR

At its simplest, the LPCR method is an iPCR assay where the nucleic acid segment coupled directly to the second Ab has been replaced with 60–400 free nucleic acid segments encapsulated inside a 100 nm diameter unilamellar liposome. The outer bilayer surface of the liposome can incorporate receptor molecules, such as gangliosides, that bind directly to the target Ag, replacing the second Ab altogether. Alternatively, biotin can be conjugated to the outer surface of the liposome and attached to a biotinylated second Ab through a streptavidin bridge, analogous to universal iPCR. LPCR links each Ag-binding event to dozens of templates for PCR (amplicons) that are measured by real-time quantitative PCR (qPCR). The output data are readily understood and quantifiable. Excepting this novel reporter, the features of sandwich ELISA are preserved in gLPCR and ILPCR. A representation of the gLPCR assay format is shown in Fig. 7.1.

LPCR presents specific binding ligands on the surface of liposomes and offers a number of improvements upon ELISA, iPCR, PCR, and other technologies. First, coupling binding ligands to reporters is simplified because the amplicon reporters and lipid-based binding ligands spontaneously incorporate into the nascent liposomes. Second, encapsulating 60–400 copies of the amplicon per liposome overcomes the effects of not only PCR inhibitors but also stochastic events at low Ag concentrations.[29,30] Third, the multiple binding moieties per liposome increase the avidity of the detection reagent. Fourth, and perhaps most importantly, encapsulation allows specific and nonspecific amplicons to be distinguished. Consequently, nonspecific DNA in the assay well can be degraded by DNase I without disturbing the specific amplicons encapsulated within the liposomes. The DNase I is inactivated by heat prior to the rupture of the liposomes by detergent, releasing the amplicons for quantification by qPCR. This approach also simplifies purification because rigorous removal of all unencapsulated DNA reporters from the liposome preparation is unnecessary. These features translate to increased signal and reduced noise.

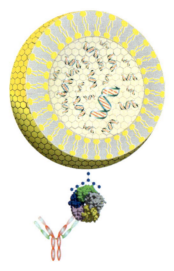

Figure 7.1   Representation of a ganglioside liposome detection reagent in cross section.[11,31] The dsDNA reporters (green with red bars) are encapsulated by the bilayer (yellow) into which a ganglioside receptor (blue) has been incorporated. The pentameric toxin subunit is shown immobilized by a capture Ab, which provides specificity to the assay. (Reprinted with permission from Ref. [11], Copyright 2006, Macmillan Publishers Ltd. http://www.nature.com/nbt/journal/v24/n5/full/nbt1201.html)

7.3.1   Ganglioside-Based Liposome-PCR

Gangliosides are ceramide-based lipids conjugated to oligosaccharides that terminate in negatively charged sialic acid residue(s) (Chapter 1, Fig. 1.7). These amphipathic molecules are ubiquitous components of biological membranes where some are cellular receptors for bacterial and other toxins. Monosialoganglioside GM1 is a ligand for cholera toxin and *Escherichia coli* heat-labile enterotoxin. Trisialoganglioside GT1B is a ligand for BoNT/A.[31] Dye-encapsulating liposomes decorated with these gangliosides have apparent dissociation constants (K_D) of approximately 10^{-8} for their respective toxins in solution.[32] Our first formulation of LPCR exposed ganglioside ligands on liposomes that encapsulated PCR amplicons.[11,33] A detection complex consisting of a GM1-liposome bound to cholera toxin β subunit (CTBS) immobilized by a capture (primary) Ab is shown in Fig. 7.1. The steps associated with this direct sandwich gLPCR assay are shown in Fig. 7.2. In the first step (Fig. 7.2a), a capture Ab specific to CTBS is added to a microtiter plate well followed by bovine serum albumin (BSA), which serves as a blocking agent. In the second step (Fig. 7.2b), the sample solution is added allowing CTBS to bind to the capture Abs. The well is then rinsed to remove the remaining solution. In the third step (Fig. 7.2c), liposomes with encapsulated nucleic acid amplicons and ganglioside GM1 embedded in the outer bilayer leaflet are added, which bind to the capture-Ab-immobilized CTBS. Small 20 nm diameter empty phospholipid vesicles, produced by sonication, are added to reduce nonspecific binding of the detection liposomes. The well is then rinsed to remove unbound liposomes and vesicles. In step four (Fig. 7.2d), nonspecific nucleic acids in the plate well are degraded by the addition of DNase I. Specifically bound amplicons are protected from degradation by virtue of their encapsulation inside the liposomes. Brief heating at 80°C inactivates the DNase I without disrupting the liposomes. The plate well is then rinsed. Nonspecific nucleic acids can arise from the sample solution, incomplete removal of amplicons during liposome purification, and liposomes that rupture prematurely in the plate well. In step five (Fig. 7.2e), the specifically bound liposomes are ruptured by detergent (Triton X-100), which serves to release the amplicons into the assay solution. In step six (Fig. 7.2f), an aliquot of the assay solution is quantified using qPCR by plotting fluorescence intensity versus cycle number followed by determination of the cycle threshold (Ct). A plot of Ct values determined from samples of known CTBS concentration allows the construction of a calibration curve from which unknown sample CTBS concentrations can be determined.

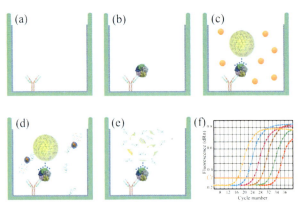

Figure 7.2 A summary of the important steps of the gLPCR assay format. (a) Addition of a CTBS-specific capture antibody to a microtiter plate well followed by the addition of bovine serum albumin (blue hatched lines) as a blocking agent. (b) Addition of the sample solution allowing immobilization of CTBS by the capture antibody followed by the removal of excess sample solution. (c) Addition of detection liposomes (yellow) with encapsulated amplicons and ganglioside GM1 (blue) embedded in the outer bilayer leaflet. The GM1 binds to CTBS immobilizing the liposome detection reagent. Empty 20 nm diameter phospholipid vesicles (orange), prepared by sonication, are added to reduce liposome nonspecific binding. (d) Nonspecific nucleic acids are degraded by the addition of DNase I. The enzyme is then denatured by heating at 80°C for 10 min and removed by rinsing of the plate well. (e) The liposomes are ruptured with detergent (Triton X-100), which releases the specifically bound amplicons into the assay solution. (f) An aliquot is taken from the plate well and the concentration of amplicons is determined by qPCR. The cycle threshold (Ct) is the cycle number corresponding to the point where the PCR amplification probe fluorescence crosses the detection threshold (orange horizontal line).

The field of gene therapy led the technology of DNA encapsulation into liposomes. Gene therapy is intended to deliver nucleic acids such as plasmids, single-stranded antisense oligodeoxynucleotides (ODN), or small interfering RNA (siRNA) to cells and organisms.[34] The specifications of most liposomes designed for gene therapy include slightly positive zeta potential (net surface charge) and efficient nucleic acid encapsulation percentages prior to purification. Liposome diameters of approximately 100 nm and coatings such as gangliosides and poly(ethylene glycol) (PEG) are intended to control the pharmacokinetics of gene transfer reagents.[35] The liposome parameters designed for gene therapy do not necessarily apply to liposomal detection reagents. What matters in LPCR is optimal signal to noise. The desired outcome is strong signal-generating reagents with maximal specific binding and minimal nonspecific binding. The qPCR reporters for LPCR liposome encapsulation are double-stranded DNA amplicons that serve only as a PCR amplification surrogate for the detection and quantification of the corresponding analyte; thus, the specific sequence is not critical. In general, the template should be less than 100 base pairs in length to maximize encapsulation into the liposomes and consist of a sequence not likely to be found in the samples being analyzed. Optimally, LPCR liposomes are formulated to maximize encapsulated amplicon after purification with a minimum of residual unencapsulated nucleic acid.[11,12,33] Liposome size must be empirically determined for optimal specific binding under various assay conditions. It is preferable that the liposomes are homogeneous in size and that their binding properties are adapted to the polystyrene microplate wells used in the gLPCR and ILPCR assays.

The first LPCR liposome detection reagents that we reported[11,33] were prepared by first assembling small unilamellar liposomes (SUVs) composed of the lipids 1,2-dioleoyl-*sn*-glycero-3-phosphocholine (DOPC) and rhodamine-1,2-dihexadecyl-*sn*-glycero-3-phosphoethanol amine (rhodamine-DHPE), which is a lipid-conjugated dye used for lipid quantification, and ganglioside in a molar ratio of 92:6:2. The SUVs were prepared by probe-tip sonication. The method of Bailey and Sullivan,[36] reminiscent of the classical calcium-phosphate method for transfection of mammalian cells, was used to encapsulate the DNA amplicons. The lipids were dried to a film, rehydrated in dilute neutral buffer, and sonicated. An 84-mer β2-microglobulin (β2m) DNA amplicon was mixed with the SUVs and 1.5 volumes of a solution of 8 mM $CaCl_2$ in 79% ethanol was carefully added. Following the removal of ethanol by dialysis, the liposomes were purified by elution from Sepharose CL-4B to remove the unencapsulated amplicons.

Characterization of the liposomes consists of determining the total lipid and DNA concentrations, the quantity of encapsulated and unencapsulated DNA, and the size of the liposomes. Rhodamine-DHPE is included in the liposomes to facilitate the determination of lipid concentration. Its concentration is measured by absorption at 560 nm following the addition of a 25 μL aliquot of the liposome solution to 1.5 mL of methanol and 20 μL of 0.1 N NaOH using an extinction coefficient of 95,000 M^{-1}/cm.[32] The total lipid concentration is then determined from the mol% rhodamine-DHPE in the lipid mixture used to prepare the liposomes. The total DNA concentration is measured by mixing a 25 μL aliquot of the liposome solution with 350 μL of 1 M NaCl and 1.125 mL of chloroform/methanol (2:1, v/v). The upper aqueous phase is removed by careful pipetting, and the absorbance of the reporter DNA is then read at 260 nm. The absorbance and the extinction coefficient of the reporter yield the total reporter concentration. The relative distribution of reporter DNA in free solution versus that encapsulated inside the liposomes is determined with a fluorescence assay using the DNA intercalating dye TO-PRO-1.[33] The fluorescence intensity I_1 of the intact liposome solution is measured at 532 nm using an excitation of 514 nm. The liposomes are then ruptured with Triton X-100 followed by incubation at 37°C for 15 min. The fluorescence intensity I_2 is measured again as described above. The ratio of the two fluorescence measurements yields the fraction of free (I_1/I_2) and encapsulated $[1 - (I_1/I_2)]$ reporters. The actual DNA concentrations are determined by combining the fractional distribution with the total DNA concentration, as determined above. The encapsulated DNA is then normalized to the total lipid concentration to yield the mmol of encapsulated reporter per mole total lipid. The hydrodynamic diameter of the liposomes is determined by dynamic light scattering.[12] Typical parameters for the ganglioside-containing liposome detection reagents are shown in Table 7.1. These values were calculated assuming that the liposomes were homogeneous, unilamellar vesicles 120 nm in diameter.[33,37]

Liposome stability during storage at 4°C is assessed by repeating the measurements described above. The TO-PRO-1 assay is used to determine the rate of leakage of amplicons from the liposomes. Dynamic light scattering is used to look for changes in liposome size, such as osmotic swelling, changes in liposome polydispersity, and the formation of liposomal aggregates. Loss of ganglioside can be assessed using a fluorescence-based assay for free sialic acid residues following their hydrolysis by neuraminidase.[33] Liposome aggregates or amplicons lost through leakage can be removed by gel filtration.[22] The ganglioside-based liposomes are stable for about 6 months when stored at 4°C.

Table 7.1   Parameters of the ganglioside-based detection liposomes[a]

Parameter	Value ± SD
Hydrodynamic diameter	115 ± 8 nm
Ganglioside receptors/liposome[b]	2,600 ± 130
Reporter amplicons/liposome	62 ± 9
Phospholipids/liposome	109,000 ± 7,600

[a]Parameters were determined using measurements from three replicate preparations of the liposome detection reagent.[33]
[b]The ganglioside concentration was measured as described by Hikita et al.[38] using *N*-acetylneuraminic acid as a standard.
SD is standard deviation.

The primary Ab intended to capture/immobilize toxin from the sample solution requires some optimization. Purchasing and evaluating different monoclonal and/or polyclonal Abs are the most costly and time-consuming tasks associated with LPCR assay development. Nonspecific protein binding is blocked with BSA. Samples and controls are added to the wells, and nonspecific liposome binding is blocked with SUVs composed of DOPC. The liposome detection reagent is then added. One hour later, the wells are washed and unencapsulated DNA is degraded with DNase I solution, followed by enzyme inactivation at 80°C for 10 min. The detection liposomes are stable during this short high-temperature incubation. Alternatively, the DNase I can be inactivated by the addition of EDTA to remove calcium from the digestion solution. Results using these two methods were found to be equivalent. Encapsulated reporters are then released by lysing the liposomes with Triton X-100 detergent. An aliquot from each microtiter plate well is added to a PCR reaction mixture, and the samples are analyzed by qPCR.

Serial dilutions of BoNT/A in deionized water were measured by gLPCR. A plot of the average Ct values for the serial dilutions versus the log of the number of BoNT/A molecules per microplate well is shown in Fig. 7.3. The LOD (defined as the average Ct value of the blank minus three times the standard deviation of the blank) is 12 ± 4 molecules of BoNT/A (0.1 attomolar or 0.02 fg/mL). The assay was linear over approximately five orders of magnitude. The slope of the linear regression fit of the data was −0.632 (r^2 = 0.998).[11,33] Thus, the gLPCR assay for BoNT/A has outstanding sensitivity but modest resolution.

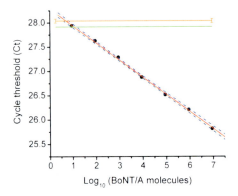

Figure 7.3   Plot of the average serial dilution cycle threshold (Ct) values versus the log of the number of molecules per plate well for triplicate measurements of BoNT/A in deionized water.[11,33] The concentration range of BoNT/A was 10^{-14} to 10^{-19} M. The solid black circles are the average Ct values. The solid red line is a linear regression fit (r^2 = 0.999) to the average Ct values, and the dashed blue lines are the upper and lower 95% confidence limits. The solid horizontal orange line denotes the average blank Ct value, with the standard deviation of the blank drawn at each end of this line. The solid horizontal green line intersecting the linear regression line indicates the LOD of the LPCR assay.

7.3.1.1   Matrix effects

Since samples are likely to be found in biological matrices, we examined matrix effects upon gLPCR detection of toxins. gLPCR assays were performed on a specimen of field runoff water collected from a local farm and spiked with CTBS. The plot for this assay is shown in Fig. 7.4. The LOD for the runoff water specimen is 377 ± 168 molecules of CTBS (0.75 fg/mL). The assay dynamic range is almost five orders of magnitude. The slope of the linear regression fit of the data is −1.02 (r^2 = 0.998).[11,33]

Since human stool is a frequent source of cholera testing in a clinical setting, we examined the effect on gLPCR quantification of a fixed concentration of toxin in different dilutions of fecal matter. In contrast to environmental water and buffer, Fig. 7.5 shows that feces significantly affected the detection of CTBS by gLPCR. This serves as a reminder that controls and standards are best prepared in the same matrix as the analyte.

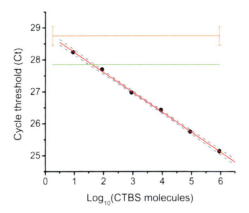

Figure 7.4   Result of a gLPCR assay of cholera toxin beta subunit in farm runoff water.[11] The lines and symbols are described in the legend to Fig. 7.3.

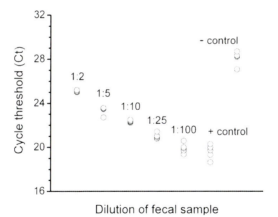

Figure 7.5   The effect of feces matrix on gLPCR quantification of CTBS [D.L. Evers and J.T. Mason, unpublished data]. With the exception of the negative controls, every sample had 100 pg/mL CTBS. Dilutions of fecal matter into buffer are indicated. For example, 1:5 corresponds to 20% (v/v) reconstituted feces in buffer. Positive control indicates buffer alone. Open circles indicate actual data points ($n = 5$).

The performance of gLPCR in biologically relevant matrices was tested in comparison to that of a standard assay for CTBS. At the time of these studies, the *Vibrio cholerae* enterotoxin and *E. coli* heat-labile enterotoxin reversed passive latex agglutination (VET-RPLA) kit (Oxoid) was the only commercially available test for CTBS. The VET-RPLA assay is the gold standard because it has been validated, its detection limits (1 to 2 ng/mL) are essentially the same as can be obtained by modern ELISAs,[39,40] and its sensitivity is equal to those of PCR and classical microbiological methods.[41,42] Table 7.2 shows the performance of gLPCR quantification of CTBS compared to that of VET-RPLA in environmental water and reconstituted fecal matter.[43]

Ganglioside-based LPCR offers several advantages over current biotoxin detection methods.[11,43] First, derivatization of the reporter or ganglioside receptors is not required; the reporter is freely encapsulated inside the liposomes as they are formed. Likewise, the ganglioside receptors, which are components of biological membranes, spontaneously partition into the bilayer as the liposomes are formed. This greatly simplifies the preparation and purification of the detection reagent. Second, the use of qPCR, rather than end point PCR, improves the quantitative accuracy of the assay; it also allows for improved precision by performing replicate measurements on the samples and applying statistical treatment to the data. Third, gLPCR displays 100–1000 times greater sensitivity than previous assays for biological toxins (Table 7.3). This is due, in part, to the multiple reporters per binding event and the low nonspecific binding of the liposome detection reagents. Fourth, sequestration of the reporters inside the liposomes offers two distinct advantages. The reporters are protected from chemical or enzymatic degradation by impurities present in the sample that are incompletely removed during the wash steps. The more important advantage of encapsulating the reporters is that DNase I can be used to degrade any contaminating DNA present in the microtiter plate wells immediately before the rupture of the liposomes by detergent. Thus, DNA contamination from the assay environment, from incomplete purification of the liposome detection reagents, from carryover by pipette tips or plate washer nozzles, or genomic DNA contamination remaining from the samples can all be eliminated. This substantially reduces the possibility of false positive results and improves the sensitivity and precision of the assay.

Table 7.2   Effect of matrix on the lower limits of cholera toxin quantified

Matrix	Dilution	gLPCR assay[a] LOD	gLPCR assay[a] FLOD[b]	VET-RPLA assay[a] LOD	VET-RPLA assay[a] FLOD[b]
Buffer alone		<1	<1	800 ± 180	600–1,000
Hydrated feces	1:100	1 ± 0.2[c]	80–120	1,400 ± 650[c]	75,000–210,000
	1:10	2 ± 0.9[c]	10–30	4,100 ± 940[c]	32,000–50,000
	1:5	3 ± 2	5–30	ND	ND
	1:2	30 ± 10[c]	40–80	9,300 ± 2,200[c]	14,000–23,000
Environmental water	9:10	< 1	< 1.1	ND	ND
	1:2	ND	ND	2,000 ± 1,800	400–7,600

[a]All parameters are in units of pg/mL.
[b]Factored LOD (FLOD) ranges are (detection limit ± SD) × dilution factor. Absolute detection amounts can be calculated as detection limit × dilution factor × assay volume (100 and 50 μL for gLPCR and VET-RPLA, respectively).
[c]Analyses of the detection limits of the 1:2, 1:10, and 1:100 dilutions of feces between the gLPCR and VET-RPLA assays were carried out using the two-tailed, homoscedastic Student's t-test, which showed $P < 0.01$.
ND is no data available.
Source: From Ref. [43].

Table 7.3   Comparison of biotoxin assay methods[a]

Assay method	Detection threshold	Assay time
Cholera toxin beta subunit		
ELISA-liposome[32]	23-70 ng/mL	24 h
Fluorescence immmunoassay[44]	10–100 ng/mL	20 min
iPCR	None identified	—
LPCR[11,33]	0.02 ng/mL	3 h
Botulinum neurotoxin type A		
ELISA-HRP[45]	4–8 pg/mL	4–6 h
Mouse lethality assay[46]	6 pg/mL	1–2 d
Flow immunoassay[47]	15 pg/mL	20 min
iPCR[48]	50 fg/mL	4–6 h
LPCR[11,33]	0.02 fg/mL	3 h

[a]Details on the performance of the listed assay methods can be found in the indicated literature references.

7.3.2 Biotin-PEG-Based Liposome-PCR

Ganglioside-based LPCR is specific to ganglioside ligands. Ab-based LPCR potentially expands the detectable ligands to any analyte for which an Ab is available. Previous studies in liposome-based drug and gene delivery provide a variety of strategies to present Abs on liposomes. Abs can be directly coupled to phospholipid anchors that spontaneously partition into the liposome bilayer. These include phosphatidylethanolamine (PE) and PE conjugated to spacers such as PEG. A number of straightforward coupling chemistries exist for linking whole Abs, or Fab' fragments, to these phospholipid anchors (Chapter 2).[49,50] Commercial biotinylated Ab can be linked to liposomes via an avidin bridge to biotin-presenting liposomes.

We developed ILPCR, a generic ultrasensitive quantitative Ag detection format, to overcome the disadvantages of iPCR and to expand upon the applications of our ganglioside-based LPCR assay format. The ILPCR detection reagent encapsulates DNA reporters and has biotin-labeled PEG phospholipid conjugates (Fig. 7.6) incorporated into the outer bilayer leaflet.

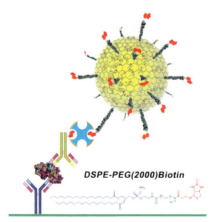

DSPE-PEG(2000)Biotin

Figure 7.6 The ILPCR assay format.[12] The Ag (purple, brown, and blue) is bound to an immobilized capture Ab (blue and red) and a biotinylated second Ab (green and red). The liposome detection reagent (yellow) is coupled to the biotinylated second Ab through a neutravidin bridge (aqua and brown). The biotin-PEG phospholipids are shown as PEG polymers (solid green) terminating in biotin molecules (red). Encapsulated DNA reporters (green with red bars) are shown inside the liposome.

The ILPCR assay follows the same sandwich ELISA format as gLPCR. The target is immobilized in microplate wells by a capture Ab followed by the addition of a biotinylated second Ab. The biotin-labeled liposome detection reagent is then coupled to the second Ab through a neutravidin bridge. This bridge is possible because avidin and its homologs, streptavidin and neutravidin, are tetrameric proteins. Each of the four subunits has its own biotin-binding site. This avidin bridge linking scheme is also employed in universal iPCR, the most widely used iPCR format.[22]

The ILPCR liposome detection reagent was prepared by a modification of the method introduced by Semple et al.[51] for the encapsulation of antisense RNA into liposomes using cationic lipids. ILPCR liposomes were formulated with 1,2-distearoyl-*sn*-glycero-3-phosphocholine (24.5 mol%), 1,2-dioleoyl-3-dimethylammoniumpropane (25 mol%), cholesterol (45 mol%), 1,2-distearoyl-*sn*-glycero-3-phosphoethanolamine-*N*-[methoxy (polyethylene glycol) 2000] (4.75 mol%), rhodamine-DHPE (0.5 mol%), and 1,2-distearoyl-*sn*-glycero-3-phospho ethanolamine-*N*-[biotinyl-(polyethylene glycol)2000] (0.25 mol%). Lipid films were taken up in pH 4.0 buffer to protonate amines, and then subjected to freeze–thaw cycles and extrusion through 0.1 micron filters. The unilamellar liposome suspension was slowly taken to 40% (v/v) ethanol, and reporter DNA (12 µg/mg total lipid) was then added. First the ethanol and then the acid were removed by dialysis against pH 7.4 buffer. Unencapsulated reporter DNA was removed by ion-exchange gel filtration on DEAE-Sepharose CL-6B. The liposomes encapsulated ~220 reporters/liposome and about 800 biotin sites/liposome were present on the bilayer surface. Parameters of the ILPCR liposomes are shown in Table 7.4. The detection liposome preparation method was reproducible, particularly when the rate, mixing, and temperature of ethanol addition were standardized.

The following components were evaluated to determine their effect on ILPCR assay performance: the type of microtiter plate, the blocking agents, capture and biotin-labeled second Abs, the Ab coating solution, the blocking reagents, the incubation and wash buffers, the type of avidin derivative used, and the properties of the liposome detection reagent.[12] Once the optimal components were identified, the following parameters were evaluated to optimize ILPCR assay performance: the concentration of all assay components, the number of blocking steps, all incubation times and temperatures, the number of wash steps and cycles performed, and the ionic strength of the wash buffers. The final concentrations of the biotin-labeled second Ab, the neutravidin, and the liposome detection reagent were optimized by the iterative method described by Wu et al.[52] for streptavidin-based iPCR assays.

Table 7.4   Parameters of the immunoliposome detection reagent[a]

Parameter	Value
Hydrodynamic diameter[b]	117 ± 20 nm
Exposed biotin/lipid molar ratio[c]	5.1 ± 0.2 mmol/mol
Reporter DNA/lipid molar ratio[d]	2.1 ± 0.4 mmol/mol
CV of liposome reagent reproducibility[e]	6%
Liposome reagent stability[f]	1.5 years at 4°C

[a]Parameters were determined using measurements from four replicate preparations of the liposome detection reagent.[12]
[b]The hydrodynamic diameter of the liposomes was determined by dynamic light scattering using a volume-weighted Gaussian size distribution.
[c]The average number of biotin molecules exposed on the surface of the liposomes was estimated using a 4'-hydroxyazobenzene-2-carboxylic acid-avidin displacement quantification assay and the total lipid concentration. The total lipid concentration was determined from the absorbance of rhodamine-DHPE.
[d]The ratio of reporter DNA to total lipid, where the reporter concentration was measured by its absorbance at 260 nm.
[e]The CV for the reproducibility of the liposome detection reagent preparation was determined from the four replicate preparations by measuring the Ct value associated with equal concentrations of total lipid.
[f]The liposome detection reagent stability was defined as the length of time the liposomes could be stored at 4°C without observing a reduction in either the LOD or dynamic range.

Various combinations of the assay components were assessed for their effect on the nonspecific background signal of the ILPCR assay with results shown in Fig. 7.7. Column A was the result of an ILPCR assay that contained all assay components except the liposome detection reagent, which was equivalent to a no-template control (Ct = 37.2). Column B reflected the nonspecific binding of the liposome detection reagent as the only components present were the capture Ab and the two blocking agents, BSA and casein (Ct = 36.1). Column C was the result of an ILPCR assay that contained all of the assay components except the second Ab. It represented the additional contribution of neutravidin to the background signal (Ct = 34.7). Column D was the result of an ILPCR assay with all of the assay components except the Ag (Ct = 31.6), which represented the true assay control (blank). Column E was a repeat of the control assay of column D, but with no DNase I digestion step (Ct = 28.2). The results of this study revealed that the nonspecific background signal of the ILPCR assay resulted from the cumulative effect of all of the assay components, with nonspecific binding of the biotin-labeled second Ab having the greatest effect. The study also revealed that the implementation of a DNA digestion step significantly reduced both the intensity and variability (standard deviation) of the nonspecific background signal.

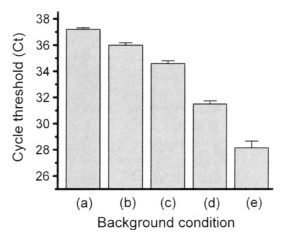

Figure 7.7 Effect of different reagents on the background of the ILPCR assay.[12] Various combinations of the assay reagents were assessed for their effect on the nonspecific background signal (noise) of the ILPCR assay. (a) All assay reagents minus the liposome detection reagent. (b) All assay reagents minus the antigen, the biotin-labeled second antibody, and the neutravidin. (c) All assay reagents minus the second antibody. (d) All assay reagents minus the antigen, which represents the true assay blank. (e) All assay reagents minus the antigen (as in d), but with no DNase I digestion step.

To demonstrate the applicability of ILPCR to clinical diagnostics, we adapted the method to measure CEA, a tumor marker used in the clinical management of gastrointestinal carcinomas.[53] A titration series was prepared by adding recombinant human CEA to CEA-negative human serum. The mean Ct value and the standard deviation of these samples, the blank, and the controls were calculated using the three replicate measurements from the qPCR analysis. Two blocking steps were used: the first (BSA) prior to the addition of Ag and the second (casein) prior to the addition of the liposomes. Controls were run for the lysis buffer, water, and PCR reaction mixture, including primers and probes, in addition to the no-template control. Desired Ct values for these controls are greater than 35. The three blanks should have a mean Ct value ≥ 30, with the preferred value being 31–32. A mean blank Ct value less than 30 could indicate contamination of one of the reagents. A standard curve was constructed from the samples by plotting the average Ct values versus the log of the Ag concentration. The linear region of the dose–response curve was identified by visual inspection and subjected to a linear regression analysis along with the calculation of the 95% confidence limits. The assay threshold, which was defined as the average Ct value of the blank minus three times the standard deviation of the blank,[52] was then determined. This value defined the minimum detectable concentration (MDC) of the assay. The assay LOD is defined as the lowest concentration of analyte that is both within the linear region of the dose–response curve and below the assay threshold.

The result of this assay is shown in Fig. 7.8, and the performance characteristics of the assay are given in Table 7.5. The linear region of the dose–response curve extended from 10^{-10} to 10^{-16} M (six orders of magnitude). The LOD was 10^{-16} M, which corresponds to 13 fg/mL of CEA or 6,023 molecules of CEA in a 100 μL serum sample. This LOD was >1,500 fold lower than the best clinically approved RIA[54-56] and ELISA[56-58] tests for CEA, while iPCR assays for CEA in serum samples[59,60] reported an LOD $\geq 900,000$ molecules and a dynamic range of 10^3. The ILPCR assay results were independent of serum dilution, demonstrating the insensitivity of the assay to matrix effects.

The dose–response curve in Fig. 7.8 flattened abruptly at the high concentration end of the curve. This was likely due to the formation of a monolayer of liposomes over the surface of the plate well, preventing further binding of liposomes to immobilized Ag.[32]

In contrast, the low concentration end of the curve did not flatten but instead displayed a second linear region with significantly reduced slope. This second linear region is characteristic of iPCR-based immunoassays,[52,61] and it defines the MDC of the ILPCR assay, which was 10^{-17} M or ~600 molecules of CEA (1.3 fg/mL).

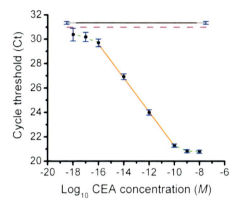

Figure 7.8   Quantitative ILPCR dose–response curve for CEA added to CEA-negative human serum.[12] A 100 μL sample volume (CEA serially diluted in CEA-negative human serum) was used for all concentrations. The black circles are the average of three replicate Ct measurements over a concentration range of 10^{-8} M to 10^{-18} M CEA; the standard deviation of the Ct values are shown as blue vertical bars. The orange line is the linear regression fit of the data. The green dotted lines are the outliers of the dose–response curve. The solid red line is the average Ct value of the blank with the standard deviation shown in blue at each end of this line. The blank Ct value was plotted as a line rather than a single point for ease of visualization. The dashed magenta line is the detection threshold of the assay, which is defined as the average Ct value of the blank minus three times the standard deviation of the blank.

The performance of this ILPCR assay was compared to that of other published high-sensitivity CEA assay formats in Table 7.6. ILPCR had an LOD eight times lower and dynamic range 1,000 times greater than the next most sensitive assay. The only published iPCR assays for CEA[59,60] had LODs that were 150 fold less sensitive than the ILPCR assay. Thus, the advantages offered by the ILPCR assay format result in overall assay performance statistics that exceed those of the iPCR assay formats.

Table 7.5   Characteristics of the ILPCR assay for CEA in human serum

Parameter	Value
CV of repeatability[a]	6% (10^{-16} M)
CV of reproducibility[a]	1.8% (10^{-16} M)
Linear regression coefficient (r^2)[b]	0.998
Dynamic range	10^{-10} M to 10^{-16} M
Detection threshold (Ct)[c]	30.99
LOD[d]	10^{-16} M (13 fg/mL)
Precision at LOD[e]	~2,850 molecules
Sensitivity[f]	87% (10^{-16} M)
Specificity[g]	100%
CV of reagent reproducibility[h]	<8%

[a]Coefficient of variance (CV).

[b]The indicated value is the linear regression coefficient resulting from the fit of the linear region of the dose–response curve shown in Fig. 7.8.

[c]The detection threshold (MDC) is a measure of the noise level of the assay and is defined as the average Ct of the blank (all assay components except the Ag) minus three times the standard deviation of the blank.

[d]The LOD is defined as the lowest concentration within the linear region of the dose–response curve that is greater than or equal to the detection threshold.

[e]The assay precision at the LOD was estimated by determining the number of molecules in the 100 µL sample (6,023) and the associated upper and lower 95% confidence limits, which yielded values of 7,498 (+25%) and 4,650 (−23%) molecules, respectively. These values were taken from Fig. 7.8. Thus, in the range of 1,000 to 10,000 molecules, the assay precision yields a minimal distinguishable difference of ~2,850 molecules.

[f]The assay sensitivity is based on the series of eleven ILPCR assays (n = 11) performed for CEA in human serum.

[g]The specificity was determined using multiple samples derived from a single CEA-negative human serum reference specimen; therefore, the specificity must be taken as preliminary.

[h]The CV of reagent reproducibility was determined by measuring the Ct associated with an equal concentration of liposomes from four identical preparations of the detection reagent.

Source: From Ref. [12].

Additional controls were performed on the CEA ILPCR assay because false positive results could arise from the failure of the DNase I treatment to digest all non-encapsulated nucleic acid. False negative results could be from the failure to rupture the liposomes, PCR inhibitors, or faulty PCR reagents. Two additional

PCR amplicons were prepared to serve as these controls: F(+), an 89 base-pair reporter from rat GRIP1 and F(−), an 81 base-pair reporter from the tobacco mosaic virus 126 kDa coat protein.[33] F(+) was employed as naked DNA. F(−) was encapsulated in liposomes formulated without biotin. Both controls are added to the assay wells of the microtiter plate immediately prior to DNase I digestion.

Table 7.6 Comparison of the dynamic range and LODs for different CEA assay formats

Assay format	Range (ng/mL)	LOD (pg/mL)[a]
Radioimmunoassay[54–56]	5–320	5000
Chemiluminescence[62,b]	1–25	500
Microarray fluorescence sensor[63,c]	0.16–9.4	400
Time-resolved fluorescence[64,d]	1–560	280
Electrochemiluminescence[65,e]	0.21–2000	200
Colorimetric ELISA[56–58]	0.05–50	20
Immuno-PCR[59,60]	0.01–100	10
Surface-enhanced Raman[66,f]	0.001–0.1	1
Nanowire sensor array[67,g]	0.001–1	0.1
ILPCR[12]	0.000013–13	0.013

[a]For the listed assays, the LOD is generally defined as the lowest CEA concentration on the dose–response curve greater than or equal to the blank minus three times the standard deviation of the blank (see the individual references for details).

[b]Flow injection chemiluminescence immunoassay using a CEA-immobilized immunoaffinity column to capture free HRP-anti-CEA Abs remaining after incubation with CEA-containing serum.

[c]Sandwich immunoassay using capture Abs immobilized on microarrays based on the self-assembly of DNA–protein conjugates. CEA is quantified using the fluorescence signal generated from fluorophores conjugated to the detection (second) Ab.

[d]Sandwich immunoassay where time-resolved fluorescence emission from a europium-labeled second Ab quantified CEA immobilized by a capture Ab.

[e]Immunoassay where a electrochemiluminescence signal measured CEA labeled with ruthenium (II) binding to capture Abs immobilized on the surface of an electrode in a competitive assay with unlabeled CEA in serum.

[f]Immunoassay in which surface-enhanced Raman scattering intensity is used to detect CEA bound to capture antibodies conjugated to hollow gold nanosphere magnetic particles.

[g]Immunoassay where a conductive signal is generated when CEA binds to capture Abs immobilized on silicon nanowires fabricated into field-effect transistor sensors.

Source: From Ref. [12].

Figure 7.9 shows that Ct values for all reporters were equivalent to the no-template control (Ct ≥ 35) when the DNase treatment was performed after the rupture of the liposomes (white bars). Normal assay conditions showed background signal for naked DNA, but amplified both encapsulated amplicons (gray bars). When the DNase I digestion step was omitted, all three reporters were amplified (dark gray bars).[12] This suggested that no obvious false positive or false negative artifacts contributed to the normal assay.

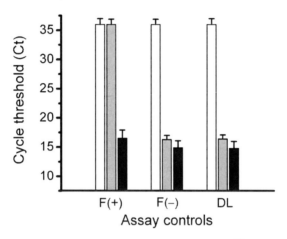

Figure 7.9 Performance of the ILPCR assay controls.[12] F(+): naked DNA GRIP1 reporter; F(−): TMV reporter encapsulated inside liposomes lacking biotin; DL: standard detection liposomes. White columns: Ct values obtained when liposomes were ruptured prior to DNase I digestion. Gray columns: Ct values obtained under normal assay conditions (DNase I digestion followed by heat deactivation) prior to rupture of the liposomes. Dark gray columns: Ct values obtained in the absence of DNase I digestion.

In order to demonstrate the applicability of ILPCR to other Ab–Ag complexes, the assay was performed using Abs to HIV-1 p24 core protein.[12] A titration series was prepared by adding recombinant HIV-1 p24 to phosphate-buffered saline (PBS). The mean Ct value and the standard deviation of the dilution series, the blank, and the controls were calculated using three replicate measurements from the qPCR analysis. The result of this assay is shown in Fig. 7.10.

The dose–response curve showed a primary linear region extending from 10^{-9} to 10^{-13} M with a slope of -1.5 ΔCt per log change in concentration, followed by a secondary linear region with a reduced slope of -0.5 ΔCt per log change in concentration that extended from 10^{-13} to 10^{-17} M. Both linear regions exhibited a dynamic range of four orders of magnitude. The LOD taken from the primary linear region was 10^{-13} M, which corresponds to 2.4 pg/mL of p24 or ~6 million molecules of p24 in a 100 μL sample. There are ~3,000 p24 molecules per HIV-1 virion particle[27]; thus, the LOD can be restated as 20,000 virions/mL. The MDC taken from the secondary linear region of the dose–response curve was 10^{-17} M, which corresponds to 0.24 fg/mL of p24 or ~600 molecules of p24 per 100 μL sample.

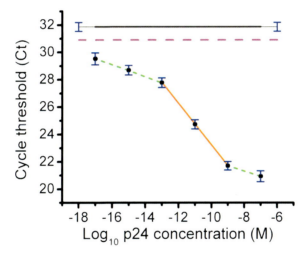

Figure 7.10 Quantitative ILPCR dose–response curve for p24 added to PBS.[12] A 100 μL sample volume (Ag diluted in PBS) was used for all concentrations. The black circles are the average of three replicate Ct measurements over a concentration range of 10^{-7} to 10^{-17} M p24; the standard deviations of the Ct values are shown as blue vertical bars. In order to be visible, the standard deviations were multiplied by the following values: 10^{-7} M (3x), 10^{-9} M (1x), 10^{-11} M (5x), 10^{-13} M (5x), 10^{-15} M (7x), and 10^{-17} M (1x). The remaining symbols and colors have the same designations as those in Fig. 7.8.

Within the limits imposed by Poisson statistics, this is sufficient to detect the p24 present in 2 virions/mL, which is 500 times more sensitive than the best ELISA assays for p24.[68,69] It remains to be seen if the performance of the ILPCR p24 assay is realized in actual clinical serum samples that require the disruption of the virion particles by acid or heat treatment to release the p24 core protein from p24 auto-antibodies typically present in patient serum samples.[69,70]

PAI-1 has been validated at the highest level of evidence as a clinical biomarker of prognosis in breast cancer.[71,72] Clinically, levels of PAI-1 and its target, urokinase-type plasminogen activator (uPA), in breast tumor tissue are used to decide whether patients with newly diagnosed node-negative breast cancer can forgo adjuvant chemotherapy. The sole validated method for quantifying uPA and PAI-1 levels in breast tumor tissue is a colorimetric ELISA assay that takes three days to complete and has an LOD of about 125 pg/mL of tissue extract.[73,74] This LOD translates into a requirement for 100–300 mg of breast tumor tissue.[74] The requirement for at least 100 mg of tissue exceeds the capabilities of most fine-needle biopsy techniques used in clinical practice and imposes a lower limit on the size of analyzable tumors that is well above the detection limit of radiological methods.

We recently developed an assay that combines pressure-cycling technology to extract PAI-1 from breast tumor tissue with an ILPCR assay for the quantification of PAI-1 in the tissue extract.[13] Following total protein extraction from 600 mg of breast tumor tissue, the validated ELISA assay (Sekisui Diagnostics, LLC, Lexington, MA) was performed on tissue extracts equivalent to 100 mg and 150 mg of breast tumor tissue. This colorimetric assay uses the binding of streptavidin-conjugated horseradish peroxidase (HRP) to a biotinylated anti-PAI-1 second Ab for quantification. The results are plotted as the two square symbols in Fig. 7.11a. ILPCR assays for PAI-1 were then carried out on tissue extracts equivalent to 100 mg, 50 mg, 5 mg, and 1 mg of breast tumor tissue. The ILPCR assay was conducted using the commercial ELISA assay by substituting neutravidin and biotin-labeled detection liposomes in place of the streptavidin–HRP conjugate followed by qPCR quantification. The results are plotted as the round symbols in Fig. 7.11a.

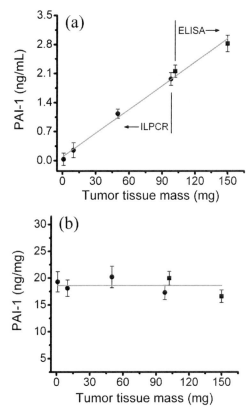

Figure 7.11 Assay of PAI-1 in human breast tumor tissue extracts.[13] (a) Conventional ELISA and ILPCR assays of PAI-1 concentration in total protein extracts equivalent to 1 to 150 mg of tumor tissue. Total protein extracts were prepared by conventional overnight stirring at 4°C for the ELISA assay and by pressure-assisted protein extraction for the ILPCR assay. (b) The PAI-1 values plotted after being normalized to the total protein concentration of the corresponding tissue extracts. Results from the ELISA assay are shown as black squares, and results from the ILPCR assay are shown as black dots. Standard deviations are shown as horizontal blue bars. The lines show the linear regression fit of the data.

The ILPCR assay reduced the required amount of breast tumor tissue for PAI-1 quantification down to 1 mg. The LOD for the ILPCR assay was 1 pg/mL and the dynamic range was 10,000; 100 fold greater than that of the ELISA assay. The PAI-1 concentrations from Fig. 7.11a were normalized to the total protein concentration of the extracts and re-plotted in Fig. 7.11b. The linearity of Fig. 7.11a,b clearly shows that the ILPCR assay can accurately quantify PAI-1 levels in tissue extracts from as little as 1 mg of breast tumor tissue. This mass is compatible with fine-needle biopsy procedures used in clinical practice and small tumors detectable by radiology. In addition, the total assay time is reduced from three days for the ELISA assay to one day for the ILPCR assay using the pressure-cycling extraction method.[13] The reduction in assay time arose from both the extraction and assay steps. Although pressure cycling did not increase the yield of extractable PAI-1, the extraction time was reduced from 18 to 2.5 h. Assay time was reduced by about 18 h because the ELISA assay required an overnight incubation of the protein extract at 4°C for optimal sensitivity. The ILPCR assay achieved satisfactory sensitivity using a 1 h incubation at 37°C.

7.3.3 Advantages of ILPCR Analytical Approach

The ILPCR assay described here was designed to mitigate the two major shortcomings of iPCR, specifically the difficulty in preparing the detection reagent conjugates and the difficulty in controlling reporter DNA contamination during the assay. The ILPCR liposome detection reagent has a long shelf-life, and its preparation requires minimal skills and equipment. In contrast to iPCR, chemical coupling of the DNA reporter to an Ab to form a conjugate is not required. The DNA reporters and biotin-labeled PEG phospholipids spontaneously incorporate into the liposomes as they form, thus simplifying the preparation of the detection reagent. The incorporation of PEG phospholipids in the outer leaflet of the liposomes also reduces nonspecific binding. The Ct values for DNA-containing liposomes applied directly to the microtiter plate are ~35. These were substantially the same values as the no-template control (Ct = 35–40). The Ct value decreased only slightly (Ct values were 30–32) in the assay blanks, which contained all of the assay components except Ag.[12] Finally, unlike gold, silver, magnetic, or carbon-tube nanoparticle-based assays, the liposomes used in ILPCR are nontoxic and biodegradable nanotechnology. The ILPCR liposome detection reagent is designed to be universal and can be adapted to detect any analyte by simply substituting appropriate capture and biotin-labeled detection reagents. Little optimization appears to be required. For example, it required only 2 weeks to optimize an ILPCR assay with an MDC of 10^{-17} M for the detection of the HIV-1 p24 viral capsid protein in buffer.[12]

In addition to minimal nonspecific binding, the use of liposomes as a detection reagent confers several additional advantages to the ILPCR assay. First, encapsulation of the DNA reporters inside the liposomes allows contaminating nonspecific DNA reporters to be degraded with DNase I prior to quantification of the encapsulated specific DNA reporters by qPCR. This unique DNase I digestion strategy also eliminates genomic DNA contamination in the test specimens that could compete with reporter amplification by nonspecific hybridization of the primers.[75] This capability, not possible with iPCR, simplifies the preparation of test specimens and significantly reduces the noise level in the negative assay controls, thus reducing the stringency required to perform the ILPCR assay. This makes the ILPCR assay format amenable to personnel without extensive experience in PCR techniques or access to PCR-compliant laboratory facilities. Second, the ability to encapsulate more than 100 DNA reporters per liposome leads to a pre-amplification factor, which increases the sensitivity of the assay and helps overcome matrix effects, including the effect of polymerase inhibitors frequently present in biological specimens.[76] This further reduces the need for extensive sample processing or dilution. Third, each liposome has more than 1,000 biotin molecules exposed on its outer bilayer surface, which increases the sensitivity of the assay by increasing the avidity of the detection reagent.[32] Above we show proof of concept that ILPCR can be conducted as a multiplex qPCR assay that allows for the inclusion of endogenous positive and negative PCR controls.[77]

In conclusion, ILPCR is a novel ultrasensitive protein assay format that successfully ameliorates the two major limitations of iPCR, which are the inherent difficulties in preparing the detection reagents and in controlling nonspecific reporter DNA contamination. ILPCR is also universal and can be readily adapted to detect any protein for which specific high-avidity binding molecules are available. Because ILPCR is easier to perform than iPCR, it is amenable to researchers in a wide spectrum of disciplines, including researchers not highly experienced in PCR. ILPCR holds particular promise as a powerful new diagnostic method for clinical medicine.

7.4 Future Perspectives

A variety of modifications to the liposome formulation are possible. Some may improve ILPCR assay performance. The current ILPCR biotin-liposomes are generic in that they can be used as detection reagents for any avidin-labeled or biotin-avidin bridged analyte. Universal liposomes tagged with avidin are an approach that conserves this feature.[78] The conjugate spacer between liposomes and biotin may be explored. Likewise, smaller amplicons may allow for greater numbers of encapsulated reporters.

Highly purified and uniform liposome-encapsulated amplicons may prove useful. Maurer et al.[79] reported predominant liposome species from the method we employed to prepare ILPCR liposomes: ~80% monolamellar vesicles with high PEG content, but low DNA concentrations and ~15% multilamellar vesicles with high DNA concentrations, but minimal PEG content. Our immunoliposome formulation may be improved by additional chromatography followed by reconstitution to achieve the optimal concentration of PEG-lipids and the greatest amount of encapsulated DNA. Others reported carefully controlled ethanol–lipid mixing, temperature, and dialysis conditions that gave reproducibly homogeneous plasmid-encapsulating liposomes on an industrial scale.[80]

For every useful sandwich Ab pair, there can be a specific ILPCR assay. Developing and perhaps benefitting from general principles for selecting candidate Abs may facilitate new assay targets. For example, Ab indicated for ELISA could often be applicable to ILPCR. Aptamers could substitute for Abs. Binding strategies other than the sandwich ELISA format may be explored. Additional multiplexing capabilities may prove useful. Assay multiplexing could be accomplished by direct attachment of Abs to the liposomes and coding these to the encapsulated DNA. Digital PCR detection may aid sensitivity and versatility to ILPCR. These and other investigations into ILPCR could enhance the dynamic range and sensitivity of protein assays.

Acknowledgments

T. J. O'Leary and J. T. Mason are listed as inventors on United States patents 7,582,430 and 7,662,568 covering the liposome detection reagent preparation and LPCR assay technology described in this chapter. The assignee on these patents is the United States of America as represented by the Secretary of the Army and/or the Secretary of Veterans Affairs. This work was supported by Veterans Health Administration Merit Review Awards VA01-0701207 (T.J.O. & J.T.M.) and 1101BX001092-01 (J.T.M.) and Army Medical Research and Material Command Grant DAMD17-02-1-0178 to J.T.M. The content of this publication does not necessarily reflect the views of the Veterans Health Administration or the Department of Defense, nor does mention of trade names, commercial products, or organizations imply endorsements by the United States Government. There was no support or involvement, financial or otherwise, by any commercial entity in the work described in this chapter.

References

1. Rusling JF, Kumar CV, Gutkind JS, Patel V. Measurement of biomarker proteins for point-of-care early detection and monitoring of cancer. *The Analyst.* 2010; 135(10): 2496–2511.

2. Brody EN, Gold L, Lawn RM, Walker JJ, Zichi D. High-content affinity-based proteomics: Unlocking protein biomarker discovery. *Expert Rev Mol Diagn.* 2010; 10(8): 1013–1022.

3. Roper MG, Guillo C. New technologies in affinity assays to explore biological communication. *Anal Bioanal Chem.* 2009; 393(2): 459–465.

4. Taitt CR, North SH, Kulagina NV. Antimicrobial peptide arrays for detection of inactivated biothreat agents. *Methods Mol Biol.* 2009; 570: 233–255.

5. Gill DM. Bacterial toxins: A table of lethal amounts. *Microbiol Rev.* 1982; 46(1): 86–94.

6. Ball HJ, Hunt NH. Needle in a haystack: Microdissecting the proteome of a tissue. *Amino Acids.* 2004; 27(1): 1–7.

7. Stoevesandt O, Taussig MJ, He M. Protein microarrays: High-throughput tools for proteomics. *Expert Rev Proteomics.* 2009; 6(2): 145–157.

8. Engvall E, Perlmann P. Enzyme-linked immunosorbent assay (ELISA). Quantitative assay of immunoglobulin G. *Immunochemistry.* 1971; 8(9): 871–874.

9. Van Weemen BK, Schuurs AH. Immunoassay using antigen-enzyme conjugates. *FEBS Lett.* 1971; 15(3): 232–236.

10. Vignati G, Chiecchio A, Osnaghi B, Giovanelli L, Meloncelli C. Different biological matrices (serum and plasma) utilization in consolidation processes: Evaluation of seven access immunoassays. *Clin Chem Lab Med.* 2008; 46(2): 264–270.

11. Mason JT, Xu L, Sheng ZM, O'Leary TJ. A liposome-PCR assay for the ultrasensitive detection of biological toxins. *Nat Biotechnol.* 2006; 24(5): 555–557.

12. He J, Evers DL, O'Leary TJ, Mason JT. Immunoliposome-PCR: A generic ultrasensitive quantitative antigen detection system. *J Nanobiotechnol.* 2012; 10(1): 26.

13. Fowler CB, Man YG, Mason JT. An ultra-sensitive immunoassay for quantifying biomarkers in breast tumor tissue. *J Cancer.* 2014; 5(2): 115–124.

14. Giljohann DA, Mirkin CA. Drivers of biodiagnostic development. *Nature.* 2009; 462(7272): 461–464.

15. Mullis KB, Faloona FA. Specific synthesis of DNA in vitro via a polymerase-catalyzed chain reaction. *Methods Enzymol.* 1987; 155: 335–350.

16. Sheehan PE, Whitman LJ. Detection limits for nanoscale biosensors. *Nano Lett.* 2005; 5(4): 803–807.

17. Ronkainen NJ, Halsall HB, Heineman WR. Electrochemical biosensors. *Chem Soc Rev.* 2010; 39(5): 1747–1763.

18. Chikkaveeraiah BV, Bhirde AA, Morgan NY, Eden HS, Chen X. Electrochemical immunosensors for detection of cancer protein biomarkers. *ACS Nano.* 2012; 6(8): 6546–6561.

19. Sano T, Smith CL, Cantor CR. Immuno-PCR: Very sensitive antigen detection by means of specific antibody-DNA conjugates. *Science.* 1992; 258(5079): 120–122.

20. Malou N, Raoult D. Immuno-PCR: A promising ultrasensitive diagnostic method to detect antigens and antibodies. *Trends Microbiol.* 2011; 19(6): 295–302.

21. Nakano S, Morizane Y, Makisaka N, et al. Development of a highly sensitive immuno-PCR assay for the measurement of alpha-galactosidase A protein levels in serum and plasma. *PLoS One.* 2013; 8(11): e78588.

22. Zhou H, Fisher RJ, Papas TS. Universal immuno-PCR for ultra-sensitive target protein detection. *Nucleic Acids Res.* 1993; 21(25): 6038–6039.

23. Adler M, Wacker R, Niemeyer CM. Sensitivity by combination: Immuno-PCR and related technologies. *The Analyst.* 2008; 133(6): 702–718.

24. Adler M. Immuno-PCR as a clinical laboratory tool. *Adv Clin Chem.* 2005; 39: 239–292.

25. Niemeyer CM, Adler M, Pignataro B, et al. Self-assembly of DNA-streptavidin nanostructures and their use as reagents in immuno-PCR. *Nucleic Acids Res.* 1999; 27(23): 4553–4561.

26. Banin S, Wilson SM, Stanley CJ. Demonstration of an alternative approach to immuno-PCR. *Clin Chem.* 2004; 50(10): 1932–1934.

27. Barletta JM, Edelman DC, Constantine NT. Lowering the detection limits of HIV-1 viral load using real-time immuno-PCR for HIV-1 p24 antigen. *Am J Clin Pathol.* 2004; 122(1): 20–27.

28. McKie A, Samuel D, Cohen B, Saunders NA. A quantitative immuno-PCR assay for the detection of mumps-specific IgG. *J Immunol Methods.* 2002; 270(1): 135–141.

29. Peccoud J, Jacob C. Theoretical uncertainty of measurements using quantitative polymerase chain reaction. *Biophys J.* 1996; 71(1): 101–108.

30. Myers LE, McQuay LJ, Hollinger FB. Dilution assay statistics. *J Clin Microbiol.* 1994; 32(3): 732–739.

31. Eidels L, Proia RL, Hart DA. Membrane receptors for bacterial toxins. *Microbiol Rev.* 1983; 47(4): 596–620.

32. Singh AK, Harrison SH, Schoeniger JS. Gangliosides as receptors for biological toxins: Development of sensitive fluoroimmunoassays using ganglioside-bearing liposomes. *Anal Chem.* 2000; 72(24): 6019–6024.

33. Mason JT, Xu L, Sheng ZM, He J, O'Leary TJ. Liposome polymerase chain reaction assay for the sub-attomolar detection of cholera toxin and botulinum neurotoxin type A. *Nat Protoc.* 2006; 1(4): 2003–2011.

34. Li W, Szoka FC, Jr. Lipid-based nanoparticles for nucleic acid delivery. *Pharm Res.* 2007; 24(3): 438–449.

35. Fenske DB, Cullis PR. Entrapment of small molecules and nucleic acid-based drugs in liposomes. *Methods Enzymol.* 2005; 391: 7–40.

36. Bailey AL, Sullivan SM. Efficient encapsulation of DNA plasmids in small neutral liposomes induced by ethanol and calcium. *Biochim Biophys Acta.* 2000; 1468(1–2): 239–252.

37. Huang C, Mason JT. Geometric packing constraints in egg phosphatidylcholine vesicles. *Proc Natl Acad Sci U S A.* 1978; 75(1): 308–310.

38. Hikita T, Tadano-Aritomi K, Iida-Tanaka N, et al. Determination of *N*-acetyl- and *N*-glycolylneuraminic acids in gangliosides by combination of neuraminidase hydrolysis and fluorometric high-performance liquid chromatography using a GM3 derivative as an internal standard. *Anal Biochem.* 2000; 281(2): 193–201.

39. Almeida RJ, Hickman-Brenner FW, Sowers EG, Puhr ND, Farmer JJ, 3rd, Wachsmuth IK. Comparison of a latex agglutination assay and an enzyme-linked immunosorbent assay for detecting cholera toxin. *J Clin Microbiol.* 1990; 28(1): 128–130.

40. Jang H, Kim HS, Kim JA, Seo JH, Carbis R. Improved purification process for cholera toxin and its application to the quantification of residual toxin in cholera vaccines. *J Microbiol Biotechnol.* 2009; 19(1): 108–112.

41. Honma Y, Higa N, Tsuji T, Iwanaga M. Comparison of a reversed passive latex agglutination and a polymerase chain reaction for identification of cholera toxin producing *Vibrio cholerae* O1. *Microbiol Immunol.* 1995; 39(1): 59–61.

42. Israil A, Balotescu C, Damian M, Dinu C, Bucurenci N. Comparative study of different methods for detection of toxic and other enzymatic factors in *Vibrio cholerae* strains. *Roum Arch Microbiol Immunol.* 2004; 63(1–2): 63–77.

43. Evers DL, He J, Mason JT, O'Leary TJ. The liposome PCR assay is more sensitive than the *Vibrio cholerae* enterotoxin and *Escherichia coli* heat-labile enterotoxin reversed passive latex agglutination test at detecting cholera toxin in feces and water. *J Clin Microbiol.* 2010; 48(12): 4620–4622.

44. Ahn-Yoon S, DeCory TR, Baeumner AJ, Durst RA. Ganglioside-liposome immunoassay for the ultrasensitive detection of cholera toxin. *Anal Chem.* 2003; 75(10): 2256–2261.

45. Ekong TA, McLellan K, Sesardic D. Immunological detection of *Clostridium botulinum* toxin type A in therapeutic preparations. *J Immunol Methods.* 1995; 180(2): 181–191.

46. Kautter DA, Solomon HM. Collaborative study of a method for the detection of *Clostridium botulinum* and its toxins in foods. *J Assoc Off Anal Chem*. 1977; 60(3): 541–545.

47. Ahn-Yoon S, DeCory TR, Durst RA. Ganglioside-liposome immunoassay for the detection of botulinum toxin. *Anal Bioanal Chem*. 2004; 378(1): 68–75.

48. Chao HY, Wang YC, Tang SS, Liu HW. A highly sensitive immuno-polymerase chain reaction assay for *Clostridium botulinum* neurotoxin type A. *Toxicon*. 2004; 43(1): 27–34.

49. Manjappa AS, Chaudhari KR, Venkataraju MP, et al. Antibody derivatization and conjugation strategies: Application in preparation of stealth immunoliposome to target chemotherapeutics to tumor. *J Control Release*. 2011; 150(1): 2–22.

50. Sawant RR, Torchilin VP. Challenges in development of targeted liposomal therapeutics. *AAPS J*. 2012; 14(2): 303–315.

51. Semple SC, Klimuk SK, Harasym TO, et al. Efficient encapsulation of antisense oligonucleotides in lipid vesicles using ionizable aminolipids: Formation of novel small multilamellar vesicle structures. *Biochim Biophys Acta*. 2001; 1510(1–2): 152–166.

52. Wu HC, Huang YL, Lai SC, Huang YY, Shaio MF. Detection of *Clostridium botulinum* neurotoxin type A using immuno-PCR. *Lett Appl Microbiol*. 2001; 32(5): 321–325.

53. Bjerner J, Lebedin Y, Bellanger L, et al. Protein epitopes in carcinoembryonic antigen. Report of the ISOBM TD8 workshop. *Tumour Biol*. 2002; 23(4): 249–262.

54. Thomson DM, Krupey J, Freedman SO, Gold P. The radioimmunoassay of circulating carcinoembryonic antigen of the human digestive system. *Proc Natl Acad Sci U S A*. 1969; 64(1): 161–167.

55. Nisselbaum JS, Smith CA, Schwartz D, Schwartz MK. Comparison of Roche RIA, Roche EIA, Hybritech EIA, and Abbott EIA methods for measuring carcinoembryonic antigen. *Clin Chem*. 1988; 34(4): 761–764.

56. Wang WS, Lin JK, Lin TC, et al. EIA versus RIA in detecting carcinoembryonic antigen level of patients with metastatic colorectal cancer. *Hepatogastroenterology*. 2004; 51(55): 136–141.

57. Wang J, Cao Y, Xu Y, Li G. Colorimetric multiplexed immunoassay for sequential detection of tumor markers. *Biosens Bioelectron*. 2009; 25(2): 532–536.

58. Liu M, Jia C, Jin Q, et al. Novel colorimetric enzyme immunoassay for the detection of carcinoembryonic antigen. *Talanta.* 2010; 81(4–5): 1625–1629.

59. Niemeyer CM, Wacker R, Adler M. Combination of DNA-directed immobilization and immuno-PCR: Very sensitive antigen detection by means of self-assembled DNA-protein conjugates. *Nucleic Acids Res.* 2003; 31(16): e90.

60. Ren J, Ge L, Li Y, Bai J, Liu WC, Si XM. Detection of circulating CEA molecules in human sera and leukopheresis of peripheral blood stem cells with *E. coli* expressed bispecific CEAScFv-streptavidin fusion protein-based immuno-PCR technique. *Ann N Y Acad Sci.* 2001; 945: 116–118.

61. Saito K, Kobayashi D, Sasaki M, et al. Detection of human serum tumor necrosis factor-alpha in healthy donors, using a highly sensitive immuno-PCR assay. *Clin Chem.* 1999; 45(5): 665–669.

62. Lin J, Yan F, Ju H. Noncompetitive enzyme immunoassay for carcinoembryonic antigen by flow injection chemiluminescence. *Clin Chim Acta.* 2004; 341(1–2): 109–115.

63. Wacker R, Niemeyer CM. DDI-microFIA—A readily configurable microarray-fluorescence immunoassay based on DNA-directed immobilization of proteins. *ChemBioChem.* 2004; 5(4): 453–459.

64. Hang JF, Wu YS, Yu WH, Huang Y, Li M. Time-resolved fluoroimmunoassay of carcino-embryonic antigen and preparation of its diagnostic reagent. *Xi Bao Yu Fen Zi Mian Yi Xue Za Zhi.* 2006; 22(1): 121–124.

65. Blackburn GF, Shah HP, Kenten JH, et al. Electrochemiluminescence detection for development of immunoassays and DNA probe assays for clinical diagnostics. *Clin Chem.* 1991; 37(9): 1534–1539.

66. Chon H, Lee S, Son SW, Oh CH, Choo J. Highly sensitive immunoassay of lung cancer marker carcinoembryonic antigen using surface-enhanced Raman scattering of hollow gold nanospheres. *Anal Chem.* 2009; 81(8): 3029–3034.

67. Zheng G, Patolsky F, Cui Y, Wang WU, Lieber CM. Multiplexed electrical detection of cancer markers with nanowire sensor arrays. *Nat Biotechnol.* 2005; 23(10): 1294–1301.

68. Wang S, Xu F, Demirci U. Advances in developing HIV-1 viral load assays for resource-limited settings. *Biotechnol Adv.* 2010; 28(6): 770–781.

69. Schupbach J. Measurement of HIV-1 p24 antigen by signal-amplification-boosted ELISA of heat-denatured plasma is a simple and inexpensive alternative to tests for viral RNA. *AIDS Rev.* 2002; 4(2): 83–92.

70. Boni J, Opravil M, Tomasik Z, et al. Simple monitoring of antiretroviral therapy with a signal-amplification-boosted HIV-1 p24 antigen assay with heat-denatured plasma. *AIDS.* 1997; 11(6): F47–52.

71. Schmitt M, Harbeck N, Brunner N, et al. Cancer therapy trials employing level-of-evidence-1 disease forecast cancer biomarkers uPA and its inhibitor PAI-1. *Expert Rev Mol Diagn.* 2011; 11(6): 617–634.

72. Harbeck N, Schmitt M, Meisner C, et al. Ten-year analysis of the prospective multicentre Chemo-N0 trial validates American Society of Clinical Oncology (ASCO)-recommended biomarkers uPA and PAI-1 for therapy decision making in node-negative breast cancer patients. *Eur J Cancer.* 2013; 49(8): 1825–1835.

73. Harris L, Fritsche H, Mennel R, et al. American Society of Clinical Oncology 2007 update of recommendations for the use of tumor markers in breast cancer. *J Clin Oncol.* 2007; 25(33): 5287–5312.

74. Schmitt M, Sturmheit AS, Welk A, Schnelldorfer C, Harbeck N. Procedures for the quantitative protein determination of urokinase and its inhibitor, PAI-1, in human breast cancer tissue extracts by ELISA. *Methods Mol Med.* 2006; 120: 245–265.

75. Chou Q, Russell M, Birch DE, Raymond J, Bloch W. Prevention of pre-PCR mis-priming and primer dimerization improves low-copy-number amplifications. *Nucleic Acids Res.* 1992; 20(7): 1717–1723.

76. Bergallo M, Costa C, Gribaudo G, et al. Evaluation of six methods for extraction and purification of viral DNA from urine and serum samples. *New Microbiol.* 2006; 29(2): 111–119.

77. Lee M, Leslie D, Squirrell D. Internal and external controls for reagent validation. In: Edwards K, Logan J, Saunders N, eds. *Real-Time PCR.* Norfolk, UK: Horizon Bioscience; 2004: 85–101.

78. Edwards KA, Curtis KL, Sailor JL, Baeumner AJ. Universal liposomes: Preparation and usage for the detection of mRNA. *Anal Bioanal Chem.* 2008; 391(5): 1689–1702.

79. Maurer N, Wong KF, Stark H, et al. Spontaneous entrapment of polynucleotides upon electrostatic interaction with ethanol-destabilized cationic liposomes. *Biophys J.* 2001; 80(5): 2310–2326.

80. Jeffs LB, Palmer LR, Ambegia EG, Giesbrecht C, Ewanick S, MacLachlan I. A scalable, extrusion-free method for efficient liposomal encapsulation of plasmid DNA. *Pharm Res.* 2005; 22(3): 362–372.

Chapter 8

Present and Potential Applications for Magnetic Liposomes in Analysis

Katie A. Edwards

Cornell University, Department of Biological and Environmental Engineering, 140 Riley-Robb Hall, Ithaca, New York 14853, USA

kae24@cornell.edu

8.1   Introduction

Particles termed magnetic liposomes or "magnetoliposomes" in the literature span the range from coating solid-core magnetic particles with phospholipid bilayers,[1,2] to encapsulation of solutions of ferromagnetic or paramagnetic materials within the aqueous core,[3,4] to the incorporation of hydrophobic magnetic species within the lipid bilayers.[5] The properties of such species, including degree of magnetization, capacity to carry encapsulants, and biocompatibility, vary significantly.[6] For iron-oxide-based liposomes, maghemite (Fe_2O_3) or magnetite (Fe_3O_4) nanoparticles coated with citrate,[3] dextran derivatives,[7] lauric acid,[8] or oleic acid[5] to improve their dispersion and stability properties are typically utilized. Other paramagnetic species such as gadolinium (Gd^{3+}) and manganese (Mn^{2+}), either encapsulated or bilayer tagged, are also termed magnetic liposomes.[9,10]

Liposomes in Analytical Methodologies

Edited by Katie A. Edwards

Copyright © 2016 Pan Stanford Publishing Pte. Ltd.

ISBN 978-981-4669-26-9 (Hardcover), 978-981-4669-27-6 (eBook)

www.panstanford.com

Liposomes incorporating magnetic species have been investigated as tissue-specific drug-delivery vehicles for chemotherapy.[11–15] In drug-delivery applications, magnetic liposomes loaded with pharmaceutical compounds have been utilized either by placing the affected site within an external magnetic field[16,17] or through implanting a magnet within a tumor in investigational studies.[14] Such liposomes localize at the tumor site directed by the magnetic field and have been successful in terms of both increasing drug efficacy and reducing systemic toxicity of chemotherapeutic agents over free drug or liposomes without encapsulated magnetite.[15] Extensive reviews of the use of magnetic species, including liposomes, in the drug-delivery realm are available.[6,18–21] Other treatment-related applications for magnetic liposomes have included the use for gene delivery[22,23] and suggestion as an affinity matrix with bilayer-embedded HIV receptor proteins to reduce circulating HIV-infected cells.[24]

However, the utility of magnetic liposomes is not limited solely to therapeutic purposes. Liposomes incorporating paramagnetic species have also been investigated as reagents for magnetic resonance imaging (MRI).[25–28] At a very basic level, in MRI, a static magnetic field is applied, followed by a radiofrequency (RF) pulse.[29–32] The static magnetic field orients protons in aqueous components toward the field, with a slightly larger proportion of the protons oriented in the parallel, rather than antiparallel direction. While the net magnetic effect of the bulk of the antiparallel and parallel protons cancels out, there exists a magnetization remaining from the unpaired protons. The RF pulse at a specific frequency causes low-energy parallel-oriented protons to flip to a high-energy antiparallel state and reduces the overall magnetization in the direction of the applied magnetic field. During this process, protons also rotate about their axes, or precess, in the X–Y direction, yielding magnetization 90° from the original field as this rotation occurs in phase. After the RF pulse, the protons return from their high-energy orientation to their low-energy orientation parallel to the magnetic field over what is known as the T1, or longitudinal, relaxation time. After the RF pulse, protons also gradually return to an out-of-phase state, which decreases magnetization in the X–Y direction, over what is known as the T2, or transverse, relaxation time. T1 and T2 relaxation times vary between tissues and are measured with receiver coils. The T1 relaxation time in water is relatively slow as the fast-moving water molecules do not efficiently transfer their energy back to their surroundings, whereas in tissues, transfer is more efficient, hence T1 is shorter. Such differences allow measurements of contrast between tissues. To improve contrast, paramagnetic MRI imaging agents, such as gadolinium (Gd), are employed. These agents contain unpaired electrons, which are influenced by the magnetic field and interact with excited protons. An improvement in transfer of energy to the surroundings results, effectively shortening T1 relaxation times. The term relaxivity refers to the inverse of the relaxation time as a function of contrast agent concentration. The above synopsis provides only a primer on the technology for the purpose of discussion. For a more thorough coverage of MRI imaging, readers are directed to several excellent sources.[29-32]

Liposomes loaded with gadolinium species offer improved MRI contrast, especially in tissues such as the liver and spleen that do not readily accumulate free imaging agents.[33,34] Hydrophilic gadolinium molecules, such as gadolinium diethylenetriamine penta-acetic acid (DTPA, commercially as Magnevist®), have been encapsulated within liposomal aqueous cores while hydrophobic conjugates, such as Gd-DTPA-distearyl ester, have been incorporated into their lipid bilayers.[10,34-36] The signal due to contrast agent encapsulation within liposomes is affected by water permeability across the lipid bilayer, which is dependent on factors such as liposome size, lipid composition, and temperature.[37-39] Increased water exchange across the bilayer yields interactions of protons with the unpaired electrons of Gd^{3+} and greater relaxivity. Chelate-based complexation of Gd^{3+} reduces its otherwise high toxicity, yet its paramagnetism, which stems from its seven unpaired electrons, remains intact. Liposome-based formulations add the benefits of a reduction in nonspecific systemic toxicity, as well as provide an option for increasing the amount of Gd through high levels of encapsulation and thus a high local concentration at the imaging site.[10,34]

While the use of liposomes as paramagnetic medical imaging agents is well established, efforts to develop liposomes capable of dual-purpose imaging are of increasing interest.[40-44] For example, the paramagnetic properties of hydrophobic Gd in the form of 1,4,7,10-tetraazacyclododecane-1,4,7,10-tetraacetic acid (DOTA) conjugated to *N,N*-distearylamidomethylamine (DSA) (Gd-DOTA-DSA) for MRI response with a lipid-based fluorescent label (DOPE-rhodamine) have extended the utility of appropriately formulated liposomes to provide both MRI and fluorescence cellular imaging (Fig. 8.1). Here, embedding the bilayer with paramagnetic species yielded a higher relaxivity than encapsulation hence was more favorable for improved MRI contrast.[40,43] Specificity toward specific targets can be afforded using bilayer-tagged recognition elements, such as antibodies or peptides. In another approach, PEGylated liposomes were prepared with hydrophobic ^{125}I and Gd-DTPA-DPPE to provide trimodal liposomes capable of yielding luminescent, positron emission tomography (PET), and MRI signals (Fig. 8.2).[45]

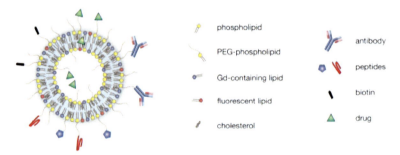

Figure 8.1   Liposome comprising fluorescent and Gd-labeled lipids with targeting possible by antibodies, peptides, or biotin.[40] Reprinted from Ref. [40], Copyright 2010, Strijkers, G., et al. http://www.ncbi.nlm.nih.gov/pmc/articles/PMC2911540/.

Other efforts take advantage of magnetic properties to achieve both imaging and delivery of contents. For example, by using an external magnet to target breast tumors in transgenic mice expressing luciferase, magnetite-encapsulating liposomes delivered the substrate D-luciferin to the tumor site allowing for its selective luminescent imaging.[46] Thermosensitive liposomes encapsulating gadolinium or manganese have been considered a means to monitor temperature changes during thermal therapies as well.[39] While these few examples provide merely an overview, several excellent review articles on magnetic liposomes in medical imaging are available.[47–51]

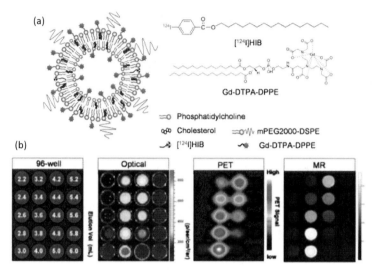

Figure 8.2 (a) Schematic of ^{124}I/Gd-labeled liposomes. (b) Fractions from size-exclusion purification of the liposomes were collected in 96-well plates and assessed using optical, PET, and MR imaging.[45] Reprinted with permission from Ref. [45], Copyright 2014, American Chemical Society. http://pubs.acs.org/doi/abs/10.1021/ml400513g.

8.2   Applications of Magnetic Liposomes in Diagnostics

Findings from the drug delivery and medical imaging realms may be taken advantage of in the in vitro diagnostics realm. A parallel between targeting specific tissue types in drug delivery and targeting specific molecules in bioanalytical applications may be drawn. Similarly, the utility of liposomes to provide a large payload of contents to cells mirrors their utility for analytical amplification. Yet, the combination of biorecognition, capacity for signaling, and ability to be influenced by a magnetic field has largely not been harnessed for in vitro diagnostics. To date, there are relatively few published studies making use of magnetic liposomes for analysis purposes. This chapter will provide a summary of the current state of the art as well as provide parallels from the findings of drug-delivery and medical imaging realms to potential untapped utility for analytical usage.

8.2.1 Controlled Release from Magnetic Liposomes

Various mechanisms have been employed to induce content release from liposomes in a controlled manner. Here, strategies for lysis involving liposomes either directly or indirectly influenced by magnetic fields will be discussed.

8.2.1.1 Thermally induced release from magnetic liposomes

Liposomes composed of a lipid composition with melting temperature slightly above body temperature can be used to deliver encapsulated drug molecules to targeted tissues under hyperthermic conditions. In such applications, it is important to formulate the lipid composition such that the liposomes are largely stable at physiological temperatures but are capable of allowing efficient content release at applied elevated temperatures that do not also cause unintended thermal injury (between 40°C and 43°C).[52] It is also critical that they can yield release within the limited time available for circulation through the elevated temperature region.[53]

Using applied heat generated through RF energy, thermal ablation—or effectively destroying dysfunctional tissue through heating—has long been employed as a strategy for tumor treatment.[54] In the 1990s, rather than drug delivery, investigations ensued using liposomes incorporating magnetic species to instead serve to mediate localized temperature. Early studies utilized phosphatidylcholine/phosphatidylethanolamine-coated magnetite, where the magnetite served to generate heat in tumor tissues in response to an applied magnetic field.[55,56] Coupled with appropriate electrostatic properties or antibody-based targeting, these particles were capable of localized heat-induced tumor cell death while minimizing thermal damage to adjacent tissues.[57-59] A similar strategy was envisioned to thermally inactivate HIV and HIV-infected cells using magnetic liposomes with bilayer-incorporated CD4 receptors.[60]

Liposomes have more recently been engineered to combine the targeting, drug-delivery, and localized-heating strategies. In one strategy, liposomes were prepared with a folic acid and PEG-coated thermosensitive lipid formulation that encapsulated both doxorubicin and iron oxide nanoparticles.[61] A permanent magnet was utilized to direct the liposomes to the target cells, with recognition and specificity conferred by folate receptors. An AC magnetic field was then used to generate hyperthermia and release of pharmaceutical contents at the target cells.

Later efforts focused on liposomal bilayers functionalized with magnetic nanoparticles. For example, oleic-acid-coated superparamagnetic iron oxide (SPIO) nanoparticles were embedded within lipid bilayers, designed to leave the internal volume available to deliver encapsulated drug molecules to tumor tissues in response to an applied alternating RF field.[5,62] Using carboxyfluorescein (CF) as a model encapsulant, Chen et al. demonstrated that the release of liposomal contents due to RF heating could be accomplished via inclusion of 5 nm oleic-acid-maghemite into a DPPC lipid formulation.[5] In their experiments, liposomes with a lipid:nanoparticle ratio of 10,000:1 yielded a marked increase in both the extent and initial rate of CF release with application of RF energy over other formulations (Fig. 8.3). The overall increase in temperature of 6°C from the ambient due to the concomitant heating of the bulk solution was not anticipated to affect DPPC bilayers, which exhibited their main transition temperature at 41.2°C; nor did they experimentally exhibit increased leakage. Here, the inclusion of the oleic acid–nanoparticle conjugates appeared to increase the stability of this formulation, evidenced by minimal CF leakage in the absence of heating and an increase in their transition temperature over DPPC liposomes alone upon heating. This was attributed to changes in the liposomal structure observed at high nanoparticle concentrations, with the appearance of smaller liposomes encapsulated within larger liposomes, and thus less exposed surface area.

Subsequently, Amstad et al. demonstrated that liposomes incorporating iron oxide nanoparticles coated with the lipid palmityl-nitroDOPA could be used to provide triggered release, but with improved stability characteristics.[63] The stability benefits of this formulation stemmed from the inclusion of PEGylated lipids, the increase in the melting temperature above that of normal body temperature, and the use of palmityl-nitroDOPA, rather than oleic acid stabilized iron oxide. The latter species, which has a more stable attachment to iron oxide, was reported to incorporate into lipid bilayers, whereas oleic acid has a tendency to dissociate from the iron oxide and form micelles.[63]

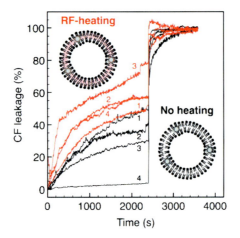

Figure 8.3 Fluorescence measurements over time of liposomes encapsulating carboxyfluorescein with (1) DPPC alone or lipid:nanoparticle ratios of (2) 25,000:1, (3) 10,000:1, and (4) 5,000:1 with RF heating at 250 A and 281 kHz. The results indicated a decrease in spontaneous leakage in the absence of heating with increasing nanoparticle incorporation (black) and an increase in the initial rate and overall release of encapsulant with a lipid:nanoparticle composition of 10,000:1 (red).[5] Once 2400 s elapsed, the surfactant Triton X-100 was added to lyse all remaining liposomes. Reprinted with permission from Ref. [5], Copyright 2010, American Chemical Society. http://pubs.acs.org/doi/abs/10.1021/nn100274v.

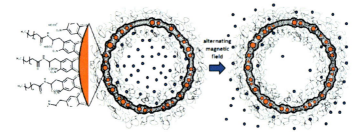

Figure 8.4 Liposome with lipid composition comprising palmityl-nitroDOPA iron oxide nanoparticles, PEGylated fluorescent and Gd-labeled lipids with which yielded release of encapsulated calcein with the application of an alternating magnetic field.[63] Reprinted with permission from Ref. [63], Copyright 2011, American Chemical Society. http://pubs.acs.org/doi/abs/10.1021/nl2001499.

With an applied alternating magnetic field of 230 kHz, liposomes loaded with self-quenching concentrations of calcein exhibited release of contents in a field time-dependent manner, whereas those without iron oxide nanoparticles remained unaffected by the applied field (Fig. 8.4). The release of contents was attributed to a transient change in bilayer permeability due to localized heating above the T_m without loss of liposome structures. By contrast, a significantly greater increase in the bulk temperature of the solution was required to elicit a similar release in the absence of applied magnetic field.

8.2.1.2 Magnet proximity-induced release from liposomes

Rather than bilayer-embedded or encapsulated magnetic species, other platforms rely on the proximity of liposomes to magnetic species. Hanuš et al. recently reported co-entrapping magnetic nanoparticles and carboxyfluorescein-encapsulating liposomes within alginate beads.[64] Investigation of the lipid formulation with respect to cholesterol content led to liposomes that could be stably entrapped within the beads, yet yield an on-demand release of content with a pulsed alternating magnetic field due to localized heating by the co-entrapped magnetic particles. In a similar embodiment, thermosensitive liposomes encapsulating a substrate were co-entrapped with magnetic nanoparticles and an immobilized enzyme within alginate beads. The application of RF energy resulted in the lysis of the thermosensitive liposomes induced by heating of the adjacent magnetic beads. Lysis of the liposomes led to the release of substrate and its subsequent enzymatic conversion.[65]

One challenge with the co-encapsulation approach in alginate beads introduced earlier, as with other lysis strategies relying on magnet-induced heating, is the requirement for a high concentration of affected particles within a limited space. Avoiding this requirement, another strategy utilized a linear chain of magnetic nanoparticles attached to doxorubicin-encapsulating liposomes, forming a ~100 nm long complex.[66] Here, the magnetic tail of the chain translated applied RF energy to mechanical deformation on the attached lipid of the liposomal bilayer, yielding content release. Supporting studies indicated no marked heat generation near the complexes, suggesting this approach yielded release as a function of mechanical oscillations, rather than thermally induced release.

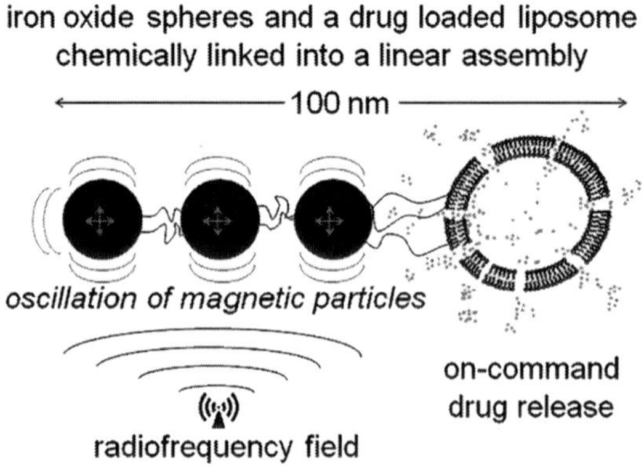

iron oxide spheres and a drug loaded liposome
chemically linked into a linear assembly

Figure 8.5 Magnetic nanoparticle–liposome chains translate RF energy to mechanical oscillation yielding release of liposome-encapsulated contents.[66] Three ~20 nm iron oxide spheres in series with a ~30 nm liposome yielded a ~100 nm assembly. Reproduced with permission from Ref. [66], Copyright 2012, American Chemical Society. http://pubs.acs.org/doi/abs/10.1021/nn300652p.

8.2.1.3 Analytical potential

These studies, among others, demonstrate that the inclusion of bilayer-incorporated magnetic nanoparticles can mediate local temperature and temperature-sensitive content release. In vivo, this approach can allow for thermal ablation and drug delivery while minimizing risk to adjacent tissues. As the magnetic nanoparticles induce local heating of the bilayer, the use of temperature-sensitive lipid formulations, which traditionally have lower T_m, can be avoided with this strategy. This minimizes the risks of nonspecific leakage at physiological temperatures, as well as greater tendency toward lysis during storage. By relying on proximity, rather than direct incorporation of magnetic particles, greater flexibility in the liposome formulation is available. Encapsulation of high concentrations of magnetic species within the interior volume or embedded in the lipid bilayer may potentially destabilize the liposome and still not provide the desired level of influence by a magnetic field for challenging applications. When considering the magnetic nanoparticle chain approach, for example, the interior volume of the liposomes remains available for encapsulation, while the magnetic tail allows for a significant degree of magnetization of the complex.

For in vitro analysis platforms, a defined region within a microfluidic device could be envisioned to receive energy sufficient to induce liposome lysis. Carefully timed release of contents could be used, for example, to deliver encapsulated reagents needed for a subsequent step or signaling reagents to a downstream detector. While liposome lysis using lasers has been accomplished,[67] this approach avoids potential photobleaching effects of fluorescent dyes. More broadly, this also would obviate the reagents needed for chemical-induced lysis, associated time for their removal, and risks associated with possible carryover for the next analysis. By using a permanent magnet for directional control and an RF field to induce release, many options for assay design are available.

8.2.2 Measurements Using Paramagnetic Encapsulants

Rather than using magnetic properties to afford content release, magnetic liposomes can serve as the species capable of providing a signal. Aside from tissue-imaging applications, liposomes encapsulating paramagnetic encapsulants have been studied as disease-specific markers in homogeneous assays. In a recent advance, hydrophilic Gd in the form of a chelate with 10-(2-hydroxy-propyl)-1,4,7,10-tetra-azacyclododecane-1,4,7-triacetic acid (gadoteridol) was encapsulated within liposomes to assess phospholipase A_2 (PLA$_2$) activity.[68] PLA$_2$ is an enzyme capable of hydrolyzing *sn*-2 acyl bonds of glycerophospholipids, such as in DPPC, in the presence of Ca^{2+}. Increases in its activity are associated with various disease states, including acute pancreatitis[69]; breast, lung, and prostate cancers[70]; and autoimmune disorders.[71,72] In practice, measure of its activity is hindered by the inability to identify an appropriate substrate representative of its in vivo behavior.[68] As a solution, rather than fluorescent or radiolabeled phospholipid substrates, Cheng and Tsourkas formulated Gd-encapsulating liposomes to serve as a more native substrate for PLA$_2$.[68] When such paramagnetic agents are encapsulated within liposomes, there exists a limited degree of water exchange across the lipid bilayer.[40] Depending on the lipid composition, this limited membrane permeability to water contributes to a limited response of these agents to the applied RF pulse in MRI.[68,73,74] PLA$_2$ served to hydrolyze the composite lipids and increase the permeability of the lipid bilayer (Fig. 8.6a), which decreased the T1 relaxation time yielding a proportional response to the PLA$_2$ concentration (Fig. 8.6b).

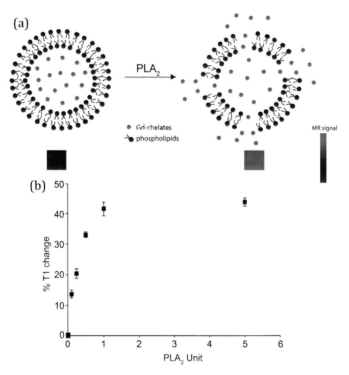

Figure 8.6 (a) Liposome-encapsulating Gd-chelates exhibit increased permeability in the presence of PLA$_2$ and consequently increased MRI response upon Gd release.[68] (b) % T1 change versus PLA$_2$ concentration. Reprinted with permission from Ref. [68], Copyright 2014, MacMillan Publishers Ltd. http://www.nature.com/srep/2014/141107/srep06958/full/srep06958.html.

In a related example, liposomes encapsulating gadoteridol and functionalized with a hydrophobically modified peptide were investigated in an assay for matrix metalloproteinases (MMPs).[75] MMPs are a class of zinc-dependent proteolytic enzymes that are involved in various functions such as wound healing and embryogenesis.[76] However, their abnormal elevation can be indicative of various disease states, including multiple sclerosis,[77] stroke,[78] and cancers.[79,80] In this approach, the hydrophilic peptide PLGLWAR served as a specific substrate for collegenase, an MMP, whereas the attached stearic acid chain served to link the peptide to the lipid bilayer. Enzymatic activity served to release the encapsulated gadoteridol yielding an increase in the relaxivity.

Aggregation formed the basis of another enzyme assay utilizing Gd-encapsulating liposomes.[74] Here, negatively charged, gadoteridol-encapsulating liposomes formed aggregates in the presence of protamine, a cationic protein with ~66 positive charges per molecule (Fig. 8.7a). These large aggregated complexes (between 2.5 μm and 7.0 μm diameter) restricted the passage of water molecules across the lipid membranes and thus yielded a negligible signal for water relaxation. The addition of trypsin, a serine protease, served to break down protamine and release intact liposomes. This restored the relaxivity signal effectively to that consistent with water permeability expected with the liposomes alone and yielded a linear response with trypsin concentration (Fig. 8.7b).

While similar strategies for enzyme activity analyses have been developed using fluorophore-encapsulating liposomes,[81,82] the advantages here with measurement of paramagnetic species include the avoidance of interferences typical to optical methods such as quenching and scattering as well as the potential to be extended to in vivo measurements. Liposomes encapsulating or bilayer tagged with magnetic species could also be envisioned to be employed in analyses relying on magnetic particles as a label. Immunoassays relying on measurement of magnetic labels, rather than optical products from enzymes, have been suggested to yield a wider dynamic range,[83] avoidance from interferences from background constituents,[84] and ability to be directed by magnetic fields.[85] In the case of lateral flow technology, magnetic measurements add the benefit of measurement of the entire depth of the capture zone rather than only the surface as with optical measurements.[83,86] Sensors relying on the measurement of inductance,[84] Hall effect,[87] and giant magnetoresistance[85] have been developed. Other assays rely on the difference in magnetic relaxation rates between bound and unbound magnetic species and hence can be employed in a homogeneous format.[88] Such strategies could readily be extended to liposome-based analyses, taking advantage of their biocompatibility and large encapsulation volume.

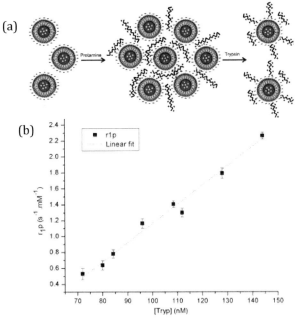

Figure 8.7   (a) Negatively charged liposomes encapsulating Gd-chelates aggregate in the presence of the cationic protein protamine.[74] In the presence of the protease trypsin, the liposome aggregates are dissociated, leading to an increase in relaxivity. (b) A linear relationship between trypsin concentration and relaxivity resulted. Reprinted with permission from Ref. [74], Copyright 2011, Elsevier. http://dx.doi.org/10.1016/j.bmc.2010.07.057.

8.2.3   Magnetic Liposomes for Analyte Isolation and Labeling

Liposomes have been widely used with magnetic beads for the purpose of immunomagnetic (or other biorecognition element-mediated) separation and subsequent detection of analytes.[89–92] However, in the analytical realm, there are comparatively few examples where liposomes themselves have been imparted with the ability to be directed by magnetic fields. Discussed below are various embodiments where liposomes that can be collected by magnetic fields served to accumulate and/or label specific analytes based on their imparted affinity characteristics.

8.2.3.1 Magnetic cell-labeling

In the early 1980s, antibody-tagged liposomes encapsulating ferromagnetic particles were investigated for the purpose of cell sorting in the presence of an applied magnetic field.[93] In one example, anti-fibronectin-tagged liposomes encapsulating ~500 Å ferrite particles were shown to successfully isolate and concentrate mouse embryo fibroblasts when situated over an electromagnet.[94] Subsequent work utilizing carboxyfluorescein and magnetic bead encapsulating immunoliposomes allowed for both concentration and labeling of specific cell types prior to magnetic activated cell sorting (MACS®).[95] In MACS®, magnetically labeled cell species are retained in a column by a magnet, while unrecognized species are removed prior to analysis, typically by flow cytometry. The antibody-mediated magnetic approach provided selective isolation of desired cell species, whereas liposomes provided a marked enhancement in signal per binding event due to the encapsulation of numerous fluorescent dye molecules versus limited labeling of antibodies with few fluorophores. This approach was subsequently applied for the analysis of antigen-presenting cells, which present peptides at physiologically relevant levels lower than that can be observed using traditional immunofluorescence methods.[96]

In a more recent study, Harjanto et al. demonstrated the utility of magnetite-tagged polydiacetylene (PDA) liposomes functionalized with the recognition peptide arginine-glycine-asparagine (RGD) for isolation and labeling of NIH 3T3 cells (Fig. 8.8).[97] Such fibroblast cells express integrins, which bind this sequence.[98] The UV light required to polymerize and consequently stabilize the PDA liposomal structures concurrently served to sterilize the preparation, efficiently also making it suitable for cell culture. This unique strategy served not only to study properties of the liposomal biomimetic material in terms of RGD coverage and cell viability but also as a cellular label owing to the colorimetric and fluorescent properties of the PDA liposomes. Here, the time course of cell adhesion and internalization of attached liposomes was monitored. The authors note a potential of such liposomes to be further investigated for the study of cellular mechanical changes as a function of force–induced PDA fluorescence.

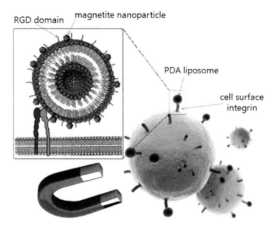

Figure 8.8 RGD-tagged, magnetite-labeled PDA liposomes for the isolation, labeling, and study of integrin-expressing cells.[97] Reprinted with permission from Ref. [97], Copyright 2013, American Chemical Society. http://pubs.acs.org/doi/abs/10.1021/la4005714.

8.2.3.2 Non-cell-based affinity applications of magnetic liposomes

Magnetic liposomes have served as affinity supports for the isolation and analysis of a variety of other analytes, taking advantage of their physiological presentation of biologically relevant molecules. For example, liposomes prepared with antigenic proteins extracted from mites were used to isolate antibodies in patients with allergies. Here, liposomes composed of DMPC and DMPE were conjugated to allergenic proteins from fungi *Dreschlera (Helminthosporium) monoceras*[99] and mites *Dermathophagoids pteronyssinus* and *Blomia tropicali.*[2] These approximately 113 nm diameter liposomes coating nanometer-sized iron oxide cores were retained in a flow-based system using an electromagnet. Serum samples from patients were passed over the magnetically retained liposomes, and the IgE from allergic patients could be differentiated on the basis of specific retention.[2] The magnetic liposome bed could be removed by turning off the electromagnet and flushing the system between analyses. A similar strategy was employed to study retention of anti-cardiolipin antibodies on magnetoliposomes prepared from cardiolipin and DMPC in patients with autoimmune disorders.[100]

A recent study combined the MACS® approach described above with affinity chromatography in a technique coined lipid-vesicle-mediated affinity chromatography (LIMACS).[101] This technique was used to study lipid–protein interactions between liposomal lipids and proteins from cell lysate. Annexin V is a 35 kDa protein that binds to phosphatidylserine (PS) in the presence of Ca^{2+}. In healthy cells, PS is situated on the inner membrane facing the cytoplasmic side, whereas this lipid becomes externalized to the outer leaflet when the cells undergo apoptosis.[102] Annexin V magnetic beads were used to capture liposomes composed of PS and lipids of interest following incubation with cell lysates to capture specific lipid-binding proteins. The complexes were then isolated by magnetic separation using an MACS column prior to SDS-PAGE and western blotting analyses. Here the magnetic influence was imparted by the Annexin-labeled magnetic beads. However, a similar approach could be taken using liposomes that are directly labeled with magnetic materials. One advantage of direct magnetization of the liposomes is additional flexibility for lipid studies if PS was not a requirement for lipid formulation. Additionally, if the magnetic liposomes were the only requirement of such assays, the potential for nonspecific interactions with magnetic beads could be avoided and the greatest similarity to physiological conditions could be ensured through removal of these secondary species.

8.2.3.3 Bacteria-derived magnetosomes

While the focus of this chapter is on magnetic liposomes that are formed synthetically, other strategies previously developed using bacteria-derived magnetic structures bear mention. Certain prokaryotic bacteria are affected by magnetic fields owing to their bioaccumulation of minerals. These "magnetotactic bacteria" contain intracellular structures known as magnetosomes, which consist of magnetite or greigite (Fe_3S_4) crystals coated with a lipid bilayer.[103] These structures range in size from 35–120 nm, though their morphology is consistent within a given bacterial species.[104–106] The composition of the lipid bilayer includes constituents such as phospholipids, fatty acids, and proteins.[106] Aside from evolutionary interest, such magnetosomes are of interest for analytical applications.[107–109] Their often-cited benefits include their chemical purity; consistent, monodisperse, and small size range; desirable magnetic properties; biocompatible membrane coating; ability to express desired surface biorecognition elements; and potentially low cost versus commercial magnetic beads.[110–113]

Several examples of the use of bacterial magnetosomes to serve as capture phases in immunoassays or DNA-based assays have been reported.[114,115] These include the quantification of mouse IgG,[115] human insulin,[116] and endocrine-disrupting chemicals.[117] Their incorporation in the technique of immuno-PCR (iPCR) serves as an example of their utility. In this report, rather than synthetic magnetic nanoparticles, bacteria-derived magnetosome particles were used as a magnetizable binding surface, akin to that in immunomagnetic separation.[112] Here these magnetosomes were functionalized with streptavidin via a biotin linkage and served as a capture surface for biotinylated antibodies against hepatitis B surface antigen (HBsAg). In the presence of the analyte HBsAg, anti-HBsAg conjugated to DNA formed the detection end of the sandwich prior to real-time PCR amplification of the attached probe (Fig. 8.9).

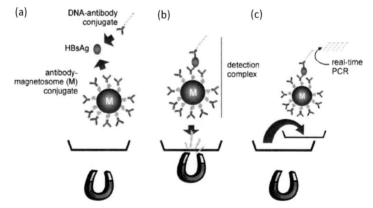

Figure 8.9 Bacteria-derived magnetosomes serving as a capture phase in immuno-PCR for the detection of hepatitis B surface antigen (HBsAg).[112] Reprinted with permission from Ref. [112], Copyright 2007, Elsevier. http://dx.doi.org/10.1016/j.bbrc.2007.03.156.

The use of these magnetosomes resulted in a 25-fold lower limit of detection and broader linear range than commercially available magnetic beads.

8.2.4 Magnetic Liposomes as Reagent Concentrators

Aside from using liposomes as biocompatible magnetic separators, the internal volume can be used to provide storage or sequestration of reagents. In an approach developed by Roman-Pizarro et al., liposomes were prepared encapsulating hydrophobic gold/iron oxide nanoparticles, also entrapping the enzyme substrate 4-methylumbelliferyl-phosphate (MUP).[118] These magnetic liposomes served as pre-concentrators in a flow-injection method for the quantification of alkaline phosphatase (ALP) (Fig. 8.10a). Here liposomes entrapping MUP and gold-coated iron oxide nanoparticles were injected into a flowing system and spatially retained by an electromagnet. Subsequently, a mixture of Triton X-100 and a sample potentially containing ALP was introduced. In the presence of ALP, the substrate released by the surfactant could be converted to a fluorescent product and detected by the downstream fluorescence detector (Fig. 8.10b).

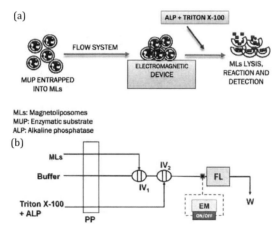

Figure 8.10 Magnetic liposomes encapsulating substrate for the determination of alkaline phosphatase (ALP) activity in milk samples.[118] (a) General reaction flow. (b) Scheme of flow-injection system where magnetic liposomes (ML) are concentrated by an electromagnet prior to the introduction of surfactant (Triton X-100) and sample containing ALP. Product generated from the enzymatic reaction then passes to the in-line fluorescence detector (FL) prior to going to waste (W). Reprinted with permission from Ref. [118], Copyright 2014, American Chemical Society. http://pubs.acs.org/doi/abs/10.1021/jf5004804.

This method was applied to the analysis of ALP in raw and pasteurized milk samples. This heat-sensitive enzyme can serve as a measure of the effectiveness of the pasteurization process. The advantage that the substrate-encapsulating magnetic liposomes provided over substrate alone was a 58-fold lower limit of detection for ALP.

Rather than substrate encapsulation, magnetic liposomes functionalized with enzymes such as cytochrome c-oxidase have also been suggested for use in bioreactors.[119,120] By taking advantage of the stability imparted by phospholipid bilayers, the activity of this membrane enzyme toward its substrate could be retained over several hours using liposomes magnetically retained within a fixed-bed bioreactor.

8.2.5 Magnetic Liposomes in Heterogeneous Sandwich Assays

Another promising application of magnetic liposomes is their use in heterogeneous assay formats. Using an ELISA as an example, it is easy to envision the mass transfer limitations that exist between analytes and signaling species in the bulk phase and species responsible for biorecognition immobilized at the binding surface. In such heterogeneous assay formats, interactions are dependent on factors such as the surface concentration of binding sites, concentration of solution-phase molecules, affinity of binding partners, reaction rate constants, and diffusion constants of the solution-phase species.[121-125] Depletion of solution-phase reagents and analytes near the solid phase upon binding and subsequent need for transport to the surface from the bulk solution[126] can result in lengthy incubation times to attain the required level of sensitivity, especially with the use of signaling based on nanoparticles.[127] Many approaches have been employed to overcome these limitations, including mixing during incubation times[127,128]; reducing diffusion times by utilizing the increased surface-area-to-volume ratio in microfluidic devices[129,130]; applying perpendicular flow to force analyte streams closer to binding surfaces in microfluidic channels[131]; and the use of magnetic microparticles as solid supports to increase reaction rate via improved diffusion throughout the solution phase.[132,133]

The advantages of liposomes for analytical applications have been introduced in Chapter 1. However, some of their key disadvantages are those which are shared with other particle-based signaling approaches, which include suboptimal binding kinetics and mass transfer limitations. To overcome these challenges, a strategy utilizing magnetic liposomes was recently developed.[134] By imparting magnetic properties and biorecognition capabilities to liposomal lipid bilayers, the interior volume could be maintained as a concentrated source of hydrophilic signaling molecules. In a simple demonstration of their potential, a 96-well magnet was placed under liposomes with and without functionalization by iron oxide–oleic acid. Only those with the iron oxide were drawn to the underlying magnet, forming a pattern consistent with the magnet shape visualized readily through the encapsulated dye (Fig. 8.11).

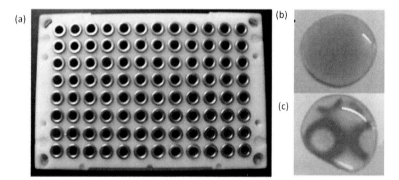

Figure 8.11 Directional control of magnetic liposomes via permanent magnets. A 96-well magnetic plate (a) was placed under a glass coverslip onto which dye-encapsulating liposomes without (b) and with (c) an iron oxide complex were pipetted.[134] Liposomes prepared with the iron oxide–oleic acid complex were drawn to the underlying magnets, whereas those without were not. Reprinted with permission from Ref. [134], Copyright 2014, American Chemical Society. http://pubs.acs.org/doi/abs/10.1021/ac501219u.

When also functionalized with a biorecognition element, such liposomes could serve as signal-enhancement reagents in heterogeneous assays, relying on their magnetic properties to allow controlled direction toward surfaces and promote binding interactions. As a representative embodiment, sulforhodamine

B-encapsulating liposomes were prepared with both iron oxide–oleic acid complexes and cholesterol-modified DNA reporter probes as part of their lipid composition.[134] These liposomes were used to provide signal enhancement for a sandwich hybridization assay in a standard 96-well microtiter plate format (Fig. 8.12a). By using an underlying magnet to overcome diffusion limitations, these liposomes could be directed from the bulk solution toward the well bottom using a permanent magnet. This served to increase interactions with the target captured by the surface-immobilized DNA probe (Fig. 8.12b). Aside from a lower limit of detection (Fig. 8.13), enhanced sensitivity, decreased assay time, and a reduction in the reagent concentrations to yield the same signal intensity were attained.

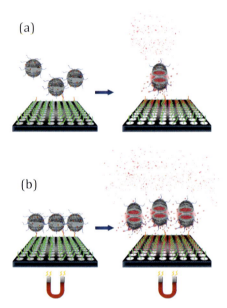

Figure 8.12 Magnetic liposomes encapsulating sulforhodamine B dye and tagged with DNA reporter probes for the quantification of target RNA in a sandwich hybridization assay. (a) In the absence of a magnet, sandwich hybridization complexes form but are subject to diffusion limitations. (b) The use of a magnet serves to draw the liposomes to the underlying surface and promote additional interactions with the captured target.[134] Reprinted with permission from Ref. [134], Copyright 2014, American Chemical Society. http://pubs.acs.org/doi/abs/10.1021/ac501219u.

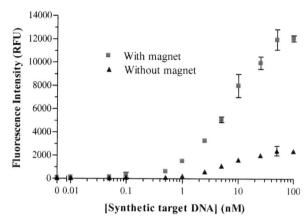

Figure 8.13 Enhancement in assay sensitivity and limit of detection in a sandwich hybridization assay when a magnet was employed for liposome-based signaling versus without.[134] Reprinted with permission from Ref. [134], Copyright 2014, American Chemical Society. http://pubs.acs.org/doi/abs/10.1021/ac501219u.

Here this strategy was successfully employed in a standard microtiter plate format, which is broadly applicable to common assays such as ELISAs. However, given challenges in magnet design, which currently do not allow for maximal attraction in the entire well volume, this strategy could be even more advantageous in microfluidic assay designs. Preliminary investigations demonstrated that a well-placed permanent magnet could be used to retain such liposomes in a microfluidic device, allowing for enhanced signal due to concentration and subsequent lysis within a defined volume (Fig. 8.14). Other applications could utilize an electromagnet to provide on-demand, timed accumulation as well as afford mixing strategies to improve interactions between biorecognition element-tagged magnetic liposomes and their corresponding analytes.

Similar to the affinity applications described earlier, another strategy could be envisioned where biorecognition element labeled liposomes could be directed to a defined location and retained by an electromagnet, then allowing analyte solution to pass through this matrix. This concentrated zone would ensure maximal interaction of analytes with their corresponding affinity partners, while simultaneously labeling them with a tag. The labeled complexes could then be released upon the removal of the magnetic field for subsequent downstream analyses.

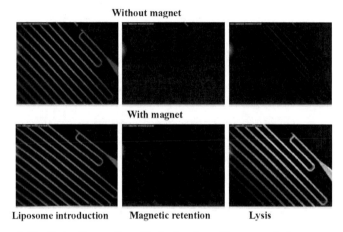

Figure 8.14 Retention of sulforhodamine B-encapsulating magnetic liposomes within microfluidic channels in the absence (top) or presence (bottom) of an underlying permanent magnet.[134] Reprinted with permission from Ref. [134], Copyright 2014, American Chemical Society. http://pubs.acs.org/doi/abs/10.1021/ac501219u.

8.3   Future Perspectives

The ability to control the motion and direction of magnetic liposomes offers many exciting, yet not fully explored, opportunities in the analytical realm. Examples were described showing the use of magnetic liposomes to specifically label and isolate cells, provide physiologically relevant surfaces for biomolecule presentation in readily renewable affinity systems, and provide a controlled source of substrates in a flow-injection analysis system for enzyme analysis. Also demonstrated within were magnetic liposomes that could be directed to underlying binding surfaces to enhance analyte detection by overcoming mass transfer limitations in a heterogeneous high-throughput assay platform. Other applications drew from medical imaging technologies and utilized liposomes encapsulating paramagnetic agents in enzyme-based assays relying on liposome lysis or aggregation to afford changes in time-weighted signals.

Findings intended for drug-delivery applications could add significant flexibility for analytical utility. An overview of release of contents from magnetic liposomes for drug delivery using RF energy was provided, as well as strategies to afford the same without directly magnetizing the liposomes. Such strategies can provide an alternative to traditional chemical or biomolecule-induced lysis and thus reduce carryover concerns. By relying on proximity, rather than direct magnetization, some of the challenges with magnetic liposomes, which can include ensuring adequate retention or direction by the magnetic field while maintaining substantial signaling ability, can be avoided. In the in vitro realm, optimization of liposome formulations for maximal analytical functionality, matrix compatibility, and stability, rather than in vivo toxicity, needs to be carried out.

Work to date has exemplified several analytical strategies for magnetic liposomes. By combining the known advantages of analytical liposomes—including large interior volume for encapsulation, ease of bilayer functionalization, and time-independent signaling—with the directional control, induced release, and unique signaling options imparted by magnetic fields, many exciting opportunities exist as their full analytical potential is explored.

References

1. De Cuyper M, Joniau M. Magnetoliposomes: Formation and structural characterization. *Eur Biophys J.* 1988; 15(5): 311–319.

2. Zollner TCA, Zollner RdL, De Cuyper M, Santana MHA. Adsorption of isotype "E" antibodies on affinity magnetoliposomes. *J Dispersion Sci Technol.* 2003; 24(3–4): 615–622.

3. Garnier B, Tan S, Miraux S, Bled E, Brisson AR. Optimized synthesis of 100 nm diameter magnetoliposomes with high content of maghemite particles and high MRI effect. *Contrast Media Mol Imaging.* 2012; 7(2): 231–239.

4. Bealle G, Di Corato R, Kolosnjaj-Tabi J, et al. Ultra magnetic liposomes for MR imaging, targeting, and hyperthermia. *Langmuir: ACS J Surf Colloid.* 2012; 28(32): 11834–11842.

5. Chen Y, Bose A, Bothun GD. Controlled release from bilayer-decorated magnetoliposomes via electromagnetic heating. *ACS Nano.* 2010; 4(6): 3215–3221.

6. De Cuyper M, Hodenius M, Soenen SJH. Magnetoliposomes: Versatile innovative nanocolloids for use in biotechnology and biomedicine. *Nanomedicine.* 2009; 4: 177+.

7. Bogdanov AA, Jr., Martin C, Weissleder R, Brady TJ. Trapping of dextran-coated colloids in liposomes by transient binding to aminophospholipid: Preparation of ferrosomes. *Biochim Biophys Acta.* 1994; 1193(1): 212–218.

8. De Cuyper M, Joniau M. Mechanistic aspects of the adsorption of phospholipids onto lauric acid stabilized magnetite nanocolloids. *Langmuir.* 1991; 7(4): 647–652.

9. Schwendener RA, Wuthrich R, Duewell S, Wehrli E, von Schulthess GK. A pharmacokinetic and MRI study of unilamellar gadolinium-, manganese-, and iron-DTPA-stearate liposomes as organ-specific contrast agents. *Invest Radiol.* 1990; 25(8): 922–932.

10. Kabalka G, Buonocore E, Hubner K, Moss T, Norley N, Huang L. Gadolinium-labeled liposomes: Targeted MR contrast agents for the liver and spleen. *Radiology.* 1987; 163(1): 255–258.

11. Kiwada H, Sato J, Yamada S, Kato Y. Feasibility of magnetic liposomes as a targeting device for drugs. *Chem Pharm Bull (Tokyo).* 1986; 34(10): 4253–4258.

12. Viroonchatapan E, Sato H, Ueno M, Adachi I, Tazawa K, Horikoshi I. Magnetic targeting of thermosensitive magnetoliposomes to mouse livers in an in situ on-line perfusion system. *Life Sci.* 1996; 58(24): 2251–2261.

13. Liburdy RP, Tenforde TS, Magin RL. Magnetic field-induced drug permeability in liposome vesicles. *Radiat Res.* 1986; 108(1): 102–111.

14. Kubo T, Sugita T, Shimose S, Nitta Y, Ikuta Y, Murakami T. Targeted delivery of anticancer drugs with intravenously administered magnetic liposomes in osteosarcoma-bearing hamsters. *Int J Oncol.* 2000; 17(2): 309–315.

15. Widder KJ, Morris RM, Poore G, Howard DP, Jr., Senyei AE. Tumor remission in Yoshida sarcoma-bearing rts by selective targeting of magnetic albumin microspheres containing doxorubicin. *Proc Natl Acad Sci U S A.* 1981; 78(1): 579–581.

16. Babincova M, Altanerova V, Lampert M, et al. Site-specific in vivo targeting of magnetoliposomes using externally applied magnetic field. *Z Naturforsch C.* 2000; 55(3–4): 278–281.

17. Mikhaylov G, Mikac U, Magaeva AA, et al. Ferri-liposomes as an MRI-visible drug-delivery system for targeting tumours and their microenvironment. *Nat Nanotechnol.* 6(9): 594–602.

18. Bakandritsos A, Fatourou AG, Fatouros DG. Magnetoliposomes and their potential in the intelligent drug-delivery field. *Ther Deliv.* 2012; 3(12): 1469–1482.

19. Mody V, Cox A, Shah S, Singh A, Bevins W, Parihar H. Magnetic nanoparticle drug delivery systems for targeting tumor. *Appl Nanosci.* 2014; 4(4): 385–392.

20. Veiseh O, Gunn J, Zhang M. Design and fabrication of magnetic nanoparticles for targeted drug delivery and imaging. *Adv Drug Del Rev.* 2010; 62(3): 284–304.

21. Soenen SJ, Hodenius M, De Cuyper M. Magnetoliposomes: Versatile innovative nanocolloids for use in biotechnology and biomedicine. *Nanomedicine (Lond).* 2009; 4(2): 177–191.

22. Zheng X, Lu J, Deng L, Xiong Y, Chen J. Preparation and characterization of magnetic cationic liposome in gene delivery. *Int J Pharm.* 2009; 366(1–2): 211–217.

23. Hirao K, Sugita T, Kubo T, et al. Targeted gene delivery to human osteosarcoma cells with magnetic cationic liposomes under a magnetic field. *Int J Oncol.* 2003; 22(5): 1065–1071.

24. Babincova M, Machova E. Magnetoliposomes may be useful for elimination of HIV from infected individuals. *Z Naturforsch C.* 1998; 53(9–10): 935–936.

25. Storrs RW, Tropper FD, Li HY, et al. Paramagnetic polymerized liposomes as new recirculating MR contrast agents. *J Magn Reson Imaging.* 1995; 5(6): 719–724.

26. Pauser S, Reszka R, Wagner S, Wolf KJ, Buhr HJ, Berger G. Liposome-encapsulated superparamagnetic iron oxide particles as markers in an MRI-guided search for tumor-specific drug carriers. *Anticancer Drug Des.* 1997; 12(2): 125–135.

27. Caride VJ. Liposomes as carriers of imaging agents. *Crit Rev Ther Drug Carrier Syst.* 1985; 1(2): 121–153.

28. Unger E, Tilcock C, Ahkong QF, Fritz T. Paramagnetic liposomes as magnetic resonance contrast agents. *Invest Radiol.* 1990; 25 Suppl 1: S65–66.

29. Schmid HH. MRI Made Easy. Germany: Schering AG; 1990: http://www.stat.columbia.edu/~martin/Tools/MRI_Made_Easy.pdf. Accessed 2/11/15.

30. Hanson LG. Introduction to Magnetic Resonance Imaging Techniques. Danish Research Center for Magnetic Resonance: http://www.drcmr.dk/Docs/MRI_English_a4.pdf. Accessed 2/12/15.

31. Weishaupt D, Köchli V, Marincek B. How does MRI work? *An Introduction to the Physics and Function of Magnetic Resonance Imaging*: Springer; 2006.

32. McRobbie D, Moore E, Graves M. *MRI from Picture to Proton.* 2nd ed: Cambridge University Press; 2007.

33. Fujimoto Y, Okuhata Y, Tyngi S, Namba Y, Oku N. Magnetic resonance lymphography of profundus lymph nodes with liposomal gadolinium-diethylenetriamine pentaacetic acid. *Biol Pharm Bull.* 2000; 23(1): 97–100.

34. Vion-Dury J, Masson S, Devoisselle JM, et al. Liposome-mediated delivery of gadolinium-diethylenetriaminopentaacetic acid to hepatic cells: A P-31 NMR study. *J Pharmacol Exp Ther.* 1989; 250(3): 1113–1118.

35. Kabalka GW, Buonocore E, Hubner K, Davis M, Huang L. Gadolinium-labeled liposomes containing paramagnetic amphipathic agents: Targeted MRI contrast agents for the liver. *Magn Reson Med.* 1988; 8(1): 89–95.

36. Tilcock C, Unger E, Cullis P, MacDougall P. Liposomal Gd-DTPA: Preparation and characterization of relaxivity. *Radiology.* 1989; 171(1): 77–80.

37. Ghaghada K, Hawley C, Kawaji K, Annapragada A, Mukundan S, Jr. T1 relaxivity of core-encapsulated gadolinium liposomal contrast agents: Effect of liposome size and internal gadolinium concentration. *Acad Radiol.* 2008; 15(10): 1259–1263.

38. Fossheim SL, Fahlvik AK, Klaveness J, Muller RN. Paramagnetic liposomes as MRI contrast agents: Influence of liposomal physicochemical properties on the in vitro relaxivity. *Magn Reson Imaging.* 1999; 17(1): 83–89.

39. Lindner LH, Reinl HM, Schlemmer M, Stahl R, Peller M. Paramagnetic thermosensitive liposomes for MR-thermometry. *Int J Hyperthermia.* 2005; 21(6): 575–588.

40. Strijkers GJ, Kluza E, Van Tilborg GA, et al. Paramagnetic and fluorescent liposomes for target-specific imaging and therapy of tumor angiogenesis. *Angiogenesis.* 2010; 13(2): 161–173.

41. Kamaly N, Kalber T, Ahmad A, et al. Bimodal paramagnetic and fluorescent liposomes for cellular and tumor magnetic resonance imaging. *Bioconjug Chem.* 2008; 19(1): 118–129.

42. Castelli DD, Terreno E, Cabella C, et al. Evidence for in vivo macrophage mediated tumor uptake of paramagnetic/fluorescent liposomes. *NMR Biomed.* 2009; 22(10): 1084–1092.

43. Mulder WJ, Strijkers GJ, Habets JW, et al. MR molecular imaging and fluorescence microscopy for identification of activated tumor endothelium using a bimodal lipidic nanoparticle. *FASEB J.* 2005; 19(14): 2008–2010.

44. Kamaly N, Kalber T, Kenny G, Bell J, Jorgensen M, Miller A. A novel bimodal lipidic contrast agent for cellular labelling and tumour MRI. *Org Biomol Chem.* 2010; 8(1): 201–211.

45. Kim J, Pandya DN, Lee W, et al. Vivid tumor imaging utilizing liposome-carried bimodal radiotracer. *ACS Med Chem Lett.* 2014; 5(4): 390–394.

46. Mikhaylov G, Mikac U, Magaeva AA, et al. Ferri-liposomes as an MRI-visible drug-delivery system for targeting tumours and their microenvironment. *Nat Nano.* 2011; 6(9): 594–602.

47. Kamaly N, Miller AD. Paramagnetic liposome nanoparticles for cellular and tumour imaging. *Int J Mol Sci.* 2010; 11(4): 1759–1776.

48. Fattahi H, Laurent S, Liu F, Arsalani N, Elst LV, Muller RN. Magnetoliposomes as multimodal contrast agents for molecular imaging and cancer nanotheragnostics. *Nanomedicine.* 2011; 6(3): 529–544.

49. Kamaly N, Miller AD. Paramagnetic liposome nanoparticles for cellular and tumour imaging. *Int J Mol Sci.* 2010; 11(4): 1759–1776.

50. Langereis S, Geelen T, Grüll H, Strijkers GJ, Nicolay K. Paramagnetic liposomes for molecular MRI and MRI-guided drug delivery. *NMR Biomed.* 2013; 26(7): 728–744.

51. Soenen SJ, Vande Velde G, Ketkar-Atre A, Himmelreich U, De Cuyper M. Magnetoliposomes as magnetic resonance imaging contrast agents. *Wiley Interdiscip Rev Nanomed Nanobiotechnol.* 2011; 3(2): 197–211.

52. Dewhirst MW, Vujaskovic Z, Jones E, Thrall D. Re-setting the biologic rationale for thermal therapy. *Int J Hyperthermia.* 2005; 21(8): 779–790.

53. Dewhirst MW, Landon CD, Hofmann CL, Stauffer PR. Novel approaches to treatment of hepatocellular carcinoma and hepatic metastases using thermal ablation and thermosensitive liposomes. *Surg Oncol Clin N Am.* 2013; 22(3): 545–561.

54. Chu KF, Dupuy DE. Thermal ablation of tumours: Biological mechanisms and advances in therapy. *Nat Rev Cancer.* 2014; 14(3): 199–208.

55. Shinkai M, Matsui M, Kobayashi T. Heat properties of magnetoliposomes for local hyperthermia. *Jpn J Hyperthermic Oncol.* 1994; 10: 168–177.

56. Shinkai M, Suzuki M, Iijima S, Kobayashi T. Antibody-conjugated magnetoliposomes for targeting cancer cells and their application in hyperthermia. *Biotechnol Appl Biochem.* 1995; 21 (Pt 2): 125–137.

57. Yanase M, Shinkai M, Honda H, Wakabayashi T, Yoshida J, Kobayashi T. Intracellular hyperthermia for cancer using magnetite cationic liposomes: An in vivo study. *Jpn J Cancer Res.* 1998; 89(4): 463–469.

58. Yanase M, Shinkai M, Honda H, Wakabayashi T, Yoshida J, Kobayashi T. Intracellular hyperthermia for cancer using magnetite cationic liposomes: Ex vivo study. *Jpn J Cancer Res.* 1997; 88(7): 630–632.

59. Yanase M, Shinkai M, Honda H, Wakabayashi T, Yoshida J, Kobayashi T. Antitumor immunity induction by intracellular hyperthermia using magnetite cationic liposomes. *Jpn J Cancer Res.* 1998; 89(7): 775–782.

60. Müller-Schulte D, Füssl F, Lueken H, De Cuyper M. A new AIDS therapy approach using magnetoliposomes. In: Häfeli U, Schütt W, Teller J, Zborowski M, eds. *Scientific and Clinical Applications of Magnetic Carriers*: Springer US; 1997: 517–526.

61. Pradhan P, Giri J, Rieken F, et al. Targeted temperature sensitive magnetic liposomes for thermo-chemotherapy. *J Control Release.* 2010; 142(1): 108–121.

62. Chen Y, Chen Y, Xiao D, Bose A, Deng R, Bothun GD. Low-dose chemotherapy of hepatocellular carcinoma through triggered-release from bilayer-decorated magnetoliposomes. *Colloids Surf B Biointerfaces.* 2014; 116: 452–458.

63. Amstad E, Kohlbrecher J, Muller E, Schweizer T, Textor M, Reimhult E. Triggered release from liposomes through magnetic actuation of iron oxide nanoparticle containing membranes. *Nano Lett.* 2011; 11(4): 1664–1670.

64. Hanus J, Ullrich M, Dohnal J, Singh M, Stepanek F. Remotely controlled diffusion from magnetic liposome microgels. *Langmuir.* 2013; 29(13): 4381–4387.

65. Ullrich M, Haufova P, Singh M, Stepanek F. Radiofrequency triggered enzymatic reaction inside hydrogel microparticles, ECAL 2013; 2013; Taormina, Italy.

66. Peiris PM, Bauer L, Toy R, et al. Enhanced delivery of chemotherapy to tumors using a multicomponent nanochain with radio-frequency-tunable drug release. *ACS Nano.* 2012; 6(5): 4157–4168.

67. VanderMeulen DL, Misra P, Michael J, Spears KG, Khoka M. Laser mediated release of dye from liposomes. *Photochem Photobiol.* 1992; 56(3): 325–332.

68. Cheng Z, Tsourkas A. Monitoring phospholipase A(2) activity with Gd-encapsulated phospholipid liposomes. *Sci Rep.* 2014; 4: 6958.

69. Aufenanger J, Samman M, Quintel M, Fassbender K, Zimmer W, Bertsch T. Pancreatic phospholipase A2 activity in acute pancreatitis: A prognostic marker for early identification of patients at risk. *Clin Chem Lab Med.* 2002; 40(3): 293–297.

70. Cummings BS. Phospholipase A2 as targets for anti-cancer drugs. *Biochem Pharmacol.* 2007; 74(7): 949–959.

71. Cunningham TJ, Yao L, Oetinger M, Cort L, Blankenhorn EP, Greenstein JI. Secreted phospholipase A2 activity in experimental autoimmune encephalomyelitis and multiple sclerosis. *J Neuroinflamm.* 2006; 3: 26.

72. Niwa Y, Miyachi Y, Sakane T, Kanoh T, Taniguchi S. Methyltransferase and phospholipase A2 activity in the cell membrane of neutrophils and lymphocytes from patients with Behcet's disease, systemic lupus erythematosus, and rheumatoid arthritis. *Clin Chim Acta.* 1988; 174(1): 1–14.

73. Terreno E, Sanino A, Carrera C, et al. Determination of water permeability of paramagnetic liposomes of interest in MRI field. *J Inorg Biochem.* 2008; 102(5–6): 1112–1119.

74. Figueiredo S, Moreira JN, Geraldes CFGC, Aime S, Terreno E. Supramolecular protamine/Gd-loaded liposomes adducts as relaxometric protease responsive probes. *Bioorg Med Chem.* 2011; 19(3): 1131–1135.

75. Figueiredo S, Terreno E, Moreira JN, Geraldes CF, Aime S. Enzymatic triggered release of imaging probe from paramagnetic liposomes. *Proc Intl Soc Mag Reson Med.* 2010; 18: 33.

76. Visse R, Nagase H. Matrix metalloproteinases and tissue inhibitors of metalloproteinases: Structure, function, and biochemistry. *Circ Res.* 2003; 92(8): 827–839.

77. Yong VW, Zabad RK, Agrawal S, Goncalves Dasilva A, Metz LM. Elevation of matrix metalloproteinases (MMPs) in multiple sclerosis and impact of immunomodulators. *J Neurol Sci.* 2007; 259(1–2): 79–84.

78. Ramos-Fernandez M, Bellolio MF, Stead LG. Matrix metalloproteinase-9 as a marker for acute ischemic stroke: A systematic review. *J Stroke Cerebrovasc Dis.* 2011; 20(1): 47–54.

79. Rundhaug JE. Matrix metalloproteinases, angiogenesis, and cancer: Commentary re: A. C. Lockhart et al., Reduction of wound angiogenesis

in patients treated with BMS-275291, a broad spectrum matrix metalloproteinase inhibitor. *Clin. Cancer Res.*, 9: 00–00, 2003. *Clin Cancer Res.* 2003; 9(2): 551–554.

80. Egeblad M, Werb Z. New functions for the matrix metalloproteinases in cancer progression. *Nat Rev Cancer.* 2002; 2(3): 161–174.

81. Sarkar N, Banerjee J, Hanson AJ, et al. Matrix metalloproteinase-assisted triggered release of liposomal contents. *Bioconjug Chem.* 2008; 19(1): 57–64.

82. Xue-Ying L, Chikashi N, Jun M. Immobilized fluorescent liposome column for bioanalysis and signal amplification. *Biological Systems Engineering.* Vol 830: American Chemical Society; 2002: 259–270.

83. Benefits of the Magnasense Technologies System. http://magnasense. com/index.php?page=benefits. Accessed 2/28, 2015.

84. Ibraimi F, Kriz D, Lu M, Hansson L-O, Kriz K. Rapid one-step whole blood C–reactive protein magnetic permeability immunoassay with monoclonal antibody conjugated nanoparticles as superparamagnetic labels and enhanced sedimentation. *Anal Bioanal Chem.* 2006; 384(3): 651–657.

85. Dittmer WU, de Kievit P, Prins MW, Vissers JL, Mersch ME, Martens MF. Sensitive and rapid immunoassay for parathyroid hormone using magnetic particle labels and magnetic actuation. *J Immunol Methods.* 2008; 338(1–2): 40–46.

86. Barnett JM, Wraith P, Kiely J, et al. An inexpensive, fast and sensitive quantitative lateral flow magneto-immunoassay for total prostate specific antigen. *Biosensors.* 2014; 4(3): 204–220.

87. Bhalla N, Chung D, Chang Y-J, et al. Microfluidic platform for enzyme-linked and magnetic particle-based immunoassay. *Micromachines.* 2013; 4(2): 257–271.

88. Chemla YR, Grossman HL, Poon Y, et al. Ultrasensitive magnetic biosensor for homogeneous immunoassay. *Proc Natl Acad Sci U S A.* 2000; 97(26): 14268–14272.

89. Shin J, Kim M. Development of liposome immunoassay for salmonella spp. using immunomagnetic separation and immunoliposome. *J Microbiol Biotechnol.* 2008; 18(10): 1689–1694.

90. DeCory TR, Durst RA, Zimmerman SJ, et al. Development of an immunomagnetic bead-immunoliposome fluorescence assay for rapid detection of *Escherichia coli* O157:H7 in aqueous samples and comparison of the assay with a standard microbiological method. *Appl Environ Microbiol.* 2005; 71(4): 1856–1864.

91. Chen CS, Baeumner AJ, Durst RA. Protein G-liposomal nanovesicles as universal reagents for immunoassays. *Talanta.* 2005; 67(1): 205–211.

92. Edwards KA, Baeumner AJ. Periplasmic binding protein-based detection of maltose using liposomes: A new class of biorecognition elements in competitive assays. *Anal Chem.* 2013; 85(5): 2770–2778.

93. Margolis LB, Namiot VA, Kliukin LM. Cell sorting using magnetoliposomes. *Biofizika.* 1983; 28(5): 884–885.

94. Margolis LB, Namiot VA, Kljukin LM. Magnetoliposomes: Another principle of cell sorting. *Biochim Biophys Acta.* 1983; 735(1): 193–195.

95. Scheffold A, Miltenyi S, Radbruch A. Magnetofluorescent liposomes for increased sensitivity of immunofluorescence. *Immunotechnology.* 1995; 1(2): 127–137.

96. Kunkel D, Kirchhoff D, Volkmer-Engert R, Radbruch A, Scheffold A. Sensitive visualization of peptide presentation in vitro and ex vivo. *Cytometry A.* 2003; 54(1): 19–26.

97. Harjanto D, Lee J, Kim J-M, Jaworski J. Controlling and assessing the surface display of cell-binding domains on magnetite conjugated fluorescent liposomes. *Langmuir.* 2013; 29(25): 7949–7956.

98. Ruoslahti E. RGD and other recognition sequences for integrins. *Annu Rev Cell Dev Biol.* 1996; 12: 697–715.

99. Zollner T, Zollner R, Gambale W, Santana M. Immunodetection of IgE antibodies against allergens using magnetoliposomes. Paper presented at: *Proceedings of XIII Brasilian Congress of Chemical Engineering* 2000.

100. de Pinho SC, Zollner RL, de Cuyper M, Santana MH. Adsorption of antiphospholipid antibodies on affinity magnetoliposomes. *Colloids Surf B Biointerfaces.* 2008; 63(2): 249–253.

101. Bieberich E. Lipid vesicle-mediated affinity chromatography using magnetic activated cell sorting (LIMACS): A novel method to analyze protein-lipid interaction. *J Vis Exp.* 2011; (50).

102. Fadok VA, Bratton DL, Frasch SC, Warner ML, Henson PM. The role of phosphatidylserine in recognition of apoptotic cells by phagocytes. *Cell Death Differ.* 1998; 5(7): 551–562.

103. Lefèvre C, Abreu F, Lins U, Bazylinski D. A bacterial backbone: Magnetosomes in magnetotactic bacteria. In: Rai M, Duran N, eds. *Metal Nanoparticles in Microbiology*: Springer Berlin Heidelberg; 2011: 75–102.

104. Schuler D. Genetics and cell biology of magnetosome formation in magnetotactic bacteria. *FEMS Microbiol Rev.* 2008; 32(4): 654–672.

105. Lower BH, Bazylinski DA. The bacterial magnetosome: A unique prokaryotic organelle. *J Mol Microbiol Biotechnol.* 2013; 23(1–2): 63–80.

106. Bazylinski DA, Frankel RB. Magnetosome formation in prokaryotes. *Nat Rev Microbiol.* 2004; 2(3): 217–230.

107. Bazylinski DA, Schubbe S. Controlled biomineralization by and applications of magnetotactic bacteria. *Adv Appl Microbiol.* 2007; 62: 21–62.

108. Yan L, Zhang S, Chen P, Liu H, Yin H, Li H. Magnetotactic bacteria, magnetosomes and their application. *Microbiol Res.* 2012; 167(9): 507–519.

109. Schuler D, Frankel RB. Bacterial magnetosomes: Microbiology, biomineralization and biotechnological applications. *Appl Microbiol Biotechnol.* 1999; 52(4): 464–473.

110. Kuhara M, Takeyama H, Tanaka T, Matsunaga T. Magnetic cell separation using antibody binding with protein a expressed on bacterial magnetic particles. *Anal Chem.* 2004; 76(21): 6207–6213.

111. Xie J, Chen K, Chen X. Production, modification and bio-applications of magnetic nanoparticles gestated by magnetotactic bacteria. *Nano Res.* 2009; 2(4): 261–278.

112. Wacker R, Ceyhan B, Alhorn P, Schueler D, Lang C, Niemeyer CM. Magneto Immuno-PCR: A novel immunoassay based on biogenic magnetosome nanoparticles. *Biochem Biophys Res Commun.* 2007; 357(2): 391–396.

113. Alphandéry E. Applications of magnetosomes synthesized by magnetotactic bacteria in medicine. *Front Bioeng Biotechnol.* 2014; 2: 5.

114. Ceyhan B, Alhorn P, Lang C, Schuler D, Niemeyer CM. Semisynthetic biogenic magnetosome nanoparticles for the detection of proteins and nucleic acids. *Small.* 2006; 2(11): 1251–1255.

115. Matsunaga T, Kawasaki M, Yu X, Tsujimura N, Nakamura N. Chemiluminescence enzyme immunoassay using bacterial magnetic particles. *Anal Chem.* 1996; 68(20): 3551–3554.

116. Tanaka T, Matsunaga T. Fully automated chemiluminescence immunoassay of insulin using antibody-protein A-bacterial magnetic particle complexes. *Anal Chem.* 2000; 72(15): 3518–3522.

117. Matsunaga T, Ueki F, Obata K, et al. Fully automated immunoassay system of endocrine disrupting chemicals using monoclonal

antibodies chemically conjugated to bacterial magnetic particles. *Anal Chim Acta.* 2003; 475(1–2): 75–83.

118. Roman-Pizarro V, Fernandez-Romero JM, Gomez-Hens A. Fluorometric determination of alkaline phosphatase activity in food using magnetoliposomes as on-flow microcontainer devices. *J Agric Food Chem.* 2014; 62(8): 1819–1825.

119. de Cuyper M, Joniau M. Binding characteristics and thermal behaviour of cytochrome-C oxidase, inserted into phospholipid-coated, magnetic nanoparticles. *Biotechnol Appl Biochem.* 1992; 16(2): 201–210.

120. De Cuyper M, Joniau M. Immobilization of membrane enzymes into magnetizable, phospholipid bilayer-coated, inorganic colloids. In: Lindman B, Rosenholm JB, Stenius P, eds. *Surfactants and Macromolecules: Self-Assembly at Interfaces and in Bulk.* Vol 82: Steinkopff; 1990: 353–359.

121. Stenberg M, Werthen M, Theander S, Nygren H. A diffusion limited reaction theory for a microtiter plate assay. *J Immunol Methods.* 1988; 112(1): 23–29.

122. Stenberg M, Stiblert L, Nygren H. External diffusion in solid-phase immunoassays. *J Theor Biol.* 1986; 120(2): 129–140.

123. Werthen M, Nygren H. Effect of antibody affinity on the isotherm of antibody binding to surface-immobilized antigen. *J Immunol Methods.* 1988; 115(1): 71–78.

124. Stenberg M, Nygren H. A receptor-ligand reaction studied by a novel analytical tool: The isoscope ellipsometer. *Anal Biochem.* 1982; 127(1): 183–192.

125. Stenberg M, Nygren H. A diffusion limited reaction theory for a solid-phase immunoassay. *J Theor Biol.* 1985; 113(3): 589–597.

126. Nygren H, Stenberg M. Rate limitation of antigen-antibody reactions: Theoretical and practical aspects. In: Butler JE, ed. *Immunochemistry of Solid-Phase Immunoassay*: CRC Press; 1991: 285–291.

127. Kusnezow W, Syagailo YV, Ruffer S, et al. Optimal design of microarray immunoassays to compensate for kinetic limitations: Theory and experiment. *Mol Cell Proteomics.* 2006; 5(9): 1681–1696.

128. Butler JE, ed. *Immunochemistry of Solid-Phase Immunoassay*: CRC Press; 1991.

129. Rossier JS, Girault HH. Enzyme-linked immunosorbent assay on a microchip with electrochemical detection. *Lab Chip.* 2001; 1(2): 153–157.

130. Zimmermann M, Delamarche E, Wolf M, Hunziker P. Modeling and optimization of high-sensitivity, low-volume microfluidic-based surface immunoassays. *Biomed Microdevices.* 2005; 7(2): 99–110.

131. Hofmann O, Voirin G, Niedermann P, Manz A. Three-dimensional microfluidic confinement for efficient sample delivery to biosensor surfaces: Application to immunoassays on planar optical waveguides. *Anal Chem.* 2002; 74(20): 5243–5250.

132. Jungell-Nortamo A, Syvanen AC, Luoma P, Soderlund H. Nucleic acid sandwich hybridization: Enhanced reaction rate with magnetic microparticles as carriers. *Mol Cell Probes.* 1988; 2(4): 281–288.

133. Hendrix PG, Hoylaerts MF, Nouwen EJ, Van de Voorde A, De Broe ME. Magnetic beads in suspension enable a rapid and sensitive immunodetection of human placental alkaline phosphatase. *Eur J Clin Chem Clin Biochem.* 1992; 30(6): 343–347.

134. Edwards KA, Baeumner AJ. Enhancement of heterogeneous assays using fluorescent magnetic liposomes. *Anal Chem.* 2014; 86(13): 6610–6616.

Chapter 9

Liposome-Based Methodologies to Assess Pharmacokinetic Parameters of Drugs

Magdalena Przybyło,[a,b] Tomasz Borowik,[b] and Marek Langner[a,b]

[a]*Laboratory for Biophysics of Lipid Aggregates Chair of Biomedical Engineering, Wroclaw Technical University, Wyb. Wyspianskiego 27, 50-370 Wrocław, Poland*
[b]*Lipid Systems Ltd, Duńska 9, 54-427 Wrocław, Poland*

marek.langner@pwr.edu.pl

Liposomes have been used in pharmacology for more than two decades now. First, they have been used as a tool for the delivery of active pharmacological ingredients. Liposomes, by providing the enclosed aqueous compartment, protect encapsulated active compounds from metabolic degradation. When properly designed, they also improve the compound biodistribution and/or reduce side effects. Liposomes are also used in the new drug development process serving as an experimental model of biological membranes. Due to the extensive legal regulations and rigorous quality requirements, the current drug discovery and development processes are a complex effort requiring large resources and taking more than 10 years to complete.[1–3] In order to reduce the amount of resources and time needed for the development of a new drug,

Liposomes in Analytical Methodologies
Edited by Katie A. Edwards
Copyright © 2016 Pan Stanford Publishing Pte. Ltd.
ISBN 978-981-4669-26-9 (Hardcover), 978-981-4669-27-6 (eBook)
www.panstanford.com

there are continuous efforts to introduce cost- and time-effective methodologies. In this chapter, the description of liposome application as a model of biological barriers is presented along with the description of experimental strategies and measurement techniques for the determination of parameters critical for a drug.

9.1 Introduction

For most pharmacological formulations, the first step in determining the drug's fate within the body is its absorption. In order to be absorbed, the drug must be in a dissolved form; thus, the *solubility* is the first critical parameter. Other factors controlling the rate of drug absorption are the *degree of ionization* (pK_a and the pH of the solution), *lipophilicity* (lipid-to-water partition coefficient $\log K$ and the apparent lipid-to-water partition coefficient $\log D$), and chemical *stability*. Once a drug has been absorbed, it has to be distributed throughout the body. In some approaches, the fate of the compound in the body is presented in terms of fluxes between various compartments. An example of such approach is schematically presented, for an orally delivered drug, in Fig. 9.1. The drug flux is reduced at barriers between compartments, and this is what limits its availability at the targeted location. Therefore, the fate of an active compound can be dissected into a series of discrete events, which can be modeled and evaluated individually. This makes possible the identification of critical descriptors, which quantitate the capacity of a compound to cross a specific barrier. The nature of barriers can be different, ranging from the metabolic transformation to a physical obstacle, i.e., biological membranes.[4] In order to assess the effect of a barrier on the quantity of the active compound available, simplified model experimental systems are needed. The recurring element of each barrier is the presence of proteins and membranes.

The flux between aqueous compartments is directly proportional to the quantity and state of a free drug. The amount of the free drug depends on the extent of binding to proteins and its capacity to cross membranes. The additional factor affecting the flux is the extent of the drug degradation and/or chemical alteration.

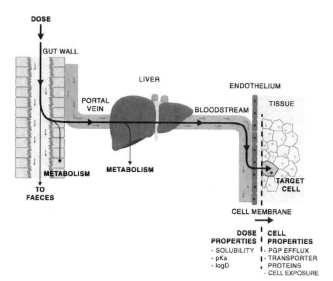

Figure 9.1   The graph demonstrates the fate of the active pharmacological ingredient (API) in the body following the oral
administration along with selected physiological barriers.
The pharmacologically relevant parameters for the barrier
are also indicated.

9.1.1   In vitro Models

It has been observed that a chemical compound is a good candidate
for an active pharmaceutical ingredient if it possesses certain
properties that can be derived from its chemical structure. Lipinski
et al. deduced from a library containing about 2000 drugs that
the compound is likely to reach its intracellular target if it has the
following properties[5]:

- Molecular weight ≤ 500 (optimally $= \sim 350$)
- # Hydrogen bond acceptors ≤ 10 (optimally $= \sim 5$)
- # Hydrogen bond donors ≤ 5 (optimally $= \sim 2$)
- $-2 < \operatorname{Log} K < 5$ (optimally $= \sim 3.0$)
- # Rotatable bonds ≤ 5.

Later, other descriptors were added, such as polar surface
area.[6] In order to quantitatively validate predictors, experimental
model systems of barriers are needed. The following discussion

is limited to the biological membrane barrier but is intended to demonstrate the methodology of other barriers quantification as well.

The reliable experimental models in vitro should account for all relevant physiological factors. Therefore, the models containing combination of proteins and lipid aggregates are constructed for the determination of a variety of descriptors, including protein binding, partition coefficient, membrane permeability, or kinetics and thermodynamics of the active compound exchange between membranes and proteins.[7] Whereas the active compound binding to proteins can be evaluated using well-established approaches, insight into its interaction with the biological membrane is not straightforward. It is believed that the pharmacological compound is effective when it is able to cross the biological membrane barrier via passive diffusion across the lipid bilayer.[8]

The first experimental model of biological membrane assumes that the lipid bilayer is a preliminary route for drug crossing the barrier and that the lipid bilayer is a uniform, hydrophobic slab covered with surface-active molecules. In practice, the lipid bilayer is modeled with a hydrophobic filter containing an inert organic solvent mixed with phospholipids (parallel artificial membrane permeability assay—PAMPA). The measurement of flux is based on the determination of the concentration buildup in the receiving chamber.[9] In traditional PAMPA, a simple diffusion at iso-pH conditions is measured.[10] Recently, a variation of the method has been introduced, known as "Double-Sink™ PAMPA". In this experiment, the pH in the donor chamber is different from that in the acceptor chamber, resulting in more than 50% of the compound being transferred. This setup is much faster than "traditional" PAMPA and may be used to simulate conditions in the gastrointestinal track.[9,11,12] Both PAMPA setups are schematically presented in Fig. 9.2.

The PAMPA model is too simplistic for many applications; therefore, a more convenient, yet realistic, experimental model of the biological membrane is needed. Liposomes, spherical structures formed from lipid bilayers, fulfill those requirements. They can be relatively easily and reproducibly produced, their composition can be well controlled, and there is a large body of experimental techniques available to quantitate their properties.[13]

All those arguments stimulate the development of theoretical, numerical, and experimental approaches, which can be used for the selection of drug candidates at the early stages of the drug discovery process.[14]

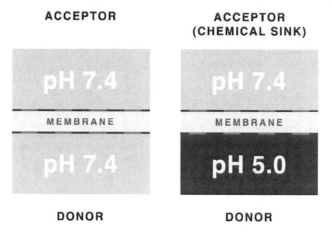

Figure 9.2 The schematic presentation of PAMPA (parallel artificial membrane permeability assay) systems for the determination of the permeability coefficient. Left panel: traditional PAMPA setup. Right panel: Double-Sink™ PAMPA setup.

9.2 Properties of Pharmacological Active Ingredients

9.2.1 Solubility

Before any adsorption/permeation tests can be performed, the compound needs to be dissolved in the aqueous phase. The solubility can be evaluated using both computational and physicochemical methods.[15-20] Computational methods are convenient, but they lack high level of certainty; therefore, experimental confirmation is required. The experimental methods of solubility determination are not straightforward, especially for amphiphilic and hydrophobic compounds. To ensure such compounds' solubility, the universal solvent (dimethyl sulfoxide or DMSO) or molecular carriers (such as cyclodextrins or albumins) are used.[15,17,21]

9.2.2 Degree of Protonation

The degree of ionization affects the solubility of the compound, as well as its partitioning into biological membranes. The thermodynamic parameter relating the pH of the solution to the protonation of a molecule is the protonation constant, pK_a, defined for weak acids ($HX \Leftrightarrow X^- + H^+$) as follows in Eq. 9.1[22,23]:

$$pK_a = pH + \log\left(\frac{[HX]}{[X^-]}\right)$$

(9.1)

where p denotes "–log" operation. These equations correlate the degree of compound protonation with its pK_a and with the pH value of the solution. Similar equations can be derived for weak bases.

9.2.3 Distribution Constant

Lipophilicity is a derivative of the Born energy and is the measure of the tendency of the compound to partition between the lipophilic organic phase and the polar aqueous phase. It shows that the charged compounds require higher energy than the neutral ones to be transferred from aqueous to hydrophobic phase. The lipophilicity can be expressed in terms of the distribution constant D. The distribution constant is defined as the ratio of concentrations of the compound X between two immiscible solutions, regardless of its level of ionization or protonation (Eq. 9.2).

$$D = \frac{[X^0]_{\text{lipophilic phase}} + [X^1]_{\text{lipophilic phase}}}{[X^0]_{\text{aqueous phase}} + [X^1]_{\text{aqueous phase}}}$$

(9.2)

where $[X^1]$ and $[X^0]$ stand for neutral and charged forms of the compound present in a solution. For weak acids and bases, the distribution constant changes with the value of pH. For non-ionizable compounds, the distribution constant reduces to the partition coefficient K_P, which is pH invariant. The value of lipophilicity most commonly refers to the logarithm of the partition coefficient K ($\log K$) or the logarithm of the distribution coefficient D ($\log D$) between the two immiscible phases, typically the octanol/water system.[24]

9.3 Determining Pharmacokinetic Parameters Depending on Lipid Bilayer Properties

When the lipid bilayer is treated as an unstructured, hydrophobic slab separating two aqueous phases, the crossing of the membrane can be represented as a series of steps, as presented in Fig. 9.3.

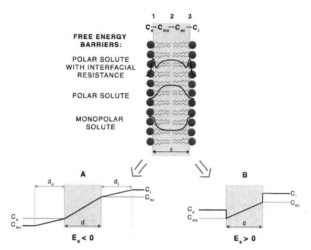

Figure 9.3 The permeation process quantitated using the energy barrier encountered by the compound entering the membrane (the upper panel). The energy barriers encountered by the nonpolar and polar solutes, with and without the interfacial resistance, are indicated. Panel A shows the concentration profile of a compound, which efficiently crosses the membrane. Panel B shows the concentration profile for a compound, which crosses membrane slowly. C_o and C_i are the concentrations of the compound in the aqueous phases, whereas C_{mo} and C_{mi} are the compound concentrations at the two surfaces of the membrane. The ratios $C_{mo}/C_o = C_{mi}/C_i$ reflect the membrane/aqueous phase partition coefficient of the compound.

In this representation, the membrane crossing requires compound adsorption onto the membrane interface, its diffusion through the hydrophobic core, and the subsequent dissociation from the membrane interface on the other side of the membrane. The energy barrier results mainly from the compound interaction with lipids at bilayer interfaces mainly by hydrogen bonds formation.[25]

9.3.1 Permeability Coefficient

The permeability coefficient (P) is defined as a constant in the flux J dependent on the concentration difference ($C_i - C_0$) between two aqueous phases separated by the membrane (Eq. 9.3):

$$J = -\frac{P}{A}(C_i - C_o) \tag{9.3}$$

where A stands for the membrane surface area.[26,27]

When the molecules equilibrate rapidly between the aqueous and membrane phases, compared to the membrane permeation process, the flux is proportional to the concentration difference of the compound at the two membrane interfaces (Fig. 9.2b) where d is the membrane thickness (Eq. 9.4):

$$J = -\frac{P}{A}\left(\frac{C_{mi} - C_{mo}}{d}\right) \tag{9.4}$$

The equilibration of molecules between the aqueous and hydrophobic phases requires that their chemical potentials in water phase (μ_w) and in the membrane (μ_m) are equal (Eq. 9.5):

$$\mu_w = \mu_w^0 + RT\ln C_w = \mu_m = \mu_m^0 + RT\ln C_m \tag{9.5}$$

Therefore, the drug concentration at the surface of the membrane C_m will correlate with the aqueous concentration C_w, according to Eq. 9.6:

$$C_m = C_w \exp\left(\frac{\mu_w^0 - \mu_m^0}{RT}\right) \tag{9.6}$$

Since the compound diffusion within the membrane is quantitated with the diffusion coefficient D, the molecular flux can be rewritten as Eq. 9.7:

$$J = -\frac{D}{d}\exp\left(\frac{\mu_w^0 - \mu_m^0}{RT}\right)(C_i - C_o) \tag{9.7}$$

Therefore, the permeability coefficient P can be determined via Eq. 9.8:

$$P = \left(\frac{D}{d}\right)\exp\left(\frac{\mu_w^0 - \mu_m^0}{RT}\right) \tag{9.8}$$

The permeability coefficient accounts for the properties of the solute and the membrane alike. The solute capacity to enter the membrane is quantitated with the experimentally determined partition coefficient (K_P). Therefore, the permeability coefficient can be rewritten as Eq. 9.9:

$$P = D\frac{K_P}{d} \tag{9.9}$$

In this membrane representation, the permeability coefficient depends on the partition coefficient of the solute and its mobility in the membrane.[26]

9.3.2 Membrane Association/Partition Testing

In principle, the membrane association/partition test is relatively simple to perform since in order to obtain quantitative data, it is sufficient to determine the amount of compound in the aqueous phase.[28] Model lipid bilayers in the form of vesicles or other lipid aggregates are the most suitable for this purpose since they have all the main features of biological membranes relevant for the membrane nonspecific association and permeabilization.[29] In order to perform the association/partition test, it is important to control precisely the surface area of the lipid aggregate; therefore, unilamellar vesicles or a single lipid bilayer deposited on a solid support, frequently in the form of solid particles, can be used.[30]

9.3.3 Determination of the Solute Intra-Membrane Location

The determination of the compound membrane-bound fraction does not provide information necessary for the differentiation between various locations within the lipid bilayer. If more detailed analysis is needed, the perception of the lipid bilayer as a uniform hydrophobic slab is insufficient. Based on experimental studies, the more realistic description of the lipid bilayer has been proposed by White et al.[31,32] and later supplemented by computer simulations.[31] In this description, the lipid bilayer is presented as a dynamic structure, arbitrary divided into four regions (organized water, interface, soft polymer, and hydrophobic core).

In order to determine the compound exact location within the lipid bilayer and/or to measure the incorporation kinetics, a dedicated molecular probe and experimental methodologies are required. Traditionally, fluorescent dyes are used to study various membrane properties and processes. In order to monitor the flux of a compound, the correlation between the probe fluorescence and the compound quantity is required. If the probe is sensitive to a specific property, such as electrostatic charge, local polarity, and/or local molecular dynamics, the passing or accumulating compound can be detected and quantified.[33,34] Specifically, electrostatically charged compounds can be detected with the pH-sensitive fluorescent dye fluorescein attached to the phosphatidylethanolamine headgroup.[35–37] Alterations in local interfacial polarity can be monitored with diphenylhexatriene (DPH) and its derivatives or lipids labeled with 7-nitrobenz-2-oxa-1,3-diazol-4-yl (NBD).[38,39] These dyes are excellent probes of membrane interface, as they exhibit weak fluorescence in aqueous mediums, but strong fluorescence in hydrophobic environments. By contrast, properties of the membrane interior can be monitored with the hydrophobic probe pyrene attached to lipid hydrocarbon chains, which undergoes fluorescence quenching due to quencher membrane partitioning, or with fluorescent molecules sensitive to the strength of the local electrostatic field, which can change upon electrostatically charged compound partitioning.[40,41] The presence of the compound can also be detected by the shift and/or smearing of the lipid thermotropic phase transition as evaluated with differential scanning calorimetry or dedicated fluorescence techniques.[42–47]

Later, more sophisticated experimental models that provide information on the water/membrane partition coefficient using lipid bilayers have been developed. For example, one application of BIACORE technology is a direct method where signal alteration is proportional to the quantity of a compound adsorbed onto immobilized liposomes.[48] Other methods frequently used for the determination of partitioning are presented later in the chapter.

9.3.4 Partition Coefficient–Membrane Localization

For a compound X being a weak base, its partition to the lipid bilayer can be described by partition coefficients for neutral and ionized species, respectively (Eq. 9.10 and 9.11):

$$\log K^0_{\text{mem}} = \log\left(\frac{[X^0]_{\text{mem}}}{[X^0]_{\text{aq}}}\right) \tag{9.10}$$

$$\log K^{\text{SIP}}_{\text{mem}} = \log\left(\frac{[XH^+]_{\text{mem}}}{[XH^+]_{\text{aq}}}\right) \tag{9.11}$$

When the compound's charged species migrate into the lipid membrane environment, the counter ion that accompanies it may be exchanged with the zwitterionic PC headgroups forming a surface ion pair.[49]

The molecular view of the partitioning of the drug molecule to the phospholipid bilayer may be divided into three major components:

(1) **Hydrophobic effect** driving the incorporation of amphiphilic and hydrophobic compounds into the membrane
(2) **Electrostatic interactions** with lipid headgroups affected by the local value of the dielectric constant
(3) **Hydrogen bond formation** via rearrangements in proton-mediated interactions at the membrane interface.

Due to the attributes related directly to lipid membrane structure and properties, such as spatial anisotropy of physicochemical parameters (lipid packing, cross-sectional dielectric constant profile), discrepancies between the results of $\log K^1$ and $\log K^1_{\text{mem}}$ for some types of molecules (including macromolecules) are observed. For example, it has been shown that charged species partition more strongly into liposomes than expected based on the $\log K^1$ values.[50] Similarly, it has been shown that neutral H-bond forming species have higher lipophilicity than determined using octanol/water system.[50] Another important factor is the free volume available for a compound in the lipid bilayer. From this point of view, permeation of the compound can be analyzed in terms of the solute molecules finding nearby cavities to fill. In particular, the degree of solute partitioning to the membrane may depend on the probability of finding free volume within the hydrophilic headgroup region.[51] Such perspective implies that both shape and size of the solute as well as lipid packing density will affect the compound's localization within the membrane and the extent of membrane partitioning.

9.4 Experimental Methods for Determining Partition Coefficient

The evaluation of the membrane partition coefficient requires the determination of the compound quantity associated with membrane and that remaining in the aqueous phase. The liposome-based experimental system differs from the octanol/water test since there are three distinctly different regions in the sample: the outer aqueous phase, the lipid phase, and the inner-vesicle aqueous phase. In order to calculate the water/membrane partition coefficient, the volume of lipid phase and inner-vesicle aqueous volume need to be known in advance. In general, hydrophobic compounds can be considered to dissolve within the whole volume of the lipid bilayer, whereas amphiphilic molecules will predominantly locate at the lipid bilayer surface. Therefore, requirements for the lipid vesicles are different for the two situations. In the case of an amphiphilic molecule, the properties of the membrane surface should be uniform, meaning that the vesicles should have similar sizes and preferentially consist of a single homogeneous membrane. It is well established that large unilamellar vesicles (LUVs) with diameters preferably equal or larger than 100 nm (ensuring equal lipid distribution within the inner and outer membrane leaflets) are the best models for partitioning studies.

There are two types of methodologies for the water/membrane partition coefficient determination: (1) methods involving physical separation of free and membrane-bound molecules and (2) methods where such physical separation is not required.

9.4.1 Determination of Partition Coefficient by Separation of Free and Membrane-Bound Molecules

When no physical signal is produced upon compound insertion into the lipid bilayer, the separation of membrane-bound and free species is required for the determination of partition coefficient. The main difficulty with these kinds of experimental methodologies is the requirement of complete separation of two coexisting populations of molecules (free and membrane bound) without perturbation of the partitioning equilibrium and preventing lipids from entering compartments containing unbound compound.

9.4.1.1 Equilibrium dialysis and ultrafiltration

Equilibrium dialysis is a standard reference technique. It was introduced by Pauletti to study drug partitioning in the membrane system formed from egg phosphatidylcholine.[52] When combined with a sensitive analytical method for drug detection, equilibrium dialysis enables determining the $\log K$ values for a wide range of compounds. The dialysis cell consists of two compartments separated by a semipermeable membrane, usually composed of porous cellulose. Pores, which work as molecular weight cut-off (MWCO) separators, are approximately 4 nm in diameter, which corresponds to 10 kDa, and are much smaller than the average diameter of liposomes (100 nm). The time of the dialysis depends on the nature of the compound, the solute properties (ionic composition and strength, osmotic pressure), lipids used, and the experimental conditions (temperature, dialysis membrane MWCO, dialysis membrane chemical composition). For example, the time needed for the equilibration of a system consisting of propranolol and egg PC liposomes was shown to be about 5 h, whereas a system study of selected water-soluble fluorophores required up to 86 h.[53-55] Once equilibrium is reached, the concentration of solute and lipids is determined in both compartments. Lipid concentration in the free solute-containing compartment should be equal to zero. The partition coefficient K is calculated based on the mass balance in the liposome-containing compartment,[56] according to Eq. 9.12:

$$K_{\text{mem}} = \frac{V_{\text{LC}}}{V_{\text{M}}} \left(\frac{[X]_{\text{LC}} - [X]_{\text{AC}}}{[X]_{\text{AC}}} \right) + 1 \qquad (9.12)$$

where V_{LC} is the volume of the liposome compartment, V_{M} is the lipid membrane volume, $[X]_{\text{LC}}$ is the concentration of compound X in the lipid compartment, and $[X]_{\text{AC}}$ is the concentration of compound X in the aqueous compartment. One has to keep in mind that in order to determine the concentration of membrane-bound species in the lipid fraction, a dedicated extraction procedure has to be used. The ultrafiltration technique is a variation of the equilibrium dialysis where the liposome-free solvent is forced through the membrane using hydrostatic pressure differences.[57]

9.4.1.2 Centrifugation

The centrifugation-based technique is a density-dependent separation process utilizing glucose-containing liposomes as model membranes. Liposomes prepared in glucose solution are diluted, centrifuged, and the resulting liposome-containing sediment is re-suspended in an aqueous buffer without glucose. The ionic strength of the buffer used is critical since the isosmotic conditions should be maintained throughout the sample preparation process so that the membrane rupture is avoided. In a typical experiment, the compound of interest is added to the suspension of glucose-containing liposomes, the mixture is left to equilibrate (20 min), and is then centrifuged at 130,000 g for 5 min.[58] Since the density of the aqueous phase inside the liposomes is higher than that of the external solution, all liposomes, including the membrane-bound fraction of the compound, are in the sediment. The partition coefficient is calculated based on the determined solute concentrations in both sediment and supernatant. The lipid quantity in the supernatant should be determined to ensure the complete liposome sedimentation.[58]

9.4.1.3 Reverse-phase high-performance liquid chromatography

The measurement is based on the assumption that the retention parameters can be converted into a $\log K$ scale. For column partitioning chromatography, a solute distributed between an aqueous mobile phase and a gel stationary phase can be expressed as a distribution coefficient (Eq. 9.13)[59]:

$$B = \frac{(V_e - V_0)}{V_s} \tag{9.13}$$

where V_e is the elution volume of the solute, V_0 is the mobile phase volume, and V_s is the stationary phase volume. This can be converted to a $\log K$ scale through the use of reference compound(s).[60]

In one variation of the method, immobilized lipids form the stationary phase—immobilized artificial membranes (IAMs). Pidgeon et al.[61,62] used PC lipids covalently attached to the surface of silica beads. In this case, the volume of the stationary phase is equal to the volume of the immobilized artificial membrane accessible for partitioning.[63,64] The main drawback of IAM chromatography is related to the uncertainty of lipid structuring.[65] Moreover, the preparation of IAM column is not a trivial task and requires a high level of expertise.

In contrast to IAM chromatography, a method developed by Yang and coworkers is based on immobilized unilamellar liposomes on gel beads via avidin-biotin binding.[66] Immobilization of intact liposomes brings the experimental system much closer to reality. The approach also enables relatively easy manipulation of the membrane composition. In this case, the stationary phase equals the volume of lipid membrane accessible for partitioning. Liu and coworkers studied the effect of liposome size, lamellarity, surface charge, and presence of cholesterol on the partitioning of 15 drug molecules determined with immobilized liposome chromatography.[67] They found differences in drug partitioning when multilamellar vesicles (MLVs), LUVs, and small unilamellar vesicles (SUVs) were used as immobilized phase. This is likely due to the differences in volumes of lipid phases accessible for partitioning (MLVs vs. LUVs) and differences in the molecular surface area between SUVs and LUVs. The method is applicable for compounds efficiently equilibrating throughout the whole membrane volume, so the kinetic factor can be safely neglected.

9.4.2 Determination of Partition Coefficient without Separation of Free and Membrane-Bound Molecules

Determination of the partition coefficient without separation of bound and unbound fractions of a compound is based on the global system signal response analysis, which is a combination of signals from free and membrane-bound species. The experiment is typically carried out at various ratios of lipid and water phases, so a large number of experimental data are available for analysis. An elegant and robust methodology ("a universal thermodynamic approach") for handling such data sets has been developed by Schwarz.[68-70] The method can be used for experimental systems as long as there is the detection method of a parameter altered as a result of the binding/partition process.[71-73]

The following sections present selected methods of binding/partition determination.

9.4.2.1 Potentiometric titrations

The titration of the ionizable compound in a biphasic system, such as an aqueous liposome suspension, may serve as an excellent example of the experimental design proposed by Schwarz,[70] which enables the partition coefficient determination for charged amphiphiles. The method is based on the effect of surface-adsorbed charged species on the proton distribution within the sample. In order to determine a compound's membrane partition coefficient, first its pK_a value in the aqueous phase is determined. Then the experiment is repeated for various membrane/aqueous phase volume ratios (r). Since the measured pK constant (pK_a^{app}) is r-dependent, the shift in pK_a^{app} is related to the compound's partitioning into the membrane phase.[49,74–76] The potentiometric titration method is restricted exclusively to ionizable compounds. The range of lipophilicity, which can be determined by this method, is smaller to that accessible by separation techniques (i.e., equilibrium dialysis) due to relatively high solute concentrations in the aqueous phase needed for titration.

9.4.2.2 Zeta-potential measurements

Determination of the membrane partition coefficient using ζ-potential measurements requires the presence of electrostatic charge on the compound and/or membrane. The partition of charged compound results in the surface charge alterations.[77] The electrophoretic mobility of charged particle, U_E, in the external electrical field depends on the ζ-potential according to Henry's relation (Eq. 9.14)[78]:

$$U_E = \frac{2\varepsilon\zeta f(ka)}{3\eta} \tag{9.14}$$

where ζ is the zeta-potential, $f(ka)$ is Henry's function, ε is the solvent dielectric constant, and η is the solvent viscosity.

To derive the value of K_{mem} using ζ-potential measurements, it is necessary to know in advance the net charge of the compound (z_X) and/or lipid (z_{cL}) along with the mole fraction of the charged lipids in the membrane (f_{cL}). The change in the value of the

ζ-potential upon compound partitioning $|\Delta\zeta/\zeta_0|$ is proportional to the fraction of the charge appearing/disappearing on the liposome surface (Eq. 9.15):

$$\left|\frac{\Delta\zeta}{\zeta_0}\right| = \frac{n_{nL}}{n_{tL}} \tag{9.15}$$

where n_{nL} is the number of charges introduced to the membrane surface or charged lipids neutralized and n_{tL} is the total number of charged lipids. Assuming 1:1 interaction between the charged compound and the charged lipid moieties, the following relation (Eq. 9.16) can be stated:

$$\left|\frac{\Delta\zeta}{\zeta_0}\right| = 1 + \frac{X_L z_X}{f_{cL}[L]z_{cL}}[X] \tag{9.16}$$

where $[L]$ and $[X]$ are lipid and compound concentrations, respectively, and X_L is the fraction of membrane-bound compound X, which is related to the membrane partition coefficient K_{mem} according to the following equation (Eq. 9.17):

$$X_L = \frac{K_{mem}\gamma_L[L]}{1 + K_{mem}\gamma_L[L]} \tag{9.17}$$

where γ_L is the molar volume of lipid.

Plotting the value of ζ-potential when compound X is titrated into the suspension of lipid membranes, a linear relationship is expected since $|\zeta/\zeta_0| = f([X])$. The membrane partition coefficient K_{mem} can be determined from the slope using Eqs. 9.16 and 9.17.

9.4.2.3 Isothermal titration calorimetry

Isothermal titration calorimetry (ITC) is a powerful technique to determine energetics of any process. It allows determination of the Gibbs free energy (ΔG), enthalpy (ΔH), and entropy (ΔS) at a given temperature T. Those quantities satisfy the following relation (Eq. 9.18)[79-81]:

$$\Delta G = \Delta H - T\Delta S \tag{9.18}$$

Whereas enthalpy change (ΔH) relates to molecular interactions, the change of ΔS is a measure of the change in the molecular arrangement within the system. These values are related to the dissociation constant K_d^{-1} according to the following equation (Eq. 9.19):

$$\Delta G = -RT \ln(K_d^{-1}) \tag{9.19}$$

where R is the universal gas constant.

The first applications of ITC to study drug–membrane interactions were performed by Seelig and coworkers.[82,83] In a typical ITC experiment, a sample in a syringe is titrated into the reaction cell, and the resulting heat flow in an isolated system is measured. There are two possible titration procedures for the evaluation of the membrane association process: type-A and type-B titrations. In type-A titration, the drug solution is titrated into the liposome suspension. In type-B titration, the liposome suspension is titrated into the drug solution.

Most ITC partitioning assays are based on the injections of the liposome suspensions into the reaction cell. The type-B titration described earlier can be utilized for this purpose as a so-called uptake protocol.[84–86] Alternatively, the release protocol can be employed based on the injection of the liposome suspension-containing compound into a large excess of water/buffer, causing the release of the compound from membranes.

The relation between heat flow ΔQ and the amount of the injected lipid, expressed as a lipid concentration $[L]$ in the cuvette, is given by Eq. 9.20.[87]

$$\Delta Q = V_C \frac{(K_d + n[L] + [T])}{2} - \frac{\sqrt{(K_d + n[L] + [T])^2 - 4n[L][T]}}{2} \tag{9.20}$$

where V_C is the reaction cell volume, n is the number of binding sites per lipid molecule, $[T]$ is the total concentration of molecules (lipids and drugs) in the reaction cell, and K_d is the dissociation constant, defined as Eq. 9.21:

$$K_d = \frac{[L]_{unbound}[X]_{aq}}{[X]_{mem}} \tag{9.21}$$

where $[X]_{aq}$ is the concentration of free drug X in the aqueous phase, $[X]_{mem}$ is the concentration of the membrane-bound drug, and $[L]_{unbound}$ is the concentration of unoccupied membrane-binding sites. The values of ΔH, K_d, and n can be determined from titration curves using the least squares fitting method. Assumptions regarding the number of binding sites per lipid molecule, n, are essential for the estimation of the membrane partition coefficient K_{mem} from the titration data. The number of lipid molecules involved in the binding of a single drug molecule may vary significantly, for example from 4 for miconazole to 45 for propranolol.[87] The value K_{mem} can be derived from the titration data using the following equation (Eq. 9.22)[87]:

$$K_{mem} = \frac{n}{aK_d} \qquad (9.22)$$

where a is the molar lipid volume. The molar lipid volume a for PC molecule is 0.755 mL/mmol.[88] Equation 9.22 shows that the membrane partition coefficient (K_{mem}), in addition to the binding constant K_d, also depends on the number of binding sites per lipid molecule and the molar lipid volume.

9.5 Membrane Permeability Determination

In contrast to membrane partitioning evaluation, the determination of the permeability coefficient is technically difficult. It requires an experimental system consisting of two aqueous compartments separated by a hydrophobic barrier. Therefore, the experimental model based on the lipid vesicle with the capability to detect the presence of the tested compound simultaneously in an outer and inner water compartment seems to be the most appropriate for permeability determination.[37,89]

9.5.1 Permeability Tests Using Liposomes as Membrane Model Systems

A uniform population of unilamellar vesicles is a well-defined model of the lipid bilayer and is frequently used as an experimental system for drug permeability studies. In this case, the permeability coefficient can be quantitatively determined using the following dependence (Eq. 9.23):

$$\frac{1}{A}\frac{dm}{dt} = \frac{P}{RT}(C_{out} - C_{in}) \qquad (9.23)$$

where A stands for the vesicle surface area, P stands for membrane permeability coefficient, and C_{in} and C_{out} are the concentrations of permeate in the inner and outer aqueous phases, respectively. In principle, the concentration asymmetry can be generated in either direction; however, the experimental setup where the higher concentration of tested compound is in the inner-vesicle compartment produces a number of difficulties resulting mainly from the small relative volume of the inner-vesicle compartment and possible leakage of the compound during sample preparation. Consequently, in typical experimental setups, the concentration of a compound is elevated in the outer compartment causing its flux toward the inner-vesicle compartment. Preferably, the compound concentration buildup in the inner-vesicle compartment is monitored. From such kinetic traces, the permeability coefficient can be calculated by fitting the experimental data to Eq. 9.23. In order to avoid changes of the inner-compartment volume, liposomes should be formed in the iso-osmotic solution, so there would be no osmotic pressure difference present across the membrane during the experiment. This seemingly simple experimental strategy is difficult to utilize since there are limited possibilities to monitor the buildup of permeate concentration in the inner-liposome compartment. In the following sections, examples of experimental designs for the evaluation of the transmembrane flux are described.

9.5.1.1 Determination of permeability coefficient with molecular probe encapsulated in vesicle inner compartment

To monitor the flux of the compound into the inner-vesicle compartment, molecular probes that are able to quantitatively detect the compound's presence are needed. In some strategies, the probe is highly hydrophilic, so it will not interact with the membrane surface and/or will not leak out of the vesicle. When the investigated compound is fluorescent, the fluorescence of the entrapped probe should be sensitive to the presence of the compound (dynamic or static quenching or distance-dependent energy transfer). Dynamic quenching can be achieved by the encapsulation of a quencher (heavy metals or chloride ions).[90,91] The main limitation of the experimental design results from the small fraction of the compound exposed to the quencher. Other detection methods for the compound's presence in the inner-vesicle compartment are based on the alteration of the local pH value. In this case, a pH-sensitive fluorescent probe is encapsulated inside vesicles and its fluorescence monitored as a function of time.[92] The main problems with such assays are difficulty ensuring that reproducible quantities of entrapped fluorophore are present and the possibility of dye leakage during the experiment.

In strategies utilizing entrapped probe, the experimental system should consist of unilamellar vesicles, so their surface area is well controlled. Additionally, the dye concentration should be below its self-quenching concentration. The value of the permeability coefficient is calculated from the fit of the diffusion model (Eq. 9.23) to the experimental kinetic curves generated in the stopped-flow experiment.[93] In the typical setup, fluorescently labeled liposomes are placed in one syringe, while solution of permeate is in the other syringe. Usually syringes are gas driven (Applied Photonics, Skipton, UK), but electronically driven motors can also be used (BioLogic, Grenoble, FR). The later design is preferred since two pistons can be driven individually with different speeds, which enables precise injection of solutions with different volume ratios. Following the injection, both solutions are mixed and pushed into the quartz measurement chamber following the hard stop of the flow. The compound/membrane interaction can be followed in time by monitoring alterations in fluorescence emission due to the compound's membrane insertion and/or penetration (Fig. 9.4).

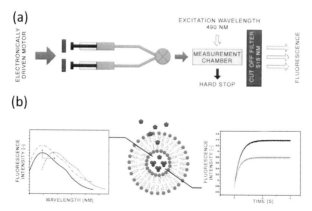

Figure 9.4 The schematic presentation of the stopped-flow method equipped with the optical detection (Panel a). The compound/membrane interaction can be followed in time by monitoring alterations in fluorescence emission in the course of membrane insertion and/or penetration (Panel b).

9.5.1.2 Determination of permeability coefficient with molecular probe covalently attached to a lipid molecule

Langner et al.[37] proposed a new approach where the hydrophilic fluorescent moiety of the probe is covalently attached to the lipid molecule, schematically shown in Fig. 9.5. This design allows for the elimination of all main problems inherent to assays based on the encapsulated hydrophilic probe. Specifically

- The quantity of the fluorescent probe is precisely controlled.
- The covalent attachment of the fluorophore to the lipid molecule results in a stable fluorophore location.
- When the fluorophore is hydrophilic (i.e., fluorescein), the inner and outer aqueous passes can be monitored simultaneously.
- When the fluorophore is amphiphilic or hydrophobic (i.e., NBD, pyrene), the membrane interface or hydrophobic core can be monitored, respectively.

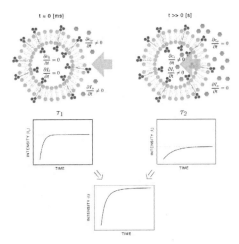

Figure 9.5 Principle of permeability determination with interfacial fluorescent dye covalently attached to a lipid molecule. This arrangement results in two dye populations on vesicle surfaces. The outer-located dye reports the kinetics of the compound association with the membrane (left panel), whereas the inner-located dyes monitor the transmembrane flux of the compound (right panel). The kinetics of the resulting fluorescence changes (lower panel) can be dissected into two curves showing the adsorption and permeability kinetics.

The experiment provides simultaneous information on the compound's association at the membrane surface and its flux into the inner aqueous compartment.[37] Consequently, the determination of the permeability coefficient is a straightforward task without the need for the independent determination of the compound intra-vesicle concentration. Specifically, after the rapid mixing of labeled liposomes with the compound solution, the fluorescence intensity change is measured as a function of time. The time course of the fluorescence intensity changes, $F(t)$, allows evaluating the membrane permeability for the compound according to the simple dependence shown in Eq. 9.24:

$$\frac{\Delta F(t)_{tot}}{F^0_{tot}} \approx \frac{\Delta F_{in}(t)}{F^0_{tot}} = A\exp(-t\tau), \qquad (9.24)$$

where A and τ are constants. Equation 9.24 is applicable to cases when the transmembrane compound flow is significantly slower than its association with vesicle surface.

9.5.1.3 Permeability determination by the association of the active compound to its molecular target

The other experimental design relies on the encapsulation of the molecular target itself. If the ligand binding (interaction) results in a change of any sample parameter (i.e., fluorescence or UV/VIS), then the kinetic curves can be generated and permeability coefficient evaluated. Using this strategy, the permeation coefficient of anthracyclines was investigated using liposomes with entrapped nucleic acids. In this case, the fluorescence intensity of anthracycline is quenched upon intercalation into the DNA. Such experiments require that the membrane crossing is the rate-limiting step for the observed fluorescence change and that the membrane integrity is not compromised during the experiment.[94]

9.5.1.4 Permeability tests with the molecular sensor located in the outer aqueous compartment

In this approach, the active compound is enclosed in liposomes and its release over time is monitored.[95] The principle of this approach can be illustrated with the example of fluorescamine, which is nonfluorescent in native state but reacts readily and rapidly ($t_{1/2} = 0.1$–0.5 s) with primary amines in a 1:1 stoichiometric ratio to yield highly fluorescent moieties that can be quantified in the nanomolar range. In this case, liposomes containing amino acids were exposed to fluorescamine and the rising fluorescence due to the reaction product in the external aqueous compartment is monitored as a function of time.[96] Assuming that the concentration of amino acid inside the liposome is much greater than that outside, the efflux can be described with the following equation (Eq. 9.25):

$$A(t)_{ex} = A(eq)_{ex}(1 - e^{-kt})$$ (9.25)

where $A(t)_{ex}$ is the exterior concentration of amino acid at time t, $A(eq)_{ex}$ is the equilibrium exterior concentration, and k is the rate constant associated with the efflux process. The plot of $\ln(([A(eq)_{ex}]-[A(t)_{ex}])/A(eq)_{ex}])$ versus t gives a slope of $-k$ (the rate constant). The permeability coefficient (P) can then be calculated using Eq. 9.26:

$$P = \frac{V_0}{A_m}k$$ (9.26)

where k is the rate constant, V_0 is the aqueous volume of the lipid dispersion, and A_m is the area of the liposome membrane.[97]

9.6 Effectiveness of Membrane-Perturbing Compounds Evaluated Using Liposomes

In some situations, the biologically active compound is targeted toward the membrane itself. In such cases, essential membrane properties such as its dynamics, topological integrity, asymmetry, or lateral homogeneity need to be monitored. There are pharmacological strategies aiming at affecting membrane-associated lipases, membrane integral proteins, or the physical membrane integrity.

Liposomes are natural substrates for lipases and any changes of the reaction progress may be indicative of the active compound's potency. Membrane-active enzymes are evaluated by the quantity of released reaction products (i.e., free fatty acids). The common experimental strategy is to monitor the quantity of the free fatty acid in the aqueous phase. For that, changing pH, surface pressure, or fluorescence signal is used.[98-100] In the early days, pH-stat was used to quantitate the released free fatty acids. In this case, the amount of released free fatty acids was quantitated by the amount of base needed to maintain the constant value of aqueous pH.[101] The other method relies on the use of labeled lipid molecules (with isotopes or fluorescent dyes).[102] The reaction progress is again correlated with the amount of free fatty acid released from liposomes, but here relying on scintillation counting or fluorescence detection of labeled fatty acid itself. In yet another approach, the released free fatty acid is measured using fluorescent free fatty acids binding protein (ADIFAB–acrylodan labeled intestinal fatty acid binding protein).[103,104] In this approach, detection of free fatty acid is based on a change in a position of acrylodan fluorophore relatively to the binding pocket of protein when it becomes occupied by fatty acid and the resulting changes in fluorescence emission. The progress of the reaction can also be followed with intrinsic fluorescence of a lipase and/or changing optical properties of the liposome suspension caused by enzyme activity.[105,106]

Other pharmaceuticals such as anesthetics are designed to change transiently global properties of biological membranes.[107-109] It would be very useful to develop an experimental model capable of delivering quantitative measures of anesthetic potency. Typically, the partition coefficient, capacity to alter membrane interface, or to modify the lipid bilayer state are used. However, the predictive capability of such studies is very limited.

Liposomes are also an indispensable experimental model for the evaluation of the effectiveness of cationic peptides, a potentially new class of antibiotics.[110-112] A cationic peptide action consists of three stages: association with the lipid bilayer, the intra-membrane reorganization, followed by the aggregation leading to the transmembrane pore formation. In order to perform its task, a cationic peptide should have a specific amino acid sequence. The selection of the amino acid sequence for an effective cationic peptide requires a quantitative evaluation of each amino acid. An experimentally determined, membrane-based, hydrophobicity scale for amino acids was first proposed by White.[113] The scale was derived directly from the measurements of the partitioning of a series of small peptides into the LUVs formed from the zwitterionic lipid POPC. ΔG values of the peptide partitioning into the lipid bilayer were compared with those obtained using the water–octanol model system. The observed linear correlation between the octanol and membrane partitioning supports the postulates that membrane partitioning is driven mainly by the hydrophobic effect.[114] However, the slope of the linear fit, as well as the deviations from the linearity, presented by some amino acids, reveals clear differences between bilayer and octanol partitioning models. In particular, aromatic residues Y, F, W are much more hydrophobic than predicted from the octanol/water scale (Fig. 9.6).

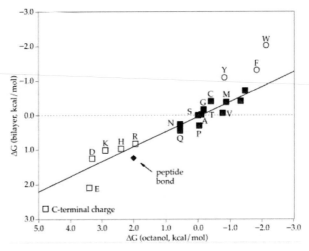

Figure 9.6 Comparisons of water-to-bilayer partitioning with water-to-octanol partitioning for AcWL-X-LL.[113] The solid line is the result of a linear regression fit of the bilayer data to the octanol data. Deviations from the line reflect the differences in free energy changes between bilayer and octanol partitioning. Reprinted with permission from Ref. [113], Copyright 1996, MacMillan Publishers Ltd. http://www.nature.com/nsmb/journal/v3/n10/abs/nsb1096-842.html.

Based on the interface- and octanol-based whole-residue hydrophobicity scales, the cationic peptide capacity to associate and penetrate the lipid bilayer can be predicted.[115] The designed peptides are then experimentally tested. The peptide association with the lipid bilayer is measured using ITC or spectroscopic methods described above.[116–118] The potency to compromise the lipid bilayer integrity is typically measured using the release of encapsulated fluorescent dye. Carboxyfluorescein or calcein is most frequently used.[92] The experimental design using encapsulated dye is capable of detecting the appearance of membrane defects, but their duration or transient character cannot be evaluated. For that purpose, the chemical or dynamic quenching of dye covalently attached to the membrane surface is more appropriate. In this case, the fluorescently labeled liposome suspension is exposed to a chemical or dynamic quencher at a specific time point and the kinetics of the resulting fluorescence change is measured.[45,46,90,91]

9.7 Perspectives

Modern pharmacology, in addition to the development of new pharmacologically active ingredients, adds new strategies, including the association of the active substance with self-organizing structures ensuring its controlled systemic distribution and or release. Such constructs are known as targeted drug-delivery systems.[119] Such an approach is used to treat infections, cancers, or inflammation, and it is a necessary vehicle for nucleic acids in various gene therapies.[120-123] Liposomes are excellent for that purpose since they can accommodate both hydrophobic and hydrophilic compounds.[124,125] Liposomes are stabilized by weak interactions; therefore, they may change their topology and/or properties in response to local conditions within the body such as pH, enzymatic activity, or the association of surface-active substances.[126,127] As a result, liposomes can serve as an excellent solvent for hydrophobic compounds,[128,129] protect the active component from enzymatic degradation,[130] and deliver and release their cargo at the desired location within the body.[131] Therefore, targeted drug-delivery systems may improve active compound performance by changing its pharmacokinetics without sacrificing its pharmacodynamics. An excellent example of a targeted delivery system is the liposomal doxorubicin (Doxil™), which reduces doxorubicin cardio-toxocity.[132]

Typically, the liposome formulation is developed for an active compound already present on the market and the main purpose of the effort is to eliminate shortcomings of its earlier formulations.[128,132-134] Physiological models help to design the liposome properties, whereas molecular dynamic simulations will provide data on the behavior of the active ingredient in the lipid aggregate as well as its performance in vivo.[14,135] Pharmacokinetics and toxicology for targeted drug-delivery systems are evaluated at the early stages of the development process, contrary to the development process of classical drugs.

For registration purposes, the liposomal formulation should be thoroughly characterized using established and validated methods, including the determination of the active compound/lipid ratio, lipid composition in the formulation, size distribution, electrostatics and lamellarity of liposomes, the kinetics of drug release during storage and when at targeted location, in vitro test of its stability, and capacity to retain the active compound following the administration.[119,128,134,136] Successful introduction of first liposomal drugs paved the way for regulatory guidelines for liposomal formulation.[132] This, in turn, stimulates the rapid growth of new pharmacological applications of various liposome systems designed for prevention, diagnostics, and pharmaco-therapies.[129,137,138] In addition, liposomes have opened new possibilities of delivering active compounds. Liposomes are tested as delivery vehicles through the skin, mucus, or to the eye.[139-142]

Acknowledgments

The work was possible thanks to the financial support from the National Centre for Research and Development grant no. WND-DEM-1-027/00. The contribution of Maciej Łukawski to the manuscript preparation is kindly acknowledged.

References

1. Italia JL, Bhardwaj V, Kumar MNVR. Disease, destination, dose and delivery aspects of cyclosporin: The state of the art. *Drug Disc Today.* 2006; 11: 846–854.

2. Hurst R, Rollema H, Bertrand D. Nicotinic acetylcholine receptors: From basic science to therapeutics. *Pharmacol Therapeut.* 2013; 137(1): 22–54.

3. Paul SM, Mytelka DS, Dunwiddie CT, et al. How to improve R&D productivity: The pharmaceutical industry's grand challenge. *Nat Rev Drug Disc.* 2010; 9: 203–214.

4. Schmidt S, Gonzalez D, Derendorf H. Significance of protein binding in pharmacokinetics and pharmacodynamics. *J Pharm Sci.* 2010; 99(3): 1107–1122.

5. Lipinski CA. Drug-like properties and the causes of poor solubility and poor permeability. *J Pharmacol Toxicol Meth.* 2000; 44: 235–249.

6. Grillo JA, Zhao P, Bullock J, et al. Utility of a physiologically based pharmacokinetic (PBPK) modeling approach to quantitatively predict a complex drug-drug-disease interaction scenario for rivaroxaban during the drug review process: Implications for clinical practice. *Biopharm Drug Dispos.* 2012; 33(2): 99–110.

7. Abreu MSC, Estronca LMBB, Moreno MJ, Vaz WLC. Binding of a fluorescent lipid amphiphile to albumin and its transfer to lipid bilayer membranes. *Biophys J.* 2003; 84: 386–399.

8. Balaz S. Does transbilayer diffusion have a role in membrane transport of drugs? *Drug Disc Today.* 2012; 17: 1079–1087.

9. Nielsen PE, Avdeef A. PAMPA—a drug absorption in vitro model 8. Apparent filter porosity and the unstirred water layer. *Eur J Pharm Sci.* 2004; 22(1): 33–41.

10. Avdeef A, Nielsen PE, Tsinman O. PAMPA—a drug absorption in vitro model 11. Matching the in vivo unstirred water layer thickness by individual-well stirring in microtiter plates. *Eur J Pharm Sci.* 2004; 22(5): 365–374.

11. Ruell JA, Tsinman KL, Avdeef A. PAMPA—a drug absorption in vitro model 5. Unstirred water layer in iso-pH mapping assays and pK(a)(flux)-optimized design (pOD-PAMPA). *Eur J Pharm Sci.* 2003; 20(4–5): 393–402.

12. Avdeef A, Artursson P, Neuhoff S, Lazorova L, Grasjo J, Tavelin S. Caco-2 permeability of weakly basic drugs predicted with the Double-Sink PAMPA pK(a)(flux) method. *Eur J Pharm Sci.* 2005; 24(4): 333–349.

13. Nagle JF, Tristram-Nagle S. Structure of lipid bilayers. *Biochim Biophys Acta.* 2000; 1469: 159–195.

14. Ying CT, Wang JT, Lamm RJ, Kamei DT. Mathematical modeling of vesicle drug delivery systems 2: Targeted vesicle interactions with cells, tumors, and the body. *J Lab Autom.* 2013; 18(1): 46–62.

15. Dai WG, Pollock-Dove C, Dong LC, Li S. Advanced screening assays to rapidly identify solubility-enhancing formulations: High-throughput, miniaturization and automation. *Adv Drug Deliv Rev.* 2008; 60: 657–672.

16. Buckley ST, Frank KJ, Fricker G, Brandl M. Biopharmaceutical classification of poorly soluble drugs with respect to "enabling formulations". *Eur J Pharm Sci.* 2013; 50(1): 8–16.

17. Elder D, Holm R. Aqueous solubility: Simple predictive methods (in silico, in vitro and bio-relevant approaches). *Int J Pharm.* 2013; 453(1): 3–11.

18. Lipinski CA, Lombarda F, Dominy BW, Feeney PJ. Experimental and computational approaches to estimate solubility and permeability in drug discovery and development settings. *Adv Drug Deliv Rev.* 2001; 46: 3–26.

19. Lipinski CA, Lombardo F, Dominy BW, Feeney PJ. Experimental and computational approaches to estimate solubility and permeability in drug discovery and development settings. *Adv Drug Deliv Rev.* 1997; 23: 3–25.

20. Jones HM, Gardner IB, Watson KJ. Modelling and PBPK simulation in drug discovery. *AAPS J.* 2009; 11(1): 155–166.

21. Wu ZM, Hassan D, Shaw JP. In-vitro prediction of bioavailability following extravascular injection of poorly soluble drugs: An insight into clinical failure and the role of delivery systems. *J Pharm Pharmacol.* 2013; 65(10): 1429–1439.

22. Perrin DD, Dempsey B, Serjeant EP. *pK$_a$ Prediction for Organic Acids and Bases.* Vol 1. London, New York: Chapman and Hall; 1981.

23. Alber A, Serjeant EP. *The Determination of Ionization Constants: A Laboratory Manual.* London: Chapman and Hall; 1971.

24. Comer J, Tam K. Lipophilicity profiles: Theory and measurement. In: Testa B, van de Waterbeemd H, Folkers G, Gay RH, eds. *Pharmacokinetic Optimization in Drug Research: Biological, Physicochemical and Computational Strategies.* Zurich: Wiley-VHCA; 2001: 275–304.

25. Goodwin JT, Conradi RA, Ho NFH, Burton PS. Physicochemical determinants of passive membrane permeability: Role of solute hydrogen-bonding potential and volume. *J Med Chem.* 2001; 44(22): 3721–3729.

26. Walter A, Gutknecht J. Permeability of small nonelectrolytes through lipid bilayer membranes. *J Membr Biol.* 1986; 90(3): 207–217.

27. Katz Y, Diamond JM. Method for measuring nonelectrolyte partition-coefficients between liposomes and water. *J Membr Biol.* 1974; 17(1): 69–86.

28. Wohnsland F, Faller B. High-throughput permeability pH profile and high-throughput alkane/water log P with artificial membranes. *J Med Chem.* 2001; 44(6): 923–930.

29. Boija E, Lundquist A, Edwards K, Johansson G. Evaluation of bilayer disks as plant cell membrane models in partition studies. *Anal Biochem.* 2007; 364(2): 145–152.

30. Coutinho A, Prieto M. Cooperative partition model of nystatin interaction with phospholipid vesicles. *Biophys J.* 2003; 84(5): 3061–3078.

31. Tieleman DP, Marrink SJ, Berendsen HJC. A computer perspective of membranes: Molecular dynamic studies of lipid bilayer systems. *Biochim Biophys Acta.* 1997; 1331: 235–270.

32. Wiener MC, White SH. Structure of a fluid dioleoylphosphatidylcholine bilayer determined by joint refinement of X-ray and neutron-diffraction data. III. Complete structure. *Biophys J.* 1992; 61(2): 434–447.

33. Gabrielska J, Przestalski S, Miszta A, Soczynska-Kordala M, Langner M. The effect of cholesterol on the absorption of phenyltin compounds onto phosphatidylcholine and sphingomyelin liposome membranes. *Appl Organometallic Chem.* 2004; 18: 9–14.

34. Hladyszowski J, Gabrielska J, Ordon P, Przestalski S, Langner M. The effect of steric constrains on the adsorption of phenyltin onto the dipalmitoylphosphatidylcholine bilayer. *J Membrane Biol.* 2002; 189: 213–223.

35. Langner M, Kubica K. The electrostatics of lipid surfaces. *Chem Phys Lipids.* 1999; 101: 3–35.

36. Olzynska A, Przybylo M, Gabrielska J, Trela Z, Przestalski S, Langner M. Di- and tri-phenyltin chlorides transfer across a model lipid bilayer. *App Organometall Chem.* 2005; 19: 1073–1078.

37. Przybylo M, Olżyńska A, Han S, Ożuhar A, Langner M. A fluorescence method for determination transport of charged compounds across lipid bilayer. *Biophys Chem.* 2007; 129: 120–125.

38. Haldar S, Chaudhuri A, Chattopadhyay A. Organization and dynamics of membrane probes and proteins utilizing the red edge excitation shift. *J Phys Chem B.* 2011; 115(19): 5693–5706.

39. Chaudhuri A, Haldar S, Chattopadhyay A. Structural transition in micelles: Novel insight into microenvironment changes in polarity and dynamics. *Chem Phys Lipids.* 2012; 165: 497–504.

40. Demchenko AP, Mely Y, Duportail G, Klymchenko AS. Monitoring biophysical properties of lipid membranes by environmental-sensitive fluorescent probes. *Biophys J.* 2009; 96: 3461–3470.

41. Andrade-Eiroa A, Canle M, Cerda V. Environmental applications of excitation-emission spectrofluorimetry: An in-depth review I. *Appl Spectrosc Rev.* 2013; 48(1): 1–49.

42. Heerklotz H, Seelig J. Correlation of membrane/water partition coefficients of detergents with the critical micelle concentration. *Biophys J.* 2000; 78: 2435–2440.

43. Afri M, Naqqash ME, Frimer AA. Using fluorescence to locate intercalants within the lipid bilayer of liposomes, bioliposomes and erythrocyte ghosts. *Chem Phys Lipids.* 2011; 164: 759–765.

44. Simrd JR, Kamp F, Hamilton JA. Measuring the adsorption of fatty acids to phospholipid vesicles by multiple fluorescence probes. *Biophys J.* 2008; 94: 4493–4503.

45. Langner M, Hui SW. Dithionite penetration through phospholipid bilayers as a measure of defects in lipid molecular packing. *Chem Phys Lipids.* 1993; 65: 23–30.

46. Langner M, Hui SW. Effect of free fatty acids on the permeability of 1,2-dimyristoyl-sn-glycero-3-phosphocholine bilayer at the main phase transition. *Biochim Biophys Acta.* 2000; 1463: 439–447.

47. Jelesarov I, Bosshard HR. Isothermal titration calorimetry and differential scanning calorimetry as complementary tools to investigate the energetics of biomolecular recognition. *J Mol Recognit.* 1999; 12: 3–18.

48. Frostell-Karlsson A, Widegren H, Green CE, et al. Biosensor analysis of the interaction between drug compounds and liposomes of different properties: A two-dimensional characterization tool for estimation of membrane absorption. *J Pharm Sci.* 2005; 94(1): 25–37.

49. Avdeef A. *Absorption and Drug Development: Solubility, Permeability, and Charge* State, 2nd ed., Hoboken, NJ: Wiley; 2012.

50. Alcorn CJ, Simpson RJ, Leahy DE, Peters TJ. Partition and distribution coefficients of solutes and drugs in brush border membrane vesicles. *Biochem Pharmacol.* 1993; 45: 1775–1782.

51. Xiang TX, Anderson BD. Influence of chain ordering on the selectivity of dipalmitoylphosphatidylcholine bilayer membranes for permeant size and shape. *Biophys J.* 1998; 75: 2658–2671.

52. Pauletti GM, Wunderli-Allenspach H. Partition coefficients in vitro: Artificial membranes as a standardized distribution model. *Eur J Pharmaceut Sci.* 1994; 1: 273–282.

53. Kramer SD, Braun A, Jakits-Deiser C, Wunderli-Allenspach H. Towards the predictability of drug-lipid membrane interactions: The pH-dependent affinity of propranolol to phosphatidylinositol containing liposomes. *Pharmaceut Res.* 1998; 15: 739–744.

54. Rawle RJ, Hughes LD, Boxer SG. Be careful when choosing your dye label: Commercial, water-soluble fluorophores often interact with lipid bilayers. *Biophys J.* 2014; 106(2): 702A–702A.

55. Hughes LD, Rawle RJ, Boxer SG. Choose your label wisely: Water-soluble fluorophores often interact with lipid bilayers. *Plos One.* 2014; 9(2).

56. van Balen GP, Caron G, Bouchard G, et al. Liposome/water lipophilicity: Methods, information content, and pharmaceutical applications. *Med Res Rev.* 2004; 24: 299–324.

57. Fugit KD, Anderson BD. Dynamic, nonsink method for the simultaneous determination of drug permeability and binding coefficients in liposomes. *Mol Pharm.* 2014; 11(4): 1314–1325.

58. Nakayama T, Ono K, Hashimoto K. Affinity of antioxidative polyphenols for lipid bilayers evaluated with a liposome system. *Biosci Biotechnol Biochem.* 1998; 62: 1005–1007.

59. Freeman DH. Interactive gel networks. I. Treatment of simple complexation and masking phenomena. *Anal Chem.* 1972; 44: 117–120.

60. Pagliara A, Khamis E, Trinh A, Carrupt PA, Tsai RS, Testa B. Structural-properties governing retention mechanisms on Rp-HPLC stationary phases used for lipophilicity measurements. *J Liq Chromatogr.* 1995; 18(9): 1721–1745.

61. Pidgeon C, Venkataram UV. Immobilized artificial membrane chromatography: Supports composed of membrane lipids. *Anal Biochem.* 1989; 176(1): 36–47.

62. Yang CY, Cai SJ, Liu H, Pidgeon C. Immobilized artificial membranes: Screens for drug membrane interactions. *Adv Drug Deliv Rev.* 1997; 23: 229–256.

63. Ong S, Liu H, Qiu X, Bhat G, Pidgeon C. Membrane partition coefficients chromatographically measured using immobilized artificial membrane surfaces. *Anal Chem.* 1995; 67: 755–762.

64. Ong S, Pidgeon C. Thermodynamics of solute partitioning into immobilized artificial membranes. *Anal Chem.* 1995; 67: 2119–2128.

65. Przybylo M, Sykora J, Humplickova J, Benda A, Zan A, Hof M. Lipid diffusion in giant unilamellar vesicles is more than 2 times faster than in supported phospholipid bilayers under identical conditions. *Langmuir.* 2006; 22: 9096–9099.

66. Yang Q, Liu XY, Umetani K, Kamo N, Miyake J. Partitioning of triphenylalkylphosphonium homologues in gel bead-immobilized

liposomes: Chromatographic measurement of their membrane partition coefficients. *Biochi Biophys Acta.* 1999; 1417: 122–130.

67. Liu XY, Yang Q, Kamo N, Miyake J. Effect of liposome type and membrane fluidity on drug-membrane partitioning analyzed by immobilized liposome chromatography. *J Chromatography A.* 2001; 913: 123–131.

68. Schwarz G. Electrical interactions of membrane active peptides at lipid/water interactions. *Biophys Chem.* 1996; 58: 67–73.

69. Schwarz G, Reiter R. Negative cooperativity and aggregation in biphasic binding of mastoparan X peptide to membranes with acidic lipids. *Biophys Chem.* 2001; 90: 269–277.

70. Schwarz G. A universal thermodynamic approach to analyze biomolecular binding experiments. *Biophys Chem.* 2000; 86: 119–129.

71. Kaminoh Y, Inoue T, Ma SM, Ueda I, Lin SH. Membrane-buffer partition coefficients of tetracaine for liquid-crystal and solid-gel membranes estimated by direct ultraviolet spectrophotometry. *Biochim Biophys Acta.* 1988; 946: 337–344.

72. Kitamura K, Imayoshi N, Goto T, Shiro H, Mano T, Nakai Y. Second derivative spectrometric determination of partition coefficients of chlorpromazine and promazine between lecithin bilayer vesicles and water. *Anal Chim Acta.* 1995; 304: 101–106.

73. de Castro B, Gameiro P, Lima JL, Matos C, Reis P. A fast and reliable spectroscopic method for the determination of membrane-water partition coefficients of organic compounds. *Lipids.* 2001; 36: 89–96.

74. Avdeef A, Box KJ. Sirius technical application notes (STAN). In: Ltd. SAI, ed. Forest Row, UK, 21995.

75. Avdeef A, Box KJ, Comer JEA, Hibbert C, Tam KY. pH-metric logP 10. Determination of liposomal membrane-water partition coefficient of ionizable drugs. *Pharmaceutical Res.* 1998; 15: 209–215.

76. Avdeef A. Solubility of sparingly-soluble ionizable drugs. *Adv Drug Deliv Rev.* 2007; 59: 568–590.

77. Kaszuba M, Corbett J, Watson FM, Jones A. High-concentration zeta potential measurements using light-scattering techniques. *Philos Trans A Math Phys Eng Sci.* 2010; 368: 4439–4451.

78. Delgado AV, Gonzalez-Caballero F, Hunter RJ, Koopal LK, Lyklema J. Measurement and interpretation of electrokinetic phenomena. *J Coll Interface Sci.* 2007; 309: 194–224.

79. Piere MM, Raman CS, Nall BT. Isothermal titration calorimetry of protein-protein interactions. *Methods.* 1999; 19: 213–221.

80. Ladbury JE. Isothermal titration calorimetry: Application to structure-based drug design. *Thermochim Acta.* 2001; 380: 213–215.

81. Wieprecht T, Seelig J. Isothermal titration calorimetry for studying interactions between peptides and lipid membranes. *Curr Topics Mem.* 2002; 52: 31–56.

82. Baeuerle HD, Seelig J. Interaction of charged and uncharged calcium channel antagonists with phospholipid membranes. Binding equilibrium, binding enthalpy, and membrane location. *Biochemistry.* 1991; 30: 7203–7211.

83. Thomas PG, Seelig J. Binding of the calcium antagonist flunarizine to phosphatidylcholine bilayers: Charge effects and thermodynamics. *Biochem J.* 1993; 291: 397–402.

84. Seelig J, Ganz P. Nonclassical hydrophobic effect in membrane binding equilibria. *Biochemistry.* 1991; 30: 9354–9359.

85. Seelig J. Titration calorimetry of lipid-peptide interactions. *Biochi Biophys Acta.* 1997; 1331: 103–116.

86. Heerklotz H, Seelig J. Correlation of membrane/water partition coefficients of detergents with the critical micelle concentration. *Biophys J.* 2000; 78: 2435–2440.

87. Osanai H, Ikehara T, Miyauchi S, et al. A study of the interaction of drugs with liposomes with isothermal titration calorimetry. *J Biophys Chem.* 2013; 4: 11–21.

88. Yang Q, Liu XY, Umetani K, et al. Membrane partitioning and translocation of hydrophobic phosphonium homologues: Thermodynamic analysis by immobilized liposome chromatography. *J Phys Chem B.* 2000; 104: 7528–7534.

89. Carley AN, Kleinfeld AM. Flip-flop is the rate-limiting step for transport of free fatty acids across lipid vesicle membranes. *Biochemistry.* 2009; 48(43): 10437–10445.

90. Langner M, Hui SW. Iodide penetration into lipid bilayers as a probe of membrane lipid organization. *Chem Phys Lipids.* 1991; 60: 127–132.

91. Geddes CD. Optical halide sensing using fluorescence quenching: Theory, simulations and applications—a review. *Meas Sci Technol.* 2001; 12: R53–R88.

92. Hashizaki K, Taguchi H, Sakai H, Abe V, Saito Y, Ogawa N. Carboxyfluorescein leakage from poly(ethylene glycol)-grafted liposomes induced by the interaction with serum. *Chem Pharm Bull (Tokyo).* 2006; 54(1): 80–84.

93. Pucihar G, Kotnik T, Miklavcic D, Teissie J. Kinetics of transmembrane transport of small molecules into electropermeabilized cells. *Biophys J.* 2008; 95(6): 2837–2848.

94. Frezard F, Garniersuillerot A. DNA-containing liposomes as a model for the study of cell-membrane permeation by anthracycline derivatives. *Biochemistry.* 1991; 30(20): 5038–5043.

95. Chakrabarti AC. Permeability of membranes to amino acids and modified amino acids: Mechanisms involved in translocation. *Amino Acids.* 1994; 6(3): 213–229.

96. Udenfriend S, Stein S, Bohlen P, Dairman W. Fluorescamine: A reagent for assay of amino acids, peptides, proteins, and primary amines in the picomole range. *Science.* 1972; 178(4063): 871–872.

97. Chakrabarti AC, Deamer DW. Permeability of lipid bilayers to amino-acids and phosphate. *Biochim Biophys Acta.* 1992; 1111(2): 171–177.

98. Mouchlis VD, Barbayianni E, Mavromoustakos TM, Kokotos G. The application of rational design on phospholipase A(2) inhibitors. *Curr Med Chem.* 2011; 18(17): 2566–2582.

99. Gaspar D, Lucio M, Rocha S, Lima JLFC, Reis S. Changes in PLA(2) activity after interacting with anti-inflammatory drugs and model membranes: Evidence for the involvement of tryptophan residues. *Chem Phys Lipids.* 2011; 164(4): 292–299.

100. Gaspar D, Lucio M, Wagner K, et al. A biophysical approach to phospholipase A(2) activity and inhibition by anti-inflammatory drugs. *Biophys Chem.* 2010; 152(1–3): 109–117.

101. Tietz NW, Astles JR, Shuey DF. Lipose activity measured in serum by a continuous-monitoring pH-stat technique: An update. *Clin Chem.* 1989; 35: 1688–1693.

102. Jorgensen K, Davidsen J, Mouritsen OG. Biophysical mechanisms of phospholipase A_2 activation and their use in liposome-based drug delivery. *FEBS Lett.* 2002; 531: 23–27.

103. Richieri GV, Ogata RT, Kleinfeld AM. Thermodynamics of fatty-acid-binding to fatty-acid-binding proteins and fatty-acid partition between water and membranes measured using the fluorescent probe ADIFAB. *J Biol Chem.* 1995; 270(25): 15076–15084.

104. Richieri GV, Ogata RT, Kleinfeld AM. The measurement of free fatty acid concentration with the fluorescent probe ADIFAB: A practical guide for the use of the ADIFAB probe. *Mol Cell Biochem.* 1999; 192(1–2): 87–94.

105. Vermehren C, Kiebler T, Hylander I, Callisen TH, Jorgensen K. Increase in phospholipase A(2) activity towards lipopolymer-containing liposomes. *Biochim Biophys Acta Biomembr.* 1998; 1373(1): 27–36.

106. Bailey RW, Olson ED, Vu MP, et al. Relationship between membrane physical properties and secretory phospholipase A2 hydrolysis kinetics in S49 cells during ionophore-induced apoptosis. *Biophys J.* 2007; 93: 2350–2362.

107. Paiva JG, Paradiso P, Serro AP, Fernandes A, Saramago B. Interaction of local and general anaesthetics with liposomal membrane models: A QCM-D and DSC study. *Colloids Surf B: Biointerfaces.* 2012; 95: 65–74.

108. Castro V, Stevensson B, Dvinskikh SV, et al. NMR investigations of interactions between anesthetics and lipid bilayers. *Biochim Biophys Acta.* 2008; 1778: 2604–2611.

109. Frangopol PT, Mihailescu D. Interactions of some local anesthetics and alcohols with membranes. *Coll Surf B: Biointerfaces.* 2001; 22: 3–22.

110. Killian JA, Nyholm TKV. Peptides in lipid bilayers: The power of simple models. *Curr Opin Struc Biol.* 2006; 16: 473–479.

111. Matsuzaki K. Control of cell selectivity of antimicrobial peptides. *Biochim Biophys Acta.* 2009; 1788: 1687–1692.

112. Beer J, Wagner CC, Zeitlinger M. Protein binding of antimicrobials: Methods for quantification and for investigation of its impact on bacterial killing. *AAPS J.* 2009; 11(1): 1–12.

113. Wimley WC, White SH. Experimentally determined hydrophobicity scale for proteins at membrane surfaces. *Nat Struct Biol.* 1996; 3: 842–848.

114. Fauchere JL, Pliska V. Hydrophobic parameters pi of amino-acid side chains from the partitioning of *N*-acetyl-amino-acid amides. *Eur J Med Chem.* 1983; 18: 369–375.

115. White SH, Wimley WC. Membrane protein folding and stability: Physical principles. *Annu Rev Biopys Biomol Struct.* 1999; 28: 319–365.

116. Matos PM, Franquelim HG, Castanho MARB, Santos NC. Quantitative assessment of peptide-lipid interactions. Ubiquitous fluorescence methodologies. *Biochim Biophys Acta Biomembr.* 2010; 1798: 1999–2012.

117. Russell AL, Spuches AM, Williams BC, et al. The effect of the placement and total charge of the basic amino acid clusters on antibacterial organism selectivity and potency. *Bioorg Med Chem.* 2011; 19(23): 7008–7022.

118. Russell AL, Kennedy AM, Spuches AM, Venugopal D, Bhonsle JB, Hicks RP. Spectroscopic and thermodynamic evidence for antimicrobial peptide membrane selectivity. *Chem Phys Lipids.* 2010; 163: 488–497.

119. Allen TM, Cullis PR. Liposomal drug delivery systems: From concept to clinical applications. *Adv Drug Deliv Rev.* 2013; 65(1): 36–48.

120. Venditto VJ, Szoka FC. Cancer nanomedicines: So many papers and so few drugs! *Adv Drug Deliv Rev.* 2013; 65(1): 80–88.

121. Sharma A, Jain N, Sareen R. Nanocarriers for diagnosis and targeting of breast cancer. *Biomed Res Int.* 2013.

122. Oh YK, Park TG. siRNA delivery systems for cancer treatment. *Adv Drug Deliv Rev.* 2009; 61: 850–862.

123. Pozzi D, Caracciolo G, Caminiti R, et al. Toward the rational design of lipid gene vectors: Shape coupling between lipoplex and anionic cellular lipids controls the phase evolution of lipoplexes and the efficiency of DNA release. *ACS Appl Mater Interfaces.* 2009; 1(10): 2237–2249.

124. Habib L, Khreich N, Jraij A, et al. Preparation and characterization of liposomes incorporating cucurbitacin E, a natural cytotoxic triterpene. *Int J Pharm.* 2013; 448(1): 313–319.

125. Langner M, Kral T. Liposome-based drug delivery systems. *Pol J Pharmacol.* 1999; 51: 211–222.

126. Holm R, Mullertz A, Mu HL. Bile salts and their importance for drug absorption. *Int J Pharm.* 2013; 453(1): 44–55.

127. Kostarelos K. Rational design and engineering of delivery systems for therapeutics: Biomedical exercises in colloid and surface science. *Adv Colloid Interface Sci.* 2003; 106: 147–168.

128. Chen ML. Lipid excipients and delivery systems for pharmaceutical development: A regulatory perspective. *Adv Drug Deliv Rev.* 2008; 60: 768–777.

129. Bunjes H. Lipid nanoparticles for the delivery of poorly water-soluble drugs. *J Pharm Pharmacol.* 2010; 62(11): 1637–1645.

130. Yoshimoto M, Yamasaki R, Nakao M, Yamashita T. Stabilization of formate dehydrogenase from *Candida boidinii* through liposome-assisted complexation with cofactors. *Enzyme Microb Technol.* 2010; 46(7): 588–593.

131. Decker C, Schubert H, May S, Fahr A. Pharmacokinetics of temoporfin-loaded liposome formulations: Correlation of liposome and temoporfin blood concentration. *J Controlled Release.* 2013; 166(3): 277–285.

132. Barenholz Y. Doxl—the first FDA-approved nano-drug: Lessons learned. *J Controlled Release.* 2012; 160: 117–134.

133. Chen JZ, Shao RF, Zhang XD, Chen C. Applications of nanotechnology for melanoma treatment, diagnosis, and theranostics. *Int J Nanomed.* 2013; 8: 2677–2688.

134. Edwards KA, Baeumner AJ. Analysis of liposomes. *Talanta.* 2006; 68: 1432–1441.

135. Li P, Zhao LW. Developing early formulations: Practice and perspective. *Int J Pharm.* 2007; 341(1–2): 1–19.

136. Gomez-Hens A, Fernandez-Romero JM. Analytical methods for the control of liposomal delivery systems. *Trends Analyt Chem.* 2006; 25: 167–178.

137. Chatterjee DK, Fong LS, Zhabg Y. Nanoparticles in photodynamics therapy: An emerging paradigm. *Adv Drug Deliv Rev.* 2008; 60: 1627–1637.

138. Huang S-L. Liposomes in ultrasonic drug and gene delivery. *Adv Drug Deliv Rev.* 2008; 60: 1167–1176.

139. Honda M, Asai T, Oku N, Araki Y, Tanaka M, Ebihara N. Liposomes and nanotechnology in drug development: Focus on ocular targets. *Int J Nanomed.* 2013; 8: 495–504.

140. Cavalla D. Predictive methods in drug repurposing: Gold mine or just a bigger haystack? *Drug Discov Today.* 2013; 18(11–12): 523–532.

141. Mulet X, Boyd BJ, Drummond CJ. Advances in drug delivery and medical imaging using colloidal lyotropic liquid crystalline dispersions. *J Colloid Interface Sci.* 2013; 393: 1–20.

142. Sant S, Tao SL, Fisher OZ, Xu Q, Peppas NA, Khademhosseini A. Microfabrication technologies for oral drug delivery. *Adv Drug Deliv Rev.* 2012; 64: 496–507.

Chapter 10

Liposomes in Capillary Electromigration Techniques

Susanne K. Wiedmer

Department of Chemistry, University of Helsinki, Helsinki, Finland

susanne.wiedmer@helsinki.fi

This chapter describes the use of capillary electromigration (CE) techniques for the study of liposomes and interactions between liposomes and compounds. Various CE techniques will be discussed and focus will be on the use of capillary (zone) electrophoresis for the investigation of physicochemical properties of liposomes. In addition, emphasis will be on the use of capillary electrokinetic chromatography (EKC), partial-filling EKC (PF-EKC), and capillary electrophoresis frontal analysis (CE-FA) as affinity electrophoretic modes for the study of liposome–analyte interactions. Finally, there will be discussion on how liposomes can be employed as either a shielding coating or as a stationary chromatographic phase in fused silica capillaries for CE. The latter technique is commonly called open-tubular capillary electrochromatography (OT-CEC). The use of CE for studying complexes between lipids or liposomes and analytes is also briefly discussed. Some practical applications, are given and the advantages and disadvantages of the different approaches are highlighted.

Liposomes in Analytical Methodologies

Edited by Katie A. Edwards

Copyright © 2016 Pan Stanford Publishing Pte. Ltd.

ISBN 978-981-4669-26-9 (Hardcover), 978-981-4669-27-6 (eBook)

www.panstanford.com

10.1   Introduction

Capillary electromigration techniques belong to the liquid phase analytical separation techniques. The popularity of the methodology has increased steadily over the years ever since the pioneering works by Hjertén on open-tubular electrophoresis in 1967.[1,2] Later, further studies by Virtanen[3] as well as Mikkers and Everaerts[4] in the 1970s resulted in the first publications on performing electrophoresis in capillaries. These groundbreaking works gave a good start to the development of commercial instruments, and the first commercial devices appeared around 1987–89.[5]

Regarding the terminology, it is worthwhile mentioning that the general term for all types of capillary electrophoretic techniques is capillary electromigration techniques.[6] Previously, the term capillary zone electrophoresis (CZE) was used for describing free zone capillary electrophoresis; however, nowadays the term capillary electrophoresis (CE) is recommended. In order to avoid confusion, the term CZE will be used in this chapter to clearly distinguish between capillary electromigration techniques and capillary zone electrophoresis. On the other hand, it should be noted that capillary electrophoresis as a collective term for all capillary electromigration techniques is sometimes misleading as many of the techniques include other separation mechanisms than pure electrophoresis.

The different CE techniques used in combination with liposomes are rather few.[7] The CE techniques are commonly divided into capillary electrophoretic and voltage-assisted capillary chromatographic techniques. Among the capillary electrophoretic techniques, CZE, capillary isoelectric focusing, capillary gel electrophoresis, and capillary isotachophoresis can be mentioned. Of these, mainly CZE has been employed in liposome research. Among the voltage-assisted capillary chromatographic techniques, capillary electrokinetic chromatography and packed and open-tubular capillary electrochromatography can be mentioned. Both the EKC and CEC techniques have been employed in liposome studies. In general, CE can bring information on specific characteristics of intact liposomes or on interactions between compounds and liposomes. Conventional CZE has been employed rather much for the determination of physicochemical characteristics, such as the electrophoretic mobility, of liposomes. The electrophoretic mobility data are needed, for example, when calculating the retention factors of analytes in liposome electrokinetic chromatography (LEKC), which actually is one of the most commonly used liposome CE techniques nowadays. It origins in the early works on micellar electrokinetic chromatography (MEKC; also called MECC) by Shigeru Terabe in the early 1980s.[8] Nowadays, with the increasing number of studies on miniaturized devices, like microchips, it is often recommended to add the term capillary in front of MEKC to emphasize that the separation is carried out in spherical capillaries and not on chips, where the separation channel often is in a square capillary format. Another closely related technique, which can be seen as a direct modification of the previous one, is partial-filling electrokinetic chromatography. In that technique, only a part of the capillary is filled with a background electrolyte (BGE) solution comprising the liposome dispersion, and the detection part of the capillary is filled with a BGE free from liposomes. The driving force behind the development of the PF-EKC technique has been the decreased detection sensitivity sometimes observed due to the presence of liposomes in the detection window. This, however, depends much on the type of liposomes dispersions that are used. A technique that resembles the PF-EKC technique is capillary electrophoresis frontal analysis. In this analysis, equilibrium between the analyte and the liposome (ligand) is established already in the sample vial before injection into the separation channel. The differences between EKC, PF-EKC, and CE-FA are illustrated in Fig. 10.1 and Table 10.1. All these techniques will be described in more detail in the following sections.

Various types of liposomes have been used in CE techniques, but most of them have been negatively charged with zwitterionic phosphatidylcholine (PC) as the main phospholipid. Typical anionic phospholipids that have been added to liposomes for CE include phosphatidylserine (PS), phosphatidylglycerol (PG), phosphatidic acid (PA), phosphatidylinositol (PI), and doubly negatively charged cardiolipin (CL). The processing of multilamellar vesicles into unilamellar vesicles is strongly recommended, and unilamellar vesicles have been adopted in most studies. The heterogeneous properties of multilamellar vesicles usually result in very noisy background when used as pseudostationary phase in EKC.[10] Also if employed in CE as a shielding coating or in OT-CEC as a chromatographic stationary phase, the lamellarity of the liposome should be considered. The most popular ways to process multilamellar vesicles into small unilamellar vesicles are to sonicate the dispersion either using a sonication bath or a probe sonicator, alternatively to use an extrusion technique. Usually the sonication of the dispersion is stopped when the nontransparent multilamellar vesicle dispersion has become clear (visual observation), which is taken as evidence for having unilamellar vesicles in the dispersion. In the extrusion technique, the multilamellar vesicle dispersion is forced several times through a membrane with a specific pore size, mechanically forcing the multilamellar vesicles to become unilamellar. Typically, liposomes with diameters in the range of 30–120 nm have been employed in CE.

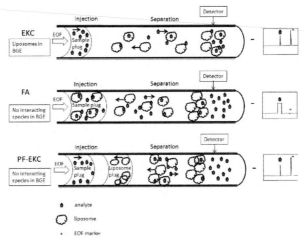

Figure 10.1 Schematic presentation of different capillary liposome affinity techniques with negatively charged liposomes in free solution (modified from Ref. [9]). In the EKC mode, the sample is injected into a capillary totally filled with a BGE solution containing liposomes (liposome-BGE); in the FA mode, a large plug containing an equilibrated analyte-ligand (liposome) sample is injected into a capillary filled with a BGE lacking liposomes; in the PF-EKC mode, a large plug of liposomes is injected into a capillary filled with a BGE without liposomes, before injection of the sample. Reproduced with permission from Ref. [9], Copyright 2012 WILEY-VCH Verlag GmbH & Co. KgaA, Weinheim. http://onlinelibrary.wiley.com/doi/10.1002/jssc.201200829/abstract.

Table 10.1   Comparison of different capillary liposome affinity techniques with liposomes in free solution

	Lipid consumption	Quantification of interaction strength/ partitioning	Advantages	Considerations
EKC	–Relatively high –Lipid dispersion present in BGE	–Binding constants derived from non-linear binding isotherm based on mobility shifts or distribution coefficient calculated from the retention factor and phase ratio	–Simple experimental set up suitable also for separations –Multiple interaction analysis in one run	–Possible high UV response –Binding stoichiometry needs to be known for binding constant determination –Non-interacting EOF marker should be carefully selected –Mobilities are affected by ionic strength and viscosity changes due to the addition of lipid dispersion to BGE–corrections are needed
FA	–Low –Filling around 10% of the capillary length	–Binding constants derived from the calibration curve and the plateau height, which is proportional to the concentration of the free analyte	–Binding stoichiometry can be directly derived –Binding constant determination is not sensitive to changes in EOF	–Mobilities of the complex and the free ligand should be almost equal and free and bound form should possess sufficiently different mobilities –Calibration curve is required –Binding constants of neutral drugs cannot be derived –Only pure samples can be processed

(Continued)

Table 10.1 *(Continued)*

	Lipid consumption	Quantification of interaction strength/ partitioning	Advantages	Considerations
PF-EKC	–Low –Plug length of 5%–45% of the capillary length	–Binding constants determination based on mobility shifts or distribution coefficient derived from the retention factor and phase ratio	–Simple experimental set up –Low sample consumption –Multiple interaction analysis in one run	–Binding stoichiometry needs to be known –The developed mathematical approach for calculating the binding constants from a single run involving only areas and migration times of peaks can be utilized only for 1:1 stoichiometry –Corrections for ionic strength and viscosity are needed

Modification of the liposomal surface with modifiers such as polyethylene glycol (PEG), polyacrylic acids (Carbopol®), poly(vinyl alcohol), *o*-palmitoylpullulan, poloxamer 338, poly(vinylpyrrolidone), carboxymethylchitin, and block copolymers (Pluronics®) has been rather frequently used in drug-delivery studies because of their liposome stabilizing and controlled drug release effect. Of these, PEG is probably the most widely used stabilizer in pharmaceutical applications because of its high solubility in aqueous solution, hydrophilicity, ability to bind a large number of water molecules, the high flexibility of its polymer chain, and most importantly, it has very low (or nonexistent) toxicity. The protective PEG layer is believed to prevent protein adsorption to the lipid bilayer and simultaneously to act as a steric barrier for inhibiting vesicle fusion. Liposome–macrophage interactions will be decreased by PEG grafting, which results in an enhancement in the blood circulation half-life of liposomes. The long-circulation ability of such grafted liposomes increases the selective accumulation of liposomes at sites of enhanced vascular permeability, such as those found in tumors and regions of infection and inflammation. However, there are reports on the occurrence of the so-called accelerated blood clearance (ABC) phenomenon; PEGylated liposomes lose their long-circulating characteristic when they are administrated twice in the same animal with certain intervals.[11] More research on the development of new strategies to avoid and/or alleviate the immunogenicity of PEG-coated liposomes without significantly limiting their in vivo performance to extend the applicability of such drug-delivery systems is thus needed. PEGylated liposomes have been used to some extent in EKC and OT-CEC (see following sections) as a carrier (pseudostationary phase) or stationary phase, and in all those studies, the PEGylated lipids have been sterically stabilized commercial lipids with covalently attached PEG chains.

10.2 Studies on Liposomes by Capillary (Zone) Electrophoresis

Individual liposomes injected as sample molecules can be investigated by CE. The liposomes are comprised of mainly PC with various amounts of negatively charged PS, PG, or PA lipids. In some studies, cholesterol has been included in the liposomes. CZE on liposomes has mainly been performed to gain information on their physicochemical characteristics. The properties that have been investigated are liposome surface charge, size, and permeability.[12] The surface charge of liposomes depends on the composition of the liposome. Since most biological membranes have a net negative surface charge, many groups working on the interaction between liposomes and analytes have preferred to use negatively charged liposomes. Actually, despite the zwitterionic character of PC, also liposomes prepared from pure PC have been shown to have a slightly negatively charged surface.[13]

The surface charge of liposomes can be obtained from the effective electrophoretic mobility (μ_{eff}) of the liposome under CZE conditions using Eq. 10.1:

$$\mu_{\text{eff}} = \mu_a - \mu_{\text{eof}},$$ (10.1)

where μ_a is the apparent liposome electrophoretic mobility and μ_{eof} is the electroosmotic mobility under a constant electric field.

Another way to describe the electrophoretic mobility of an ion is by Eq. 10.2:

$$\mu_{\text{eff}} = \frac{qD}{fRT},$$ (10.2)

where q is the total charge of the particle, D is the diffusion coefficient, f is the friction coefficient, R is the Rydberg constant, and T is the temperature. This equation assumes that the particle migrates through the capillary as a spherical particle and that there are no particle relaxation or retardation effects.

According to classical electrokinetic theory, the electrophoretic mobility of particles with ζ-potentials ≤ 25 mV can, on the other hand, be given by Eq. 10.3 (Henry equation):

$$\mu_{\text{eff}} = \frac{2\varepsilon\zeta}{3\eta} f(\kappa r),$$ (10.3)

where η is the viscosity of the medium, ε is the permittivity, and $f(\kappa r)$ is the so-called Henry function, in which κ is the Debye–Hückel parameter, which is the reciprocal of the electric double layer thickness and r stands for the radius of the particle.[14] This means that the Henry function depends on the shape, size, and orientation of the particle. The value of κ, in units of nm^{-1}, can be calculated from the ionic strength (I) of the background electrolyte solution according to Eq. 10.4:

$$\kappa = 3.288 \sqrt{I}$$ (10.4)

The value of κr determines what equation (i.e., Smoluchowski, Henry, or Debye–Hückel) should be applied to calculate the electrophoretic mobilities of particles. The function $f(\kappa r)$ lies in the range of 1–1.5, in such a way that for $\kappa r \ll 1$, the value approaches 1, whereas for $\kappa r \gg 1$, the value of the function approaches 1.5. For charged liposomes, the κr is typically $\gg 1$, meaning that a value of 1.5 can be used as a good approximation.

More details on the Overbeek–Booth electrokinetic theory can be found in the publications by Radko et al.[15,16] and in the references therein.

Usually, it has been observed that the electrophoretic mobility of the liposome increases linearly with an increase in the molar concentration of added negatively charged phospholipid, up to a certain concentration, after which the electrophoretic mobility becomes more or less constant. This effect is due to the saturation of the liposome with negatively charged phospholipids, and often this maximum concentration is around 30 mol% of negatively charged phospholipid. A further increase in the molar concentration results often in the disruption or rearrangement of the liposome.

An important aspect to keep in mind is the properties of the fused silica capillaries typically used in capillary electrophoresis. The silanol groups on the fused silica capillary surface will dissociate at pH values above approximately 2. In practice, this means that under typical experimental conditions, the fused silica capillary will be negatively charged and hence eager to interact electrostatically with positively charged molecules. As long as interactions between liposomes and the fused silica wall are assumed to be negligible or nonexisting, the method discussed earlier can be used for determining liposome electrophoretic mobilities. Direct analysis of liposomes has mainly been carried out in uncoated fused silica capillaries. However, due to liposome–wall interactions, it is obvious that cationic liposomes, much used as vehicles for DNA delivery to cells, cannot be investigated with uncoated fused silica capillaries. The liposome–wall interactions would be very strong, resulting in either no detectable peaks or highly unrepeatable results. For such liposome studies, the use of dynamic, semipermanent, or permanent surface coatings is recommended; e.g., polyacrylamide- or Brij 35-coated capillaries have been employed to some extent. These neutral coatings result in very low electroosmotic flow (EOF) values and in general they have very low interactions with the charged liposomes.

Actual liposome size determinations by CE have rarely been done, and there are only a few examples of the relationship between the electrophoretic mobilities of liposomes and their corresponding sizes. An indirect method is to add a fluorescence marker to the liposome and calculate the liposome size from the volume of the encapsulated fluorophore. Taylor dispersion analysis is an old approach for calculating the hydrodynamic radius of a particle. The methodology was introduced already in 1953 by Sir Geoffrey Taylor.[17] The method is based on the effect of band broadening of a plug of sample introduced in a cylindrical tube. The hydrodynamic radius of the particle can be determined from the measured particle diffusion coefficient. Recently, CE instrumentation has been used for such Taylor dispersion analysis, however not under CE conditions (no electric field applied).[12,18] Typically, a fused silica capillary with a total length of ca. 100 cm (75 μm ID) with two detection windows along the capillary, located after 30 and 50 cm, respectively, is used for the dispersion measurements. The UV traces of a compound to be determined are recorded at a specific wavelength. The sample is introduced into the capillary by applying a pressure (e.g., 50 mbar for 5 to 10 s) followed by a mobilization pressure of 50 mbar (flow rate 0.98 mm/s) to force the sample plug through the capillary. Apparent diffusion coefficients of the analytes are determined from the peak appearance times and the variances of the Gaussian-shaped peaks, and the hydrodynamic radii of the analytes are subsequently calculated from the Stokes–Einstein equation.

The permeability of liposomes is crucial when using liposomes as models of biological membranes for interaction studies with analytes and also when applying these as drug vehicles. The main factors affecting the permeability of liposomes are physical factors such as temperature or pressure, as well as chemical factors such as pH, ionic strength, and type of buffer solutions employed. The transition temperature of the liposome is important because usually drug leakage is higher at temperatures above the transition temperature, i.e., in the fluid liquid state than in the gel state at lower temperatures. Since the transition temperature depends on the type of phospholipid and can vary between −60°C and 80°C, it is very important to carefully select the lipids in order to have liposomes with appropriate characteristics. Maximum liposome permeability has been observed at temperatures very close to the phase transition temperature of the liposome. Typically, the transition temperature depends on fatty acid chain lengths, degree of unsaturation, chain branching, and structure of the polar headgroup; the transition temperature increases with chain length and degree of saturation of the fatty acid residues. In addition, cholesterol usually decreases membrane fluidity and broadens the temperature range of the transition.[19]

Some liposome permeability studies have been conducted by CE, and usually these have involved fluorescence or chemiluminescence detection of dyes such as calcein, fluorescein, carboxyfluorescein, Eosin Y, and Rhodamine B.[20] The permeability of the liposome has been judged according to the leakage of the dye. From the electrophoretic separation of the free and encapsulated dye, and by relating the peak area ratios, the permeability can be quantitatively measured. The most commonly used detection mode in CE is still UV detection, simply because most commercial CE instruments are equipped with UV- or diode array detectors. This means that the method development in the future will most probably bring up new good CE-UV approaches for easy physicochemical characterization of liposomes.

The use of liposomes for the delivery of drugs has forced the pharmaceutical industry to consider good methodologies, e.g., for the determination of encapsulated and non-encapsulated drugs. Among other techniques, CE has been applied to some extent to the characterization of such drug-delivery systems.[12] As a practical example, the utilization of CE in combination with inductively coupled plasma mass spectrometry for the separation of free cisplatin or oxaliplatin from liposome-encapsulated drug systems can be mentioned.[21,22] This methodology is still new but might be a promising alternative for novel industrial applications.

10.3 Liposomes as Pseudostationary Phase in Electrokinetic Chromatography

The use of liposomes as a pseudostationary phase in electrokinetic chromatography was demonstrated for the first time in 1995.[23] However, there was only one other publication on the topic during the 1990s, and then the next one appeared in 2000. After that, the number of papers on LEKC has slowly been increasing.[9] The most commonly used liposomes in LEKC are those based on PC.

The electrophoretic mobility of an analyte in EKC describes the migration of the analyte in the presence of a moving or nonmoving pseudostationary phase under the influence of electric field strength. However, the electrophoretic mobility does not describe the chromatographic partitioning of the analyte into the aggregates or particles comprising the pseudostationary phase. For obtaining a more quantitative description of the interaction between the analytes and the pseudostationary phase, the mass distribution (or retention) factor can be calculated.

10.3.1 Calculating Retention Factor

The retention factor k is widely used for the quantification of interactions between analytes and liposomes. However, retention factors are highly dependent on the phase ratio (the volume ratio between the liposome and the aqueous phase) and hence are restricted to a specific liposome concentration. The retention factor k can be calculated according to Eq. 10.5 using the effective electrophoretic mobility of the analyte in the LEKC mode (μ_{eff}), the effective electrophoretic mobility of the analyte in CE (with no liposome present in the BGE, i.e., by CZE) (μ_0), and the electrophoretic mobility of the liposome (μ_{LIP}):

$$k = \frac{\mu_{eff} - \mu_0}{\mu_{LIP} - \mu_{eff}} \tag{10.5}$$

The effective electrophoretic mobilities (μ_{eff}) can be calculated using Eq. 10.6:

$$\mu_{eff} = \frac{l_c \, l_d}{U} \left(\frac{1}{t} - \frac{1}{t_{eo}} \right), \tag{10.6}$$

where l_c is the total length of the capillary, l_d is the length of the capillary to the detector, U is the applied voltage, t is the migration time of an analyte, and t_{eo} is the migration time of an EOF marker.

Choosing a good EOF marker is necessary but not always a straightforward task.[24] The marker should be uncharged and have a strong UV absorbance. The most commonly used EOF markers are methanol, dimethyl sulfoxide, formamide, and acetone. Methanol and acetone are good because many analytes are easily solubilized in these solvents; however, they suffer from low UV absorbance. Formamide and dimethyl sulfoxide have a good

UV absorbance and can be added in only small amounts to the sample solution. Other popular EOF markers are thiourea, *N,N*-dimethylformamide, acetonitrile, propan-1-ol, and tetrahydrofuran.

In most publications, a single marker compound that is completely retained in the pseudostationary phase is employed for the determination of the migration time or the electrophoretic mobility of the dispersed phase (i.e., of the electrophoretic mobilities of the liposomes (μ_{LIP})). The marker compounds can be divided into large azo-compounds, polyaromatics, alkylbenzenes, and alkyl phenyl ketones, except for the piperidinium-analogue timepidium bromide.[25] Of these, the most commonly used are Sudan III and dodecanophenone, the latter being the most popular during the last 10 years.

In many cases, organic modifiers are included in the BGE solution in order to increase the solubility and improve the selectivity of hydrophobic analytes in aqueous BGE. However, under such conditions, the electrophoretic mobility of the pseudostationary phase using single compounds as markers for the dispersed phase is no longer reliable because the marker compound will, to some extent, migrate together with the bulk solution. One solution to this problem is to use an iteration procedure for the determination of the migration time of the pseudostationary phase, based on the retention factors of members of a homologous series of different hydrophobicities.[26,27] Various types of series of homologous compounds of different hydrophobicities have been employed as markers for the iterative process. Of the most commonly used, *n*-alkyl phenyl ketones and *n*-alkylbenzenes can be mentioned. However, series of alkyl phenyl alcohols, dansylated *n*-alkylamines, *n*-parabens, and 1-nitroalkanes have also been successfully used.

The method is based on the constant contribution of each methylene unit to the free energy change (ΔG) that is related to the transfer of the analyte from the aqueous phase to the pseudostationary phase. The logarithms of the retention factors for the members of a homologous series are linearly related to the number of the methylene units in the alkyl chain (N_c), as described by Eq. 10.7 (Martin equation):

$$\log k_{EKC} = a + b \cdot N_c \qquad (10.7)$$

To calculate the time of the pseudostationary phase (t_{ps}; in this case, the liposome), the migration times for members of a homologous series and the migration time of the EOF marker have to be determined. In the first step of the iteration procedure, the migration time of the compound with the highest carbon number is assumed to be equal to the migration time of the pseudostationary phase. The retention factors for all other members of the homologous series are calculated according to Eq. 10.8:

$$k_{EKC} = \frac{t_m - t_{eo}}{t_{eo}\left(1 - \dfrac{t_m}{t_{ps}}\right)} \tag{10.8}$$

The logarithm of the retention factor (log k_{EKC}) is plotted against the carbon number (N_c) of the alkyl group. If we assume a linear relationship between log k_{EKC} and N_c according to the Martin equation, then a new estimation of log k_{EKC} can be calculated by extrapolation of a regression line to the member of the homologous series having the highest carbon number. This k_{EKC} value is transformed into a new estimate of t_{ps} according to Eq. 10.9:

$$t_{ps} = \frac{t_m}{1 - \dfrac{t_m - t_{eo}}{k_{EKC}t_{eo}}} \tag{10.9}$$

Using the new estimated t_{ps} value, the log k_{EKC} values for all the members of the homologous series are recalculated and plotted against the carbon number, which will result in a new value of t_{ps}. The iteration procedure is repeated several times until the difference between consecutive values for t_{ps} is less than 0.1% or 0.001 min, or the correlation coefficient (R^2) exceeds 0.9999. This typically requires 30–50 iterations.

Other, but less common, approaches to determine the electrophoretic mobility of the pseudostationary phase are available, and these mainly rely on the direct determination of liposomes by CZE, using either UV absorbance or fluorescence detection. In the latter case, the liposome needs to be labeled with a fluorescent marker that is assumed to not affect the electrophoretic mobility of the liposome itself. There are different types of fluorescent markers, but the most appropriate for this approach are believed to be those that have the fluorescent probe covalently linked to either the acyl chains or the polar headgroup of the lipid. This labeled lipid will be added to the liposome at very low concentrations (less than 1 mol%).

10.3.2 Calculating Distribution Constant

Once the retention constant has been calculated, the distribution constant (K_D) can be calculated. The distribution constant describes the distribution of an analyte between two phases, and it is equal to the ratio of the molar concentration of the analyte in the (pseudo)stationary phase to the molar concentration of the analyte in the mobile phase. Calculation of distribution constants considers the phase ratio (Φ). Therefore, K_D is suitable for comparison of analyte–liposome interactions in systems with various concentrations of liposomes in the BGE solution. The distribution constant, which quantifies the interaction between the analytes and the liposomes studied, can be calculated according to Eq. 10.10:

$$K_D = \frac{k}{\Phi}, \tag{10.10}$$

where k is the retention factor and Φ is the phase ratio.

The phase ratio can be calculated from the partial molar volumes of the lipids according to Eq. 10.11:

$$\Phi = \frac{V_{lip}}{V_{aq}} = \frac{v_{spec,vol}M(c_{lip} - CAC)}{1 - v_{spec,vol}M(c_{lip} - CAC)}, \tag{10.11}$$

where V_{lip} is the volume of the liposome phase, V_{aq} is the volume of the aqueous phase, $v_{spec,vol}$ is the partial specific volume of the lipid, and M is the molar mass of the lipid. In many studies, it has been assumed that the partial specific volume of the lipids is equal to that of water and a value of $v_{spec,vol} = 1$ mL/g has been used. The concentration of the liposomes is represented by c_{lip}, and CAC is the critical aggregation concentration of the lipid. For most used phospholipids, the CAC is very low (in the nM range) and can thus be neglected. In many LEKC cases, the analyte can be assumed to only partition into the lipid bilayer of the liposome vesicle. Hence, the entire volume of the pseudostationary phase, V_{lip}, can then be calculated using the volume of the lipids, i.e., only the shell of the liposome. The volume of the aqueous phase is calculated by subtracting the liposome volume from the total capillary volume.

The main disadvantage of LEKC is that both running buffer vials must be filled with the liposome solution. Due to the rather high cost of pure phospholipids, the working volumes of liposomes are typically rather low (less than 1 mL). This is a bit challenging when working with commercial CE instruments, which often require buffer solution volumes in the low milliliter range. The use of lower volumes (couple of hundreds of microliters) of buffer solutions (e.g., utilizing the sample vials as electrolyte vials) is possible in most instruments, but then the buffer solutions must be renewed more frequently.

10.4 Liposomes in Partial-Filling Electrokinetic Chromatography

In PF-EKC, only a part of the capillary is filled with the pseudostationary phase (in this case with the liposomes). This means in practice that the detector noise is decreased because there are no liposomes in the detection window when the analytes of interest are detected. In addition, the distribution constants of analytes that are very strongly interacting with liposomes can be determined because lower interaction will result in a smaller change in the electrophoretic mobilities of the analytes. Since pure phospholipids are expensive, another main advantage of PF-EKC is the low amount of liposomes needed.

In the method, the liposome plug is injected to the capillary before injection of the sample. The sample plug will migrate through the liposome plug, and a binding equilibrium is reached as the analyte migrates through the liposome zone. Typically, the injection lengths of liposome plugs are 5–45% of the whole capillary length.

An example of the use of CE for studying liposome–analyte interactions is related to studies performed on human β2gpI, which is a phospholipid- and heparin-binding plasma glycoprotein.

The physiological role of the protein in normal blood coagulation is still unresolved as well as its role in autoimmune diseases. It is believed that quantitative binding data on interactions between β2gpI and some of its ligands may help to shed some light on the underlying mechanisms of these diseases. In addition, the development of new approaches for diagnostics, prevention, and therapy is one of the targets. Interactions between β2gpI and anionic liposomes were investigated by means of PF-EKC.[28]

10.5 Liposomes in Capillary Electrophoresis Frontal Analysis

Capillary electrophoresis frontal analysis was originally introduced for studying interactions between the drug warfarin and bovine serum albumin.[29] Later on, the technique has also been applied to study drug–plasma bindings and interactions between analytes and liposomes.[12,30] The primary prerequisite in CE-FA is the requirement of sufficiently different electrophoretic mobilities between the free and bound forms of one of the species studied. Otherwise, determination of the free ligand concentrations is not feasible. In the CE-FA method, the equilibrium between the analyte and the ligand is established in the sample vial. A large plug (typically about 10% of the capillary length) containing the equilibrated sample (i.e., free analyte, liposome, and complex) is injected into a capillary filled with buffer, and the free and bound analyte forms are separated. The different mobilities of the ligand and the free analyte will result in peaks as plateaus. The stability constant can then be calculated from the plateau height of the free analyte, which is proportional to the concentration of the free analyte in the original sample.

The sample volumes are typically 10–50 times higher in CE-FA than those used in EKC. The CE-FA injection length and set up resemble much the PF-EKC technique (see Fig. 10.1). The analytes and the dispersed pseudostationary phase are present only in the injected plug, which avoids a large background electrolyte detector response. Though the background noise is lowered in CE-FA, the lack of sensitivity of detection systems is one of the main drawbacks of CE-FA. The calculation of the binding affinity is based on the determination of the concentration of free ligand in CE-FA, whereas in EKC the migration shifts are observed. CE-FA is more robust when compared to EKC because the height and thus the calculated binding constant are not affected by changes in migration times, EOF mobility, and the peak shapes, because the plateau regions are constituted of the nondispersed zone. However, CE-FA is limited to systems where the mobility of the complex is equal to that of one interacting species, while the EKC technique can only be applied to systems where the mobilities of the drug and the complex are different.

10.6 Immobilization of Phospholipids

In many studies, phospholipids or liposomes have been immobilized on fused silica capillaries. The aim has been either to shield the capillary wall from unwanted interactions or to use the liposome coating as a model cell membrane for studying analyte interactions.

10.6.1 Phospholipids as Wall Modifiers

A common reason for coating silica capillaries for CE is to prevent the adsorption of large molecules, such as proteins, on the capillary inner surface. Especially with hydrophobic, positively charged biomolecules, this is of great importance. Another reason for coating capillaries is to modify, or even reverse, the EOF. Positively charged surfactants and polyelectrolytes have been used to a great extent for changing the negatively charged fused silica surface (dissociated silanol groups) into a positively charged surface. If the EOF flow is not of importance for the separation, neutral or zwitterionic additives are preferred. The coating serves as a protective layer for not only minimizing analyte adsorption, but also controlling the migration of analytes. By adjusting the EOF flow, the separation of analytes can be sped up and/or the selectivity can be improved. Finally, the next section will discuss coating of capillaries for capillary electrochromatographic (CEC) studies, i.e., for creating a stationary phase with affinity for certain analytes.

In general, CE coatings are classified as dynamic, semipermanent, or permanent (static) coatings. The discrimination between dynamic and permanent coatings is typically such that when using dynamic coatings, the additive must be present in the BGE solution, whereas using permanent coatings, there are no coating additives in the BGE solution. When the coating agent is included in the BGE solution, the additive molecules will compete with the analyte for adsorption sites on the capillary wall. However, since their binding affinity to the capillary wall is rather low, they are slowly washed away during electrophoresis and thereby the coating is constantly renewed.

The so-called semipermanent coatings are strongly attached to the fused silica wall simply by rinsing, and no coating additives are needed in the BGE solution during electrophoresis. The main advantage of such coatings is that they can be easily renewed and changed to another type of coating, but the disadvantage is the often observed slow leakage of the coating out of the capillary. These coatings are discussed in more detail in Section 10.6.2.

Permanent coatings, on the other hand, will remain on the capillary surface and hence no coating additives are needed in the BGE solution. Polymerized phospholipid bilayers with good stability have also been demonstrated.[31] The polymerizable lipid 1,2-bis(10,12-tricosadiynoyl)-*sn*-glycero-3-phosphocholine (Diyne PC) was utilized for preparing coatings by photochemical reaction (254 nm, $\sim 1.65 \times 10^{16}$ photons/s/cm^3 for 15 min) (Fig. 10.2). The Diyne PC coatings can withstand organic solvents, which makes them suitable for nonaqueous capillary electrophoretic separations.

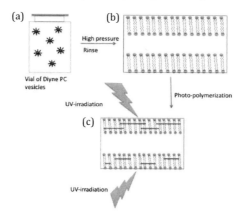

Figure 10.2 Schematic presentation of in situ preparation of photo-polymerized Diyne PC coatings.[31] Reprinted with permission from Ref. [31], Copyright 2012, Elsevier. http://dx.doi.org/10.1016/j.chroma.2012.07.017.

The main advantage of permanent coatings is the improved stability as compared with dynamic or semipermanent coatings. Some of the developed coatings are restricted to certain types of phospholipids. For example, phospholipids with primary amino groups (optimally phosphatidylserine) can be covalently linked, by the aid of glutaraldehyde, to aminopropylsilylated fused silica capillaries.[32] A typical reaction scheme is illustrated in Fig. 10.3.

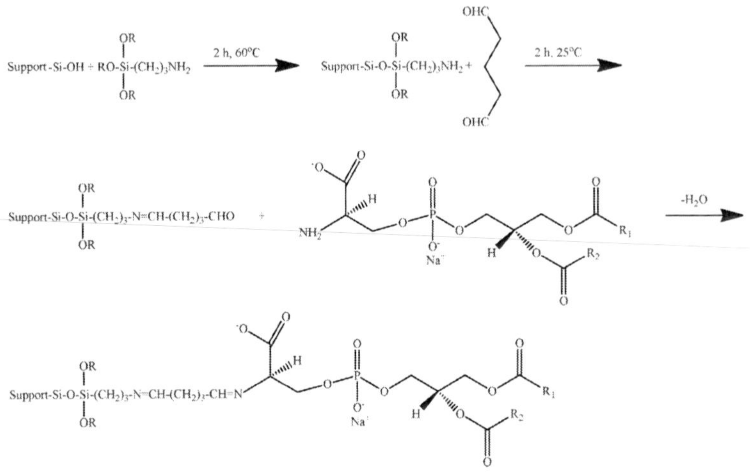

Figure 10.3 Reaction scheme on the covalent binding of phospholipids (PS in the figure) on fused silica capillaries. The aminopropylsilylation step was carried out with 3-(aminopropyl)triethoxy silyl (APTES).[32] Adapted from Ref. [32] with permission of The Royal Society of Chemistry. http://dx.doi.org/10.1039/C1SM05372H.

Surfaces terminating with zwitterionic groups have been shown to be rather resistant to protein adsorption—a finding that is in accordance with the well-known protein resistance of erythrocytes and platelets.[33,34] There are several studies where this phenomenon has been used to suppress analyte–wall interactions in capillary electrophoretic protein separation. The first study was made in 2002, and in that work, physical adsorption of zwitterionic 1,2-dilauroyl-*sn*-glycero-3-phosphocholine (DLPC) was used for the separation of both anionic and cationic proteins. The capillaries were stable over a wide pH range (3–10) and the migration times for analytes highly repeatable and reproducible. The coating was also suitable for the analysis of egg white proteins.

In addition to separation of proteins, phospholipid coatings have also been utilized in the separation of inorganic anions by CE. However, by far, zwitterionic phosphatidyl choline layers have been the most commonly adopted phospholipid layers for CE capillaries. Main emphasis has been on the development of stable coatings suitable for CE–mass spectrometry (MS) analysis.

When MS is used as a mass-sensitive detector in CE, the coating must be non-leachable and the BGE solution more or less volatile. The actual coupling of CE with MS is not straightforward mainly due to the very low flow rates (nanoliter per minute range) in CE and the need to establish a closed electrical circuit to maintain the high voltage across the capillary necessary for CE separation. This necessitates the assembly of proper interfaces. Electrospray ionization (ESI) has been the predominant ionization technique used for CE-MS so far. There are two main approaches for coupling CE with ESI-MS, i.e., using a sheath–liquid interface or a sheathless interface. The sheath–liquid interface is most widely used for CE-MS, mostly because it is commercially available.

A stable CE-MS method is crucial to obtain repeatable and reproducible results. Good stability of migration times is essential, and a constant EOF is often needed to achieve satisfactory and reproducible spray conditions for efficient analyte ionization. This put great demands on the method development, and if phospholipid coated capillaries are used, these should preferably be semipermanent or permanent.

10.6.2 Phospholipids as Stationary Phase in Open-Tubular Capillary Chromatography

Liposomes and phospholipid aggregates have been used as models to study the behavior of membranes and membrane-bound macromolecules since the early 1980s.[35] Over the years, many methods have been developed to study different types of analyte–membrane interactions. CEC, which can be regarded as a hybrid of HPLC and CE, has been one of them. In CEC, phospholipids are immobilized onto the capillary wall as supported phospholipid bilayers or as intact liposomes. Analytes of interest migrate through the capillary, and the retardation of the electrophoretic mobility is monitored. The first work on open-tubular CEC using liposomes as stationary phase was published in 1998. In that work, the affinity between avidin and biotin was utilized and biotinylated small and large unilamellar egg PC-based liposomes were immobilized onto an amidated capillary, containing avidin. The study was clearly a pioneering work in the field and later on many groups have worked in the field of OT-CEC with biomimicking and biomimetic stationary phases.

In OT-CEC the retention factor of an analyte is based on the electrophoretic mobility of the analyte in free solution, i.e., under CZE conditions, and on its interaction with the stationary phase. Therefore, the retention factor can be determined using both OT-CEC and CZE data according to Eq. 10.12:

$$k_{CEC} = \frac{t_m(1 + k_e) - t_{eo}}{t_{eo}}, \tag{10.12}$$

where t_m is the migration time of the analyte in the OT-CEC mode, t_{eo} is the migration time of the (unretained) EOF marker in the coated capillary, and k_e is the ratio of the migration times of the analyte and the EOF marker under CZE conditions (uncoated capillary). In the case of neutral (uncharged) analytes, the equation is simplified to the conventional equation for the retention factor, which is typically used in chromatography (Eq. 10.13):

$$k_{CEC} = \frac{t_m - t_{eo}}{t_{eo}} \tag{10.13}$$

In order to calculate the phase ratio, the volume of the lipid phase is needed (see aforementioned discussion; Eqs. 10.10 and 10.11). This can, for example, be done by determining the mass distribution of liposome per area by quartz crystal microbalance (QCM). Considering the inner surface of the capillary and the ratio between the liposome internal water volume and the volume of the liposomal shell (using the known bilayer thickness of 5 nm and density of the dry lipid, 0.95 g/mL[36]), the volume of the lipid phase can be calculated. Actually, it is worth mentioning here that liposomes do not always disrupt into bilayers on silica surfaces, but intact truncated liposomes have been observed as well (Fig. 10.4).[36-38]

There are several aspects that should be considered when aiming at stable phospholipid coatings applicable for OT-CEC. The first task is to select the appropriate phospholipid mixture and other constituents such as proteins or cholesterol. In many cases, the addition of proteins to liposomes is preferred to be done after the preparation of unilamellar vesicles in order to maintain the characteristics of the proteins. This has to do with the rather harsh conditions employed when preparing unilamellar vesicles either by extrusion (rough shaking and filtration through membranes of specific pore size; often 50–100 nm) or by using probe sonication (ultrasound radiation, which would alter protein structure[39]).

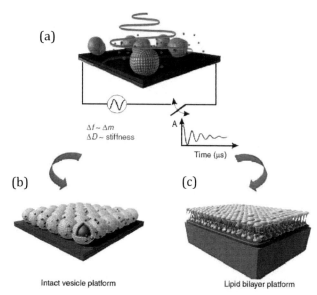

Figure 10.4   Schematic representation of the QCM-D principle (a); the adsorption of a monolayer of adsorbed, unruptured vesicles (b); the formation of a supported lipid bilayer platform through surface-mediated vesicle fusion (c).[38] Reprinted by permission from MacMillan Publishers, Ltd: *Nat Protocols.* 2010; 5(6): 1096–1106, Copyright 2010. http://www.nature.com/nprot/journal/v5/n6/full/nprot.2010.65.html.

However, in the case of poor attachment, the protein can easily leak out of the capillary. On the other hand, good results have also been obtained by mixing phospholipids and proteins before preparation of unilamellar vesicles.[40] Selection of the best procedure is highly dependent on the type of protein and other experimental conditions.

10.6.2.1   Specific coating conditions

After selecting the desired phospholipid mixture for coating, the second important aspect is to choose an appropriate BGE solution. This is strongly connected also to the preconditioning of the capillary. Piperazine-type buffers have been shown to act as linkers between negatively charged liposomes and the fused silica capillaries at neutral pH values.[41] Just by changing the buffer from phosphate to 4-(2-hydroxyethyl)-1-piperazineethanesulfonic acid (HEPES), which is a zwitterionic organic buffering agent, great improvement in the adsorption of liposomes to the fused silica capillary was obtained. Most probably the piperazine moiety serves as a linker between the fused silica capillary wall and the phospholipids. As mentioned earlier, also other types of piperazine-type buffering agents, such as N-(2-hydroxyethyl)piperazine-N'-(2-hydroxypropanesulfonic) acid (HEPPSO), piperazine-N,N'-bis(2-ethanesulfonic acid) (PIPES), and piperazine-N,N'-bis(2-propanesulfonic acid) (POPSO), can be well employed as linkers. All these zwitterionic buffers belong to the series of Good (or Good's) buffers, originally described by Norman Good and colleagues during 1966–80.[42-44] However, short linear diamines, like 1,2-ethylenediamine and 1,3-diaminopropane, can be utilized as binding agents as well, demonstrating that the degree of protonation of the amino group is one of the crucial aspects.[45]

Calcium has, since the early 1970s, been known to induce fusion of biological membranes,[46] and this effect has been utilized for attaching liposomes to fused silica capillaries. The influence of calcium on coatings of anionic liposomes made from POPC and PS coatings was measured under various experimental conditions where the calcium concentration, buffer composition, capillary temperature, and preconditioning were varied.[47] The results showed that even though the influence of calcium on the phospholipid-coating stability was pronounced, as well as on the separation of neutral model steroids, the effect of preconditioning and temperature had only slight effect on the capillary performance. An additional finding was that the influence of calcium varied depending on the structure of the anionic phospholipid in the liposome.[48] Liposomes comprising POPC in combination with the anionic phospholipids phosphatidic acid (PA), phosphatidylglycerol (PG), phosphatidylinositol (PI), and phosphatidylserine (PS) were compared. The results showed that calcium had the strongest interactions with the PA-containing liposomes, as evidenced from retention data on some model neutral steroids—the interaction of the analytes with the stationary phase clearly decreased with the addition of calcium to the system. A mechanism involving binding of calcium to the phospholipid phosphate group was suggested. The effect of other divalent metal ions (magnesium and zinc) on phospholipid membranes was studied by coating a fused silica capillary with a liposome dispersion containing calcium, magnesium, or zinc. All metal ions improved the stability of the PC-coated capillary. Increased rigidity, induced by metal ions immobilized into the membrane, is suggested to be the major reason for the improvement. Calcium appeared to improve the stability of the coating most. To sum up the results of phospholipid-coating stabilization studies, it seems that calcium and the use of piperazine-buffers (e.g., HEPES) have the most profound effect on the coating performance.

In most CE studies on analyte–liposome interactions, the pH has been around the physiological pH of 7.4. The ionization of phospholipids as well as buffer components is strongly dependent on the selected pH value. Studies have demonstrated that the pH of a lipid dispersion can affect the size of the liposomes and thereby their structure, which may strongly influence the formation and stability of phospholipid coatings.

In studies on the effect of pH on the stability of phospholipid coatings made from anionic liposomes, the conclusion is that the coating formation is influenced by pH, but the addition of calcium to the BGE solution outweighs the influence of pH.

Due to the specific transition temperature of lipids, the effect of the gel vs. fluid state should not be overlooked when using phospholipid coatings for separations in OT-CEC. Generally, phospholipid coatings are more stable when used at temperatures below the T_m, i.e., in the gel state; however, under those circumstances, interactions with compounds are also decreased compared to the interactions when the lipid membrane is in its fluid state. Adding cholesterol to a liposome dispersion of DPPC or DPPC and SM broadens the main phase transition and eventually eliminates it at higher (>30 mol%) cholesterol concentrations. Addition of cholesterol to a fluid DPPC coating makes the coating more gel like and more stable by increasing the orientation of the phospholipids. In general, it has been observed that the retention of analytes decreases when the concentration of cholesterol in the liposomes used for coating of the capillary increases. The same trend has been observed in LEKC when cholesterol-rich liposomes have been compared with liposomes lacking cholesterol in the separation of neutral analytes.[49]

10.7 Studies on Liposome–Analyte Complexes by Capillary (Zone) Electrophoresis

Studies by CE on molecular interactions between analytes and lipids or liposomes have been carried out to some extent. For instance, CE with laser-induced fluorescence (LIF) detection and CIEF with whole column imaging detection have been employed for investing interactions between phospholipids and proteins. In addition, complexes between plasmid DNA and cationic lipid/ cholesterol liposomes have been investigated with the use of CE and neutral coated capillaries with entangled acrylamide polymer solution as separation buffer. Successful separation of linear, supercoiled, and open-circle conformers of DNA in plasmid DNA and in the liposome complex was obtained.

Liposomes have shown several-fold increase in the uptake of a model 25-mer DNA-based phosphorothiate (or S-oligo) antisense drug in cells, in comparison to plain antisense. The antisense molecule was delivered to the cells through incubation and by using a cationic liposome called Cytofectin GS 3815™. In addition, the antisense activity was much enhanced in the presence of liposomes. A CE-LIF methodology was employed for the investigation of the delivery of the antisense molecule to the cells through the formation of a complex between the negatively charged antisense and Cytofectin GS 3815™.[50] CE-LIF has also been employed for the determination of the specific attachment of a human rhinovirus serotype 2 to receptor-decorated liposomes.[51] Liposomes were prepared from standard lipids, including the Ni^{2+} salt of 1,2-dioleoyl-*sn*-glycero-3-[(*N*-(5-amino-1-carboxypentyl) iminodiacetic acid) succinyl] (Ni^{2+}-NTA-DOGS). A recombinant soluble receptor containing a hexa-histidine tag (his6-tag) at its C-terminus was attached via the Ni^{2+}-NTA-lipid to the liposome surface. As a result, a receptor-decorated liposome was formed. The specificity of the method was demonstrated by testing another rhinovirus that did not attach to the liposomes.

For the intracellular derivatization of amino acids in cells, red blood cells were fused with liposomes, and the fusion efficiency was studied by CE-LIF. As a fluorescence marker, FITC was incorporated into sonicated liposomes comprising PC and cholesterol, thereafter mixed with PEG 6000 buffer solution and red blood cells. Under optimal fusion conditions, 10 amino acids could be detected; however, all of them were not baseline resolved.

10.8 Conclusion

Capillary electromigration techniques can be widely used for the determination of physicochemical properties of liposomes, as well as for liposome or lipid interactions with analytes. CE has shown to be a promising technique for the prediction of interactions between lipid membranes and analytes, e.g., in human drug absorption and skin permeability studies, for analysis of drug–liposome complexes and their stability (including drug leakage studies), as well as for the direct analysis of the characteristics of liposomes. There are several factors affecting the choice of method, such as the available amount of lipids (an important economical aspect), the type of lipids, the separation conditions (type of buffer, pH, and addition of salts), the acquired separation selectivity, and the correct selection of the dimension and type of separation channel.

When studying the general properties of liposomes or liposome–analyte complexes, it is important to select a capillary surface material having very little interaction with the liposomes or to use running conditions by which the interactions can be minimized. In the case of investigation of liposome–analyte interactions by LEKC, it is usually preferred to have a rather inert capillary surface in order to avoid a separation principle, which is a combination of LEKC and OT-CEC (i.e., pseudostationary and stationary phases).

Several immobilization or frontal analysis affinity studies have been carried out, and there are some promising features of the methodology that might be of interest for the pharmaceutical industry in the future. The main advantages of CE techniques, in comparison with other conventional separation techniques, are the speed of analysis, the low amount of samples needed, and the broad range of compounds that can be analyzed. The current limitations are mainly due to the limited sensitivity and the precision of the technique. However, nowadays special methodologies have been developed, which can be employed in order to improve the detection limits (e.g., various online sample stacking methods or the use of MS detection) and migration time repeatability and reproducibility. CE will never exceed the popularity of HPLC techniques in industry; however, it might become an important complimentary technique.

References

1. Hjertén S. *Free Zone Electrophoresis* [PhD thesis]. Almqvist and Wiksells Boktryckeri AB, Uppsala; 1967.

2. Hjertén S. Free zone electrophoresis. *Chromatographic Reviews.* 1967; 9(2): 122–219.

3. Virtanen R. Zone electrophoresis in a narrow-bore tube employing potentiometric detection: Theoretical and experimental study. *Acta Polytech Scand Chem Technol Ser.* 1974; 123: 1–67.

4. Mikkers FEP, Everaerts FM, Verheggen TPEM. Concentration distributions in free zone electrophoresis. *J Chromatogr.* 1979; 169(0): 1–10.

5. Sekhon BS. An overview of capillary electrophoresis: Pharmaceutical, biopharmaceutical and biotechnology applications. *J Pharm Ed Res.* 2011; 2(2): 2–36.

6. Riekkola M-L, Jönsson JA, Smith RM. Terminology for analytical capillary electromigration techniques: (IUPAC recommendations 2003). *Pure Appl Chem.* 2004; 76(2): 443–451.

7. Wiedmer SK, Shimmo R. Liposomes in capillary electromigration techniques. *Electrophoresis.* 2009; 30(S1): S240–S257.

8. Terabe S, Otsuka K, Ichikawa K, Tsuchiya A, Ando T. Electrokinetic separations with micellar solutions and open-tubular capillaries. *Anal Chem.* 1984; 56(1): 111–113.

9. Wiedmer SK, Lokajová J. Capillary electromigration techniques for studying interactions between analytes and lipid dispersions. *J Sep Sci.* 2013; 36(1): 37–51.

10. Wiedmer SK, Holopainen JM, Mustakangas P, Kinnunen PKJ, Riekkola M-L. Liposomes as carriers in electrokinetic capillary chromatography. *Electrophoresis.* 2000; 21(15): 3191–3198.

11. Ishida T, Kiwada H. Accelerated blood clearance (ABC) phenomenon upon repeated injection of PEGylated liposomes. *Int J Pharm.* 2008; 354(1–2): 56–62.

12. Franzen U, Østergaard J. Physico-chemical characterization of liposomes and drug substance–liposome interactions in pharmaceutics using capillary electrophoresis and electrokinetic chromatography. *J Chromatogr.* 2012; 1267(0): 32–44.

13. Wiedmer SK, Hautala J, Holopainen JM, Kinnunen PKJ, Riekkola M-L. Study on liposomes by capillary electrophoresis. *Electrophoresis.* 2001; 22(7): 1305–1313.

14. Hunter RJ. *Zeta Potential in Colloid Science: Principles and Applications.* London: Academic Press; 1981.

15. Radko SP, Stastna M, Chrambach A. Size-dependent electrophoretic migration and separation of liposomes by capillary zone electrophoresis in electrolyte solutions of various ionic strengths. *Anal Chem.* 2000; 72(24): 5955–5960.

16. Radko SP, Stastna M, Chrambach A. Capillary zone electrophoresis of sub-mu m-sized particles in electrolyte solutions of various ionic strengths: Size-dependent electrophoretic migration and separation efficiency. *Electrophoresis.* 2000; 21(17): 3583–3592.

17. Taylor G. Dispersion of soluble matter in solvent flowing slowly through a tube. *Proc R Soc Lond A.* 1953; 219(1137): 186–203.

18. Jensen SS, Jensen H, Cornett C, Møller EH, Østergaard J. Insulin diffusion and self-association characterized by real-time UV imaging and Taylor dispersion analysis. *J Pharm Biomed Anal.* 2014; 92(0): 203–210.

19. Yeagle PL, ed. *The Structure of Biological Membranes.* 2nd ed. Florida: CRC Press LLC; 2005.

20. Torchilin VP, Volkmar W, eds. *Liposomes: A Practical Approach.* 2nd ed. Oxford: Oxford University Press; 2003.

21. Nguyen TTN, Østergaard J, Stürup S, Gammelgaard B. Metallomics in drug development: Characterization of a liposomal cisplatin drug formulation in human plasma by CE–ICP–MS. *Anal Bioanal Chem.* 2013; 405(6): 1845–1854.

22. Nguyen T, Østergaard J, Stürup S, Gammelgaard B. Investigation of a liposomal oxaliplatin drug formulation by capillary electrophoresis hyphenated to inductively coupled plasma mass spectrometry (CE-ICP-MS). *Anal Bioanal Chem.* 2012; 402(6): 2131–2139.

23. Zhang YX, Zhang R, Hjerten S, Lundahl P. Liposome capillary electrophoresis for analysis of interactions between lipid bilayers and solutes. *Electrophoresis*. 1995; 16(8): 1519–1523.

24. Fuguet E, Rafols C, Bosch E, Roses M. Solute-solvent interactions in micellar electrokinetic chromatography: IV. Characterization of electroosmotic flow and micellar markers. *Electrophoresis*. 2002; 23(1): 56–66.

25. Wiedmer SK, Lokajová J, Riekkola M-L. Marker compounds for the determination of retention factors in EKC. *J Sep Sci*. 2010; 33(3): 394–409.

26. Bushey MM, Jorgenson JW. Separation of dansylated methylamine and dansylated methyl-D3-amine by micellar electrokinetic capillary chromatography with methanol-modified mobile phase. *Anal Chem*. 1989; 61(5): 491–493.

27. Bushey MM, Jorgenson JW. Effects of methanol-modified mobile phase on the separation of isotopically substituted compounds by micellar electrokinetic capillary chromatography. *J Micro Sep*. 1989; 1(3): 125–130.

28. Bohlin ME, Kogutowska E, Blomberg LG, Heegaard NHH. Capillary electrophoresis-based analysis of phospholipid and glycosaminoglycan binding by human beta(2)-glycoprotein. *J Chromatogr*. 2004; 1059(1–2): 215–222.

29. Kraak JC, Busch S, Poppe H. Study of protein drug-binding using capillary zone electrophoresis. *J Chromatogr*. 1992; 608(1–2): 257–264.

30. Østergaard J, Heegaard NHH. Capillary electrophoresis frontal analysis: Principles and applications for the study of drug-plasma protein binding. *Electrophoresis*. 2003; 24(17): 2903–2913.

31. Pei L, Lucy CA. Polymerized phospholipid bilayers as permanent coatings for small amine separations using mixed aqueous/organic capillary zone electrophoresis. *J Chromatogr*. 2012; 1267(0): 80–88.

32. Lokajová J, Tiala H, Viitala T, Riekkola M-L, Wiedmer SK. Covalent binding of phospholipid vesicles on fused silica capillaries for electrochromatography. *Soft Matter*. 2011; 7(13): 6041–6050.

33. Holmlin RE, Chen XX, Chapman RG, Takayama S, Whitesides GM. Zwitterionic SAMs that resist nonspecific adsorption of protein from aqueous buffer. *Langmuir*. 2001; 17(9): 2841–2850.

34. Chapman D. Biomembranes and new hemocompatible materials. *Langmuir*. 1993; 9(1): 39–45.

35. Watts TH, Brian AA, Kappler JW, Marrack P, McConnell HM. Antigen presentation by supported planar membranes containing affinity-purified I-Ad. *Proc Natl Acad Sci U S A.* 1984; 81(23): 7564–7568.

36. Viitala T, Hautala JT, Vuorinen J, Wiedmer SK. Structure of anionic phospholipid coatings on silica by dissipative quartz crystal microbalance. *Langmuir.* 2007; 23(2): 609–618.

37. Jing Y, Trefna H, Persson M, Kasemo B, Svedhem S. Formation of supported lipid bilayers on silica: Relation to lipid phase transition temperature and liposome size. *Soft Matter.* 2014; 10(1): 187–195.

38. Cho N-J, Frank CW, Kasemo B, Höök F. Quartz crystal microbalance with dissipation monitoring of supported lipid bilayers on various substrates. *Nat Protocols.* 2010; 5(6): 1096–1106.

39. Stathopulos PB, Scholz GA, Hwang Y-M, Rumfeldt JAO, Lepock JR, Meiering EM. Sonication of proteins causes formation of aggregates that resemble amyloid. *Protein Sci.* 2004; 13(11): 3017–3027.

40. Wiedmer SK, Bo T, Riekkola M-L. Phospholipid-protein coatings for chiral capillary electrochromatography. *Anal Biochem.* 2008; 373(1): 26–33.

41. Wiedmer SK, Jussila M, Hakala RMS, Pystynen KH, Riekkola M-L. Piperazine-based buffers for liposome coating of capillaries 1for electrophoresis. *Electrophoresis.* 2005; 26(10): 1920–1927.

42. Good NE, Winget GD, Winter W, Connolly TN, Izawa S, Singh RMM. Hydrogen ion buffers for biological research. *Biochemistry.* 1966; 5(2): 467–477.

43. Good NE, Izawa S. Hydrogen ion buffers. In: Anthony San P, ed. *Methods in Enzymology.* Vol 24: Academic Press; 1972: 53–68.

44. Ferguson WJ, Braunschweiger KI, Braunschweiger WR, et al. Hydrogen ion buffers for biological research. *Anal Biochem.* 1980; 104(2): 300–310.

45. Varjo SJO, Hautala JT, Wiedmer SK, Riekkola M-L. Small diamines as modifiers for phosphatidylcholine/phosphatidylserine coatings in capillary electrochromatography. *J Chromatogr.* 2005; 1081(1): 92–98.

46. Feigenson GW. Calcium ion binding between lipid bilayers: The four-component system of phosphatidylserine, phosphatidylcholine, calcium chloride, and water. *Biochemistry.* 1989; 28(3): 1270–1278.

47. Hautala JT, Wiedmer SK, Riekkola M-L. Anionic liposomes in capillary electrophoresis: Effect of calcium on 1-palmitoyl-2-oleyl-sn-glycero-3-phosphatidylcholine/phosphatidylserine-coating in silica capillaries. *Anal Bioanal Chem.* 2004; 378(7): 1769–1776.

48. Hautala JT, Riekkola M-L, Wiedmer SK. Anionic phospholipid coatings in capillary electrochromatography binding of Ca^{2+} to phospholipid phosphate group. *J Chromatogr.* 2007; 1150(1–2): 339–347.

49. Wiedmer SK, Jussila MS, Holopainen JM, Alakoskela JM, Kinnunen PKJ, Riekkola M-L. Cholesterol-containing phosphatidylcholine liposomes: Characterization and use as dispersed phase in electrokinetic apillary chromatography. *J Sep Sci.* 2002; 25(7): 427–437.

50. Malek AH, Khaledi MG. Monitoring liposome-mediated delivery and fate of an antisense drug in cell extracts and in single cells by capillary electrophoresis with laser-induced fluorescence. *Electrophoresis.* 2003; 24(6): 1054–1062.

51. Bilek G, Kremser L, Wruss J, Blaas D, Kenndler E. Mimicking early events of virus infection: Capillary electrophoretic analysis of virus attachment to receptor-decorated liposomes. *Anal Chem.* 2007; 79(4): 1620–1625.

Chapter 11

Fluorescent Dye-Encapsulating Liposomes for Cellular Visualization

Agnes Csiszár and Rudolf Merkel

Forschungszentrum Jülich GmbH,
Institute of Complex Systems (ICS-7): Biomechanics,
52425 Jülich, Germany

a.csiszar@fz-juelich.de

11.1 Introduction

The membranes of eukaryotic cells are highly diverse and dynamic entities. They are formed from thousands of different molecules, many of which undergo fast chemical turnover and modification. Moreover, biomembranes are liquid crystalline structures, with liquid properties in plane and astonishing softness perpendicular to it.[1] This extreme pliability enables fast shape changes as well as rapid fission and fusion events of small membrane fragments. Obviously, such dynamic membrane processes must be studied in living cells. For this purpose, light microscopy offers excellent and often unique possibilities (see Fig. 11.1).

In its simplest form, microscopy relies on the absorption of light to achieve contrast. However, biomembranes absorb little light, so they are almost invisible in amplitude contrast. The

Liposomes in Analytical Methodologies
Edited by Katie A. Edwards
Copyright © 2016 Pan Stanford Publishing Pte. Ltd.
ISBN 978-981-4669-26-9 (Hardcover), 978-981-4669-27-6 (eBook)
www.panstanford.com

invention of ingenious optical techniques such as phase contrast[2] or differential interference contrast[3] that convert minute phase changes of light into well-contrasted micrographs enabled visualization of membranes and paved the way to the observation of dynamic processes in living cells, such as cytoskeletal streaming, transport of organelles,[4] or formation of adhesion complexes.[5]

Fluorescent liposomes   **Live cell staining**   **Advanced microscopy**

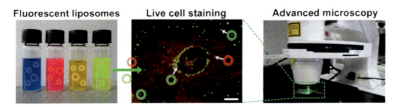

Figure 11.1   Fluorescently labeled lipid molecules as well as fluorescent lipophilic membrane sensor molecules can be incorporated into liposomes. Upon incubation with living cells, fluorescent molecular reporters may incorporate into cellular membranes enabling the visualization of membrane processes in vivo.

Unfortunately, all these techniques are not able to image the distribution of a specific molecule in cells. This formidable challenge has been partially solved in fixed cells by immunofluorescence microscopy[6] and in living cells by transfection with genetic vectors encoding proteins that comprise the molecule of interest and a fluorescent molecule[7,8] or by liposomal delivery of fluorescent membrane sensors or fluorescently tagged lipid molecules.[9] These fluorescence-based microscopy methods are at present a mainstay of cell biology. Their analytical power is progressively increased, on one hand, by the development of light microscopy techniques such as stimulated emission depletion (STED),[10,11] photoactivated localization microscopy (PALM),[12] stochastic optical reconstruction microscopy,[13] or structured illumination microscopy[14,15] that break the resolution limit of light microscopy. Other techniques of advanced fluorescence microscopy[16] such as fluorescence recovery after photobleaching,[17,18] fluorescence correlation spectroscopy,[19,20] or fluorescence lifetime microscopy[21,22] enable local measurements of molecular binding, diffusivity, or environmental polarity. Moreover, fluorescence microscopy is benefiting tremendously from the invention of novel synthetic fluorescent probes with improved properties[23-25] and novel labeling strategies.[26,27]

Despite these breathtaking advancements, microscopic analysis of cell membranes is still a formidable task. Decades of research on biomembrane organization[28-32] with sometimes conflicting results has shown that membrane molecules exhibit a pronounced heterogeneity on molecular and nanometric scales. It appears that real cell membranes are mixtures of thousands of molecules whose thermodynamic state is close to a critical point.[33] In the vicinity of such points, lateral structure formation (or dissolution) costs little free energy, which might be exactly the reason why evolution has shaped membrane composition in this singular way. Moreover, here small differences in the physicochemical properties of molecules might result in substantially different behavior.

Because few natural biomembrane components of animal cells are fluorescent, membrane scientists must resort to fluorescently labeled analogs of natural membrane lipids or membrane proteins. Now, a plethora of fluorophores, in other words synthetic molecular groups with often amazing fluorescence properties, are available and can be covalently coupled to membrane molecules to convert them into fluorescent reporters. Yet all these fluorophores exhibit molecular weights of a few hundreds of grams per mole, that is, on the same order of magnitude as ordinary membrane-forming lipids. Thus, attaching a fluorescent moiety certainly alters basic physicochemical properties of a lipid. Moreover, almost all fluorophores are of amphiphilic nature giving rise to often surprising behavior in membranes. The point we want to make is that while molecular reporters offer great and often unique possibilities in biomembrane research, they have to be used with utmost care to sidestep the pitfalls associated with them.

After having chosen the right fluorophore and successfully conjugated it to the molecule of interest, the fluorescent product has to be incorporated into living cells to subsequently get information about the biological, physical, or chemical state of cell membranes. At present, there are several delivery strategies for molecule incorporation into living cells depending on the chemical character of the reporter molecule. Most of them need a transporter system, so-called carrier particles. Lipid vesicles, called liposomes, are frequently used for these purposes due to their high bioavailability and low toxicity.[34] Moreover, liposomes can be loaded with lipophilic as well as hydrophilic cargos. For example, fluorescently conjugated lipids can be easily incorporated into the lipid bilayer of liposomes producing stable carrier particles. Upon contact of such loaded liposomes with cells, the fluorescent molecules can enter into the cells in one of four ways: adsorption, endocytosis (phagocytosis and pinocytosis), material exchange, or fusion.[35,36] In all cases, besides the uptake efficacy, the controlled and efficient release of the cargo is the most crucial factor for an efficient cellular delivery.

In this chapter, we will give a short introduction to liposomes as carriers for fluorescent probes for investigating living cells. We start out with a short description of the photophysics of fluorescent probes. We also summarize the most popular and useful fluorophores for lipid conjugation as well as fluorescent sensor molecules with their advantages and disadvantages and give a short overview about liposomal delivery of such molecules. Additionally, we present some application fields where this analytical technique will be used.

11.2 Excursion into Photophysics of Fluorophores

First, an excursion into the photophysics of fluorophores is necessary to better understand the later described fluorescence phenomenon and its importance in cell biological analysis. Readers unsatisfied with the following cursory introduction may find the referenced books helpful.[37-40] In a nutshell, fluorescence comprises absorption of a photon of visible light by an atom or molecule, followed by the emission of a photon with slightly lower energy. While fluorescence by atoms or ions is best understood, molecules containing large π-electron systems, that is, extended networks of conjugated multiple bonds, are the mainstay for fluorescence microscopy. Here absorption of light results in the excitation of electrons from the ground state into higher excited states. The quantum mechanical states of molecules comprise a hierarchy: Most important is the state of the electrons, that is, the orbitals. In addition to electronic excitation, figuratively speaking the "lifting of one electron from one orbital into another one," vibrational and rotational excitations of molecules exist, albeit at much lower energies. Thus, each excited state possesses a whole spectrum of vibrational excitations. Because in condensed matter molecular collisions occur on picosecond time scales, vibrational excitation of molecules relaxes extremely fast. In general, transitions between different electronic states occur either with or without emission of radiation. Basic considerations show that the rates of radiationless transitions decay extremely fast with increasing energy gap.[41] As the energetic distances between the different electronic states progressively decrease for higher excitations, virtually all fluorophores relax within picoseconds after photon absorption to the vibrational ground state of the first excited electronic state. An instructive counterexample to this rule is azulene. This molecule exhibits an exceptionally large energy gap between the first and the second excited states resulting in a population of both states. Thus, with the exception of azulene and related molecules, all fluorescence emission occurs from the vibronic ground state of the first excited electronic state irrespective of the initial state of excitation. The most important implication of this fact is that the spectrum of fluorescence emitted by a fluorophore does not depend on the wavelength of excitation (Kasha's rule).

Three different decay routes are possible from the first electronically excited state: (1) emission of a photon, (2) radiationless decay to the electronic ground state, and (3) intersystem crossing to the triplet state. Only the minor fraction of light-absorbing molecules (i.e., dye molecules), where process 1 can compete with the others, emits fluorescence. This process exhibits lifetimes on the order of a few nanoseconds.

Following intersystem crossing to the triplet state, again vibrational relaxation occurs. As transitions from the triplet to the singlet state or vice versa contain a change in electronic spin, which is quantum mechanically forbidden, the triplet state exhibits an extremely long lifetime. Therefore, the probabilities of photon emission from the triplet state, that is, phosphorescence, are extremely low. All these processes are conveniently summarized in the so-called Jablonski diagram (see Fig. 11.2).

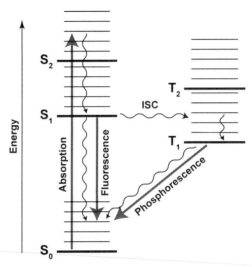

Figure 11.2 Jablonski diagram with important photophysical processes indicated. S_n: nth electronically excited state with paired spins (singlet manifold); T_n: nth electronically excited state with parallel electron spins (triplet manifold). Each electron state (fat horizontal lines) is shown with vibrational excitations (thin horizontal lines). Wavy arrows: radiationless transitions (here energy is dissipated as heat); bold arrows: transitions involving photons. ISC: intersystem crossing.

In the following, some important characteristics of fluorescent molecules are summarized:

- **Absorption coefficient** ε measures the probability of photon absorption by a molecule. It is defined via the Lambert–Beer law $I(x) = I_0 \exp(-\varepsilon c x)$, which describes the attenuation of light passing a solution of fluorophore. Here, c denotes the molecular concentration, x the path length, and I_0 the impinging light intensity. Note that ε strongly depends on wavelength and forms the absorption spectrum of the dye. In good fluorophores, peak values of ε are of the order of 10^5 L/(mol cm).

- **Fluorescence quantum yields** Φ_F are defined as the probability of photon emission per photon absorbed. In synthetic fluorophores, Φ_F may closely approach 1, whereas even in optimized, genetically engineered fluorescent proteins, values from 0.2 to 0.7 are found.[42]

- **Fluorescence lifetime** τ is the time constant of the fluorescence intensity decay measured following a sudden excitation. All processes depopulating the first electronically excited state contribute to τ. In complex environments and especially in fluorescent proteins, measured fluorescent decays are often multi-exponential. Most fluorophores display fluorescence lifetimes in the range from ≈ 0.1 ns to ≈ 10 ns.
- **Phosphorescence quantum yields** Φ_P are the probability of photon emission from the triplet state per photon absorbed. Even in the best phosphorescent dyes, Φ_P rarely exceeds 10%.
- **Phosphorescence lifetimes** are extremely high (some 10 µs and above) because transitions involving spin flips are quantum mechanically forbidden.

Please note that all processes mentioned so far are of quantum mechanical nature, that is, they are sudden transitions occurring stochastically with certain rates. Because molecules strongly couple with their environment, all these rates depend on the local environment of the excited molecule. This environmental sensitivity is mostly due to the relative longevity of the excited state. Moreover, as many physicochemical properties of a molecule, such as polarity, dipolar moment, or even geometry, are entirely dependent on the configuration of the electrons, a given molecule may exhibit vastly different physicochemical properties depending on its state of electronic excitation. In summary, fluorescence is often strongly dependent on the environment of the fluorescent molecule. If one uses fluorescence to measure local concentrations of molecules, this environmental sensitivity is a severe complication. However, it can be also exploited to measure a great number of different parameters such as temperature, pH, solvent polarity, or ion concentrations on a very local scale. The interested reader should refer to the current and rapidly expanding literature on these aspects. Good starting points for reading are the monographs of Lakowicz[43] and Jung.[8]

Finally, we have to mention photobleaching. In fluids at room temperature, all fluorophores are slowly destroyed by light. This phenomenon is a severe limitation in all techniques where very high excitation intensities are needed (e.g., fluorescence microscopy and, even more so, confocal microscopy). Unfortunately, the process is extremely dependent on the molecular environment; therefore, measurements, especially on living cells, are often of very poor reproducibility. As a result, the photochemical degradation pathways involved are not well characterized. However, it is clear that bleaching can be slowed down by the removal of molecular oxygen through the addition of chemical compounds that scavenge radicals. Unfortunately, the reaction products generated upon bleaching are often harmful to cells.

In most research applications, it is almost impossible to predict which fluorophore will perform best. Most often several candidates have to be tested and experimental conditions have to be optimized to achieve reliable results.

11.2.1   Fluorescent Membrane Probes

Although some biological molecules are weakly fluorescent, natural lipids do not exhibit any noteworthy fluorescence. Fortunately, there are several techniques established in experimental biology to render a nonfluorescent biomolecule fluorescent. For example, fluorescently tagged antibodies can visualize distinct proteins based on the highly specific antibody–antigen interaction.[6] Yet, in lipid research, this antibody-based strategy is of limited power due to the marginal number of selective anti-lipid antibodies with the notable exceptions of anti-phosphoserin[44] or anti-cardiolipin.[45] Another well-established strategy for protein visualization is the fluorescent protein technology.[7,8] Unfortunately, the molecular weights of fluorescent proteins amount to about 27 kDa.[46] In contrast to this, the average molecular weight of lipids is only 600–1000 g/mol (0.6–1 kDa). Obviously, the properties of a lipid tagged with a fluorescent protein would be entirely dominated by the large protein moiety. Moreover, while it is straightforward in genetic engineering to fuse a fluorescent protein to the protein of interest, comparable technologies for covalent lipid–protein bonds are still missing.

Therefore, another strategy is needed to visualize cellular membranes. Natural lipids can be easily conjugated with a synthetic fluorophore to also become fluorescent. These modified molecules can be visualized by light microscopy techniques. In the last decades, a wide range of fluorophores have been developed for fluorescent labeling of lipids as well as for membrane interaction monitoring.[47] Some fluorophores commonly used for lipid labeling are summarized in Fig. 11.3.

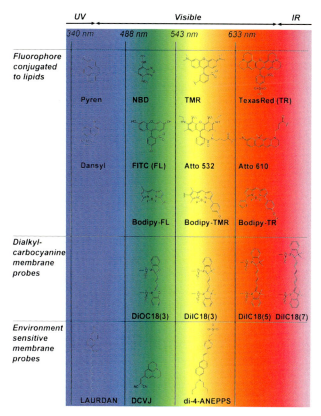

Figure 11.3 Some frequently used fluorophores conjugated to membrane lipids and fluorescent membrane sensors. For abbreviations, please see the list of abbreviations in Appendix.

Many other fluorescent membrane sensors are not natural lipid molecules subsequently conjugated with a fluorophore, but amphiphilic molecules containing a large delocalized electron system. Due to their amphiphilic molecular character, they can be easily inserted into the lipid bilayer. Similar to their natural analogs, such molecules also comprise a lipophilic aliphatic chain region that anchors the probe to the membrane and a polar molecular moiety that localizes the probe at the membrane surface. The chromophores are usually positioned in this polar headgroup range. Some prominent fluorescent membrane sensors are shown in Fig. 11.3.

Because such sensor molecules are not based on natural membrane components, they cannot be used to study cellular lipid trafficking, but they yield very useful information about overall membrane characteristics, such as membrane organization, microdomain formation, or membrane polarization. Without aspiring to cover all of the fluorophores used for lipid conjugation, we give a short overview over the most frequently used fluorophores and additionally discuss the basic principles of lipid conjugation.

11.2.1.1 Synthetic fluorescent lipids

The first generation of lipid-tagged fluorophores such as fluorescein (FITC), nitrobenz-2-oxa-1,3-diazol-4-yl (NBD), and, to some extent, rhodamine, had many drawbacks. Low fluorescence intensity, high rate of photobleaching, low quantum yield, pH-sensitive fluorescence, and relatively broad emission spectra made the visualization of tagged lipids difficult.[48] In the beginning of the 1990s, new fluorophores with improved fluorescence properties were developed. For example, the fluorophore 4,4-difluoro-4-bora-3a,4a-diaza-s-indacene, better known as Bodipy, became the most widely used fluorophore for membrane lipid studies within a relatively short time period[49-52] due to its superior photostability and unique spectral properties.[48] Later on, a complete fluorophore family was established based on Bodipy[53] using the fact that an increase in the extent of the π-electron system (i.e., degree of conjugation) led to a shift in the adsorption and fluorescence spectra to longer wavelengths.[37-40] The fluorescence spectrum of Bodipy-FL corresponds to that of FITC (FL). By adding molecular groups to the parent Bodipy structure, the new fluorophores Bodipy-TMR, a possible replacement for tetramethyl-rhodamine (TMR), and Bodipy-TR, a replacement for Texas Red (TR), were developed (see Fig. 11.3). The main advantage of these Bodipy-based fluorophores is that they are relatively nonpolar and electrically neutral around pH 7, therefore appropriate for lipid chain conjugation.

In a similar line of investigation, new members of the rhodamine family with improved fluorescence characteristics were developed.[25] Some of these molecules are now part of the commercially available line of Atto dyes. Based on their highly hydrophilic character, they are suitable for lipid headgroup conjugation.[54,55] However, a detailed photophysical description of them is still missing.

As already mentioned, lipid molecules of interest can be tagged routinely with a fluorescent moiety to visualize them. However, a lipid cannot be tagged with a fluorophore without changing its molecular characteristics. Due to the necessity for molecular probes, the visualization of cellular lipid membranes is an invasive analytical method, and like other invasive methods, it is to be applied with care. Still keeping in mind some basic chemical principles, one can avoid the main pitfalls of fluorescence lipid conjugation.

Criteria for fluorescent lipid conjugation:

- The chemical characteristics of lipid probes have to be preserved as far as possible.
- Biologically active reactive groups of the lipid molecules must not be blocked by chemical conjugation.
- Fluorophore hydrophobicity has to fit to that of the lipid moieties to conjugate.
- The physical lipid properties have to remain mainly unchanged.
- Fluorophores should not excessively increase the overall size.
- Fluorophores should not significantly influence the rotational and translational molecular motions of lipids in the bilayer.

Not all listed criteria will be discussed here; instead we will elucidate the most important rules in more detail.

In lipid structures (see Fig. 11.4), a fluorophore can be covalently conjugated to two molecular moieties. The first is the amino group in the polar lipid head, and the other is the apolar long fatty acid chain range.[56] In reality, the fluorophore replaces one of the natural fatty acids by attaching with a long-chain fatty acid (C_5 or C_{12}) through esterification. The first molecules are called head-labeled lipids, and the second molecules are called chain-labeled (Fig. 11.4a). Which one will be used in a specific study depends on the research focus. For analyzing membrane processes in which the molecular interactions in the lipid head group range play a key role, chain-labeled lipids should be chosen. Such processes are e.g. protein-lipid interactions, lipid sorting, trafficking and metabolism.[56] On the other hand, in the analysis of the lipid phase transitions, headgroup-labeled lipids are better choices because such thermotropic or lyotropic phases are strongly influenced by the packing order in the chain region and any small influences of the fluorophores in this range will change the results.

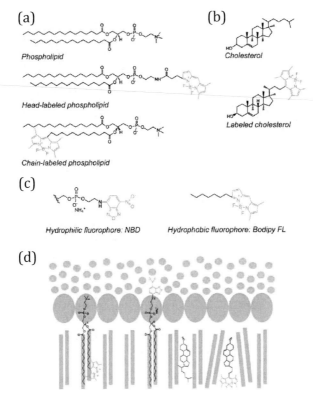

Figure 11.4 Structural lipid changes induced by (a) fluorescent-labeling site (here Bodipy-labeling site on DHPE-head and $PC_{12}PC$-chain) or (b) fluorophore size relative to lipid size (here Bodipy size to that of cholesterol) and (c) fluorophore hydrophobicity (here the polar NBD conjugated to the polar lipid head, while the apolar Bodipy to the apolar alkyl chain). (d) Schematic representation of the insertion of some fluorescently labeled lipid molecules in a lipid monolayer.

Besides the site of attachment, the fluorophore's hydrophobicity has also to be considered. In general, the overall rule is also valid here: the labeling molecule should be as hydrophobic or hydrophilic as the basic molecule. Therefore, the best choices are to take lipid molecules tagged with a polar fluorophore in the polar head region or an apolar fluorophore in the apolar chain region (see Fig. 11.4c,d). For example, the relatively apolar Bodipy is a good choice for chain labeling of any kind of lipids such as phospholipids,[57] sphingomyeline,[50-52] gangliosides,[58,59] or phosphoinositol,[60,61] while the more polar fluorophores such as NBD, TMR, or the Atto dyes are better suited to label the lipid headgroup mimicking the membrane behavior of their natural counterparts, respectively.

Last but not least, the influence of the fluorophore size in relation to the parent molecule has also to be discussed here. Natural lipid molecules are packed in cellular membranes in a highly ordered environment. The incorporation of additional components could perturb the sensitive membrane order, especially in the hydrophobic membrane core, and would need high-energy input. Therefore, keeping the fluorophore size as small as possible is the best strategy for all labeling processes. Some lipid molecules, such as phospholipids or glycolipids, are reasonably large compared to fluorescent dyes such as Bodipy, Dansyl, or NBD, while other lipids, such as sterols, are smaller molecules. Their sizes are comparable with that of the mentioned fluorophores. Upon conjugation, molecular weights of sterols double and their enlarged sizes strongly influence their spacing in the bilayer (see Fig. 11.4c,d).[62-65]

Nevertheless, even if all guidelines are followed and the best fitting fluorophores are used, it should be borne in mind that the resulting tagged molecules are at best fluorescent molecular reporters with properties close, but never identical, to those of the lipid under study.

11.2.1.2 Synthetic fluorescent lipid analogs

Synthetic lipophilic molecules are frequently used for intracellular membrane labeling. The highly lipophilic dialkylcarbocyanine dyes (Di*X*) are preeminent examples of them (see Fig. 11.3).[66-70] Using the same strategy as described for the Bodipy fluorophore family, the spectral properties of the *Di*-family members have also been adjusted by varying the heteroatoms or the substituent groups in the terminal ring system or by enlarging the delocalization in the chromophore, in this case elongating the connecting bridge containing alternating double bonds between the terminal rings. The lengths of the alkyl chains do not influence the spectral properties. All these derivates have high extinction coefficients and a good fluorescent quantum yield in the membrane environment, similar to those of dyes in octanol, whereas their fluorescence in a polar solvent such as water is quite weak.[71] These properties make the Di-family especially appropriate for long-term membrane staining spanning the visible spectral range from green ($DiOC_{18}(3)$) over red ($DiIC_{18}(3)$) to deep red ($DiIC_{18}(5)$), completing the series with a near-infrared active member ($DiIC_{18}(7)$). Even though the alkyl chain length does not markedly influence the basic fluorescent properties such as quantum yield or fluorescence lifetime, it plays a key role in staining procedures (see also Section 11.4) and in molecular localization, correspondingly. Carbocyanines with short alkyl tails (C_6) immediately insert from a DMSO- or ethanol-containing medium through the cellular plasma membrane into the mitochondria and endoplasmic reticulum (ER) membranes,[72–74] while those with longer alkyl tails (more than C_{12}) are more lipophilic and need a carrier system for efficient membrane staining.[57]

11.2.2 Environment-Sensitive Fluorescent Sensor Molecules

Fluorescent sensor molecules with photophysical properties depending on local environment can be embedded in model and cell membranes. By measuring fluorescence intensity, lifetime, wavelengths of emission, or fluorescence polarization of such molecules, information about environmental properties such as microviscosity, polarity, level of lipid order and structural changes, or hydration and surface potential can be retrieved. Readers more interested in this field may find references[43,75,76] helpful.

Similar to the application of fluorescently conjugated lipids, one should keep in mind some important rules using environment-sensitive fluorophores as well:

- The precise orientation, location, and depth of the sensor in the bilayer should be known. Please note that structural changes in the membrane may cause reorientation of the sensor molecule.[75]

- Probes with broad local membrane distribution should be avoided.

- Measuring two or more membrane parameters by simultaneously applying several sensors does not necessarily result in reliable data.

- In the case of fluorescent probes that are sensitive to several environmental parameters, special care is required and environmental parameters and their changes should be controlled precisely.

The first molecules designed for environmental sensitivity, in this case to polarity, were Laurdan and Prodan,[77] two naphthalene derivatives. The molecular structure of LAURDAN, for example, is shown in Fig. 11.3. These molecules possess a dipole moment due to a partial charge separation between the 2-dimethylamino and the 6-carbonyl residues. The energy required for solvent reorientation decreases the excited state energy of the sensor molecules resulting in a continuous red shift of their emission spectra in a polar solvent and a blue shift in an apolar solvent.[78] Due to this spectral shift, environment polarity became detectable in model membranes[78-80] or even in cellular systems.[81,82]

Other molecules, called molecular rotors or solvatochromic dyes, exhibit strong variations in their fluorescence quantum yield depending on intramolecular rotations, which are in turn strongly influenced by solvent viscosity.[76] Typical examples are di-4-ANEPPS or DCVJ[75] (see Fig. 11.3). If such solvatochromes are embedded in a lipid membrane, they yield information about the local membrane viscosity, which is largely determined by the lipid phase state. For example, crystalline, gel, or liquid-ordered phases are characterized by high lipid order and high viscosity, while fluid crystalline or liquid-disordered phases are more fluid with low viscosity. Such sensors can be used to visualize different lipid domains in the bilayer.

Depending on the phase state of the lipid bilayer, its hydration state changes as well. If reporter molecules are sensitive to the distribution of water molecules across the bilayer or to their relaxations, such as, di-4-ANEPPQ[83] or 3HC F2N8[84], membrane surface mapping by fluorescent ratiometric imaging can be carried out.

11.3   Fluorophore Incorporation into Living Cells

The main advantage of using fluorescence microscopy and spectroscopy in membrane studies is the potential to collect spatially resolved information about complex membrane systems such as biological cell membranes. In some cases, the incorporation of fluorescent sensor molecules into cellular membranes is a challenging issue, while fluorescent labeling of model membranes is easily achieved by standard preparation techniques. Therefore, we will focus on the labeling of cell membranes.

There are three different strategies how fluorescent membrane sensors can be incorporated into living cells using liposomes as carriers:

- They are capable of spontaneously diffusing from the liposomal membrane into the plasma membrane.
- Liposomes containing fluorescently labeled lipids or serum proteins complexed with fluorophores will be taken up by endocytosis.
- They can be incorporated into fusogenic liposomes whose membranes merge with the plasma membrane inserting the sensor molecules directly into the cellular plasma membrane.

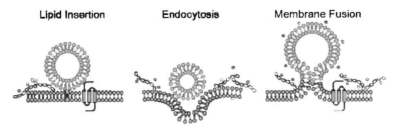

Figure 11.5   Fluorescent dye incorporation into live cells by spontaneous lipid insertion into the cellular plasma membrane (left), liposomal endocytosis (middle), and membrane fusion between liposomal and cellular plasma membrane (right).

All three pathways are schematically illustrated in Fig. 11.5. Prior to liposomal sensor delivery, only small and slightly lipophilic molecules, such as $DiOC_{2-6}(3)$, could be delivered into living cells using a small amount of ethanol or DMSO. The disadvantage of both organic solvents is their toxicity for live cells.

Independent of the route of uptake, it is possible that the fluorophore is later detached from its lipid part by biochemical degradation pathways within the cell. Unfortunately, these processes seem to be insufficiently understood. Because of the high relevance of fluorescence imaging and sensing of cell membranes, this is an important question for future research.

11.3.1 Uptake Pathway I: Lipid Insertion and Transbilayer Lipid Translocation

When liposomes containing fluorescently labeled phosphoserin (NBD-PS) were incubated with cell cultures, spontaneous transfer of the NBD-PS from the liposomes to the cells occurred, resulting in prominent labeling of the plasma membrane.[85] Such inward movement of phosphoserin is usually achieved by an integral membrane protein, aminophospholipid translocase, acting as lipid transporter.[54,86] Unfortunately, only aminophospholipids are substrates for this transporter with a preference of phosphatidylserine, while other cholin-containing phospholipids are not transported.

Besides translocase, which is only responsible for unidirectional lipid transport, lipid scramblase facilitates the bidirectional movement of all phospholipid classes across cellular membranes.[85,87–89] This protein family is not only responsible for the outside/inside transport of lipids but also for the molecular traffic between internal organelle membranes.[90] While many of the commercially available fluorescent lipids can be spontaneously taken up from the exterior environment, experimental protocols have to be optimized for each lipid because the achieved fluorescent intensities usually remain relatively low requiring highly sensitive detection.

11.3.2 Uptake Pathway II: Endocytosis of Liposomes and BSA–Lipid Complexes

Besides phosphoserin and phosphoethanolamine, other fluorescently labeled lipid molecules, such as phosphocholine or sphingomyeline, have to be inserted into living cells for analytical purposes. These molecules do not translocate spontaneously from the culture medium into the cellular plasma membrane. They can be incorporated easily into artificial liposomes made of, for example, phosphocholines. Subsequently, these labeled liposomes are incubated with living cells over several hours to days.[9,85,91] During this time, they are taken up by endocytosis. The hallmark of this process is active inward budding of plasma membrane vesicles containing the molecules taken up from the environment. Therefore, the easiest way to test whether a fluorescent lipid is taken up by endocytosis or not is blocking the endocytotic pathway with the metabolic inhibitors 2-deoxyglucose and sodium azide[92] and comparing of the fluorescent signals with and without inhibitors.

Liposomal uptake can be boosted using a special incubation procedure involving different temperatures.[9,91] Here, cells are incubated first with the liposomes at low temperatures (around 4°C). The incubation at low temperature slows down cell functions and activates protective cell mechanisms. Subsequently, the temperature is increased again to 37°C. With increasing temperature, cell functions, including the endocytotic uptake of labeled liposomes, are accelerated again. Still fluorescent intensity can remain below the detection limit, especially when the inserted molecules are sorted into cell organelles according to their chemical properties and biological functions. This molecular distribution can gravely reduce fluorescence intensity, rendering fluorescent detection unreliable.

Increases in additional fluorescence intensity can be achieved when the conjugated lipids are complexed with serum proteins such as bovine serum albumin (BSA) instead of being incorporated into liposomes.[49-51,85] This method exploits serum protein uptake by the more specific and effective receptor-mediated endocytosis. This is an active transport process in which the molecules to be incorporated, here the serum protein, will be recognized by another membrane protein, which initiates the molecular transport across the plasma membrane. Due to the complexation of the fluorescent lipids with these proteins, they will also be effectively internalized. The invention of this method by Pagano and coworkers made it possible for the first time to examine the translocation of fluorescent lipids in living cells by high-resolution fluorescent microscopy and to correlate these data with the results of classical biochemical investigations[49,93-95] as will be discussed in Section 11.4: *Application fields.*

11.3.3 Uptake Pathway III: Membrane Fusion

Fusion between cellular plasma membrane and the membrane of a carrier particle containing dye molecules is an even more effective pathway for fluorescent sensor delivery into living cells than endocytosis. Membrane fusion is a well-described and frequently observed process in cell biology.[96-98] Material transport processes such as endocytosis or exocytosis, autophagy, mitochondrial fusion[99] as well as viral entry into host cells[55] are only some examples of many relevant biological events where membrane fusion occurs. They all share the basic molecular fusion mechanism induced by the so-called fusion protein or fusion peptides. Indeed, liposomes surface conjugated with fusion peptides (e.g., TAT)[100,101] or proteins[102] (e.g., SNAREs) also became fusogenic. Even the biomolecular association mechanism of DNA base pairing can be used to render lipid membranes fusogenic.[103]

All these methods rely on chemically conjugated biomolecules on the liposomal surface to enhance the delivery efficiency of the fluorophore. In contrast, the fusogenic liposomes developed by Csiszár et al.[104] for dye incorporation into live cells function via a purely physicochemical mechanism. The authors demonstrated that positively charged liposomes containing a distinct amount of fluorescent dye spontaneously fuse with the cellular plasma membrane inserting the dye molecules directly into the target membrane regardless of whether these membranes belong to artificial giant vesicles, single cells in culture or tissues. Even several fluorescent lipids and lipid analogs with different emission spectra can simultaneously be delivered to live cells,[57] as shown in Fig. 11.6.

In this approach, membrane fusion processes occur within minutes (1–10 min) with extraordinary high delivery efficiencies. Cell damage is minimal; therefore, long-time observation of fluorescent molecules can yield biologically relevant information about cellular lipid trafficking with the caveat that the decoupling of lipid and fluorophore molecule is also possible here, as in many other cases.

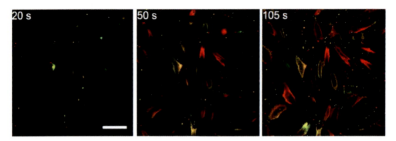

Figure 11.6   Chinese hamster ovary (CHO) cells simultaneously incubated with three different types of fusogenic liposomes containing the fluorescent carbocyanines DiO, DiI, and DiD, respectively. Liposomes diffused first to the plasma membrane surface (20 s). After membrane adhesion, the first membrane fusion events occurred in the next minutes (50 s). Efficient multicolor staining of plasma membrane was recorded over 10 min. Scale bars, 50 μm.

Successful membrane fusion can be easily tested using fluorophores. Between them, radiationless energy transfer, so-called Förster or fluorescence resonance energy transfer (FRET), can occur. The fluorophores NBD and rhodamine form a common FRET pair,[105,106] while other fluorophore combinations are also possible.[56,107] When complete membrane mixing brings these two molecules close enough together, the emission of the donor (here NBD) will vanish due to radiationless transfer to the receiving fluorophore, the acceptor (here rhodamine). Using fluorescence spectroscopy or microscopy, a reduced donor emission and a simultaneously increased acceptor emission can be detected. Fusogenic liposomes have been successfully tested for fusion efficiency by Dutta et al. using the method describe earlier.[108]

11.4   Application Fields

After incorporation, fluorescent molecules can be easily observed by fluorescent microscopy. Their localizations, intensity changes, or binding behavior yield useful information about the biological systems under investigation. In this section, we collected some applications of fluorescent or fluorescently labeled biomolecules successfully used in the life science, making no claim to be complete.

11.4.1 Cell and Organelle Staining

One of the main functions of cellular membranes is to separate the interior of the cell from the external environment to ensure physiological conditions in the interior. Cellular organelles such as plasma membrane, ER, Golgi apparatus (GA), and mitochondria are also separated from each other and the cell cytoplasm by biological membranes. Despite the fact that the basic membrane structure is similar in all biological membranes, significant differences exist and certain fluorescent lipid derivatives display a preference for particular membrane compartments of living cells. This fact has first been used in cell biology to identify cellular organelles, as shown in Fig. 11.7. Moreover, a major problem in cell biology of lipids is to understand how newly synthesized lipids are sorted into various intracellular compartments, and how these molecules are translocated to various destinations inside and outside the cell.[89,109] To elucidate these questions, fluorescently labeled lipids have been successfully used over the last decades. Here, we summarize some prominent fluorophore examples for subcellular organelle staining.

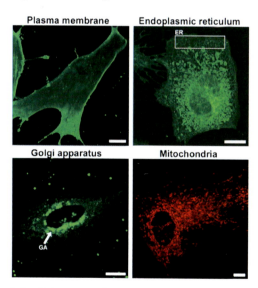

Figure 11.7 Subcellular organelle stainings of CHO cells: plasma membrane staining by $DiOC_{18}(3)$, endoplasmic reticulum staining by $DiOC_6(3)$, Golgi apparatus staining by Bodipy-ceramide, and mitochondria staining by MitoTracker. Scale bars, 10 μm.

11.4.1.1 Plasma membrane

The first cellular membrane barrier is the plasma membrane. Its in vivo staining is an experimental challenge due to the permanent lipid exchange between the plasma membrane and other organelle membranes. First NBD-PC[110] and NBD-PE[85,110] were reported as staining molecules for the plasma membrane, although NBD exhibits an unfortunate sensitivity to photobleaching. Later on, the more photostable Bodipy-sphingomyeline (Bodipy-SM) was also proposed for these purposes as Pagano and his coworkers realized that this molecule has been sorted back from the GA into the plasma membrane of Chinese hamster fibroblasts.[50–52,89]

Using membrane fusion as staining method, almost all fluorescent or fluorescently labeled lipophilic molecules can be incorporated into the plasma membrane.[104] Their persistence in the plasma membrane depends on their molecular structures. For example, the aforementioned Bodipy-SM directly inserted into the plasma membrane by fusion remains within it for 24 h similar to Bodipy-cholesterol or some long-chain carbocyanines (e.g., $DiOC_{18}(3)$ or DiR). Other molecules whose chemical characters and biological functions promote their translocation from the plasma membrane to other organelles, like in the case of Bodipy-ceramide or Bodipy-GM1, remain there no longer than a few minutes.[57] Such molecules are more appropriate for staining of other organelles.

11.4.1.2 Endoplasmic reticulum

The ER, a network of membrane tubes, sheets, and cisterna, is a prominent organelle in eukaryotic cells.[111,112] Its main function is to synthesize proteins and membrane lipids, such as structural phospholipids and cholesterol, and transport them to their functional place. Because the ER is a network containing membrane tubes, its staining using lipophilic dyes suffers from two main drawbacks: First, it cannot be reliably stained after permeabilization and fixation because such procedures require detergent or organic solvent treatments, which generally destroy the delicate ER network. Second, due to its connections to the outer nuclear membrane and the permanent rapid lipid exchange between most organelles, an exclusive ER staining is almost impossible,[113] as can be seen in Fig. 11.7 as well.

Keeping this information in mind, we can still find some fluorescent membrane dyes for ER visualization. For example, many short-chain dialkylcarbocyanines such as $DiO_2(3)$, $DiO_3(3)$, $DiO_4(3)$, and $DiO_6(3)$ were screened for this purpose by Terasaki et al.[114–116] (see Fig. 11.7), who identified $DiO_6(3)$ as the best choice. This positively charged lipophilic dye spontaneously permeates the plasma membrane. After membrane penetration, it accumulates in all cellular membranes, among others in the ER membranes. In the respective fluorescence micrographs, the ER network can be easily identified as a thin peripheral region.

11.4.1.3 Golgi apparatus

The GA is a cellular organelle involved in macromolecular modifying, sorting, packaging, and trafficking within cells.[111] Significant levels of lipid synthesis, especially sphingolipid synthesis, occur in the GA.[117] In contrast to the ER, the GA has a unique lipid composition characterized by high concentrations of cholesterol and sphingolipids such as sphingomyeline or ceramide. The latter molecules are actively enriched in the GA as part of the natural lipid flow within cells. Therefore, the GA can be stained by fluorescently labeled ceramide, such as NBD-ceramide[89] or Bodipy-ceramide[95,118,119] (see Fig. 11.7). Neither the more polar NBD, nor the more apolar Bodipy interferes with the accumulation of ceramides in the GA. These labeled molecules do not even need a special delivery system as already simple incubation of labeled ceramides with mammalian cells results in a vital staining of the GA. Please note that the fluorescence spectrum of Bodipy is concentration dependent: at low concentrations, the probe emits green light, while at high concentrations, for example upon accumulation in the GA, this green emission is partially quenched and a red-shifted signal is observed.[51,119] Using Bodipy-ceramide staining, an exclusive Golgi signal can be detected in the red channel, while a simultaneous ER and Golgi staining appears in the green channel; the latter is shown in Fig. 11.7.

11.4.1.4 Mitochondria

Mitochondria are found in almost all eukaryotic cells, but their shape and number vary according to cell type. Most of the cellular chemical energy is generated in these organelles. In addition, they are also involved in other tasks such as cell signaling, differentiation, control of the cell cycle, as well as cell growth and apoptosis.[111]

Due to the exceptionally high negative potential of the outer mitochondrial membrane, the lipophilic and cationic dialkylcarbocyanine dyes with short chains (C_1–C_4) accumulate almost exclusively in the mitochondrial membrane. When used at higher concentrations (>1 μM), carbocyanine dyes with longer chains (e.g., C_5–C_7) stain mitochondria of live cells as well as the ER.[113] These dye molecules work fast and can be applied directly to live cells without any carrier particles. Because mitochondria-specific interaction of such molecules is dependent on the highly negative transmembrane potential maintained by functional mitochondria, dissipation of the mitochondrial transmembrane potential by ionophores or inhibitors of electron transport eliminates the selective mitochondrial association of these compounds. The application of such potential-dependent probes in conjunction with fluorescence microscopy enables the monitoring of mitochondrial membrane potential in individual living cells.[120,121]

11.4.2 Microdomain Monitoring

The famous fluid mosaic model of Singer and Nicholson[29] describes the plasma membrane as a two-dimensional mosaic structure in which integral proteins "swim" in fluid lipid bilayer regions. While the vast majority of lipid molecules are arranged in a bilayer structure with their polar headgroups in contact with the aqueous phase, some are more intimately associated with integral proteins. Based on this assumption, Simons and Ikonen developed their hypothesis about functional lipid arrangements, called lipid rafts, in the membranes of living cells. These arrangements were described to contain sphingolipids and cholesterol in high concentrations.[122] Moreover, in their interior, the lipid-packing density is higher than in the surrounding regions that are mostly composed of phosphatidylcholine. Therefore, these assemblies are more rigid than their surroundings. In a highly intuitive picture, these objects were described as rafts on the sea that transport membrane associated or transmembrane proteins within the membrane.

The proof of existence of functional lipid microdomains turned out to be a challenging issue due to their short lifetimes (10–20 ms) and nanoscopic size.[123] As Dietrich and coworkers could, for the first time, microscopically visualize microdomain-like structures in model membranes composed of glycosphingolipid and cholesterol,[79] the scientific community focused on this simple model system to learn more about the infinitely complex original system. Lipid raft-like microdomains form in supported lipid monolayers and bilayers as well as in giant unilamellar vesicles (GUVs). Such microdomains can be reconstituted using an equimolar mixture of a phospholipid with low phase transition temperature, cholesterol, and a sphingolipid with high phase transition temperature. Because the partitioning coefficient of fluorescently labeled lipids such as FITC-DPPE, NBD-DPPE, or Bodipy-FL-DHPE depends on phase state, two distinct lipid phases can be identified in fluorescence micrographs: the liquid-ordered (L_o) and the liquid-disordered (L_d) phases.[124] Figure 11.8 shows this phase separation phenomenon in the ternary lipid mixture of DOPC/SM/cholesterol (1/1/1 mol/mol).

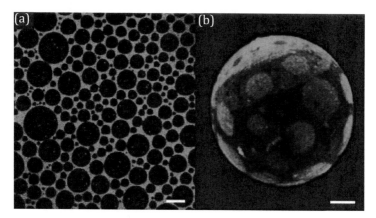

Figure 11.8 Phase separation in the ternary lipid mixture of DOPC/SM/cholesterol (1/1/1 mol/mol). (a) Two-dimensional supported lipid monolayer and (b) a three-dimensional giant unilamellar vesicle visualized by Bodipy-FL-DHPE. The fluorophore Bodipy-FL-DHPE is enriched in both cases in the L_d phase. Scale bars, 10 μm.

Most fluorescently labeled lipids show strong preference for the L_d phase, such as Bodipy-PC or -SM, while just a few fluorescent sensors such as naphtopyrene or terrylene enrich in the L_d phase. Using supported lipid bilayers,[125] GUVs,[126-132] or even giant plasma membrane vesicles[133,134] as model biomembranes, domain formation, temperature and composition dependence, as well as phase separation dynamics have been intensively studied to better understand the biological plasma membrane. With the help of the environment-sensitive fluorescent sensor molecule LAURDAN, membrane regions with low order of lipid alkyl chain alignment, called liquid-disordered phase (L_d), and regions with high order, called liquid-ordered phase (L_o), could be distinguished.[79,80,123] The phase diagram of the ternary "raft mixture" was also mapped exploiting fluorescent spectroscopic markers.[135]

Even though these in vitro liquid-ordered domains have some similarities with microdomains existing in cell membranes in vivo, cellular microdomains are infinitely more complex concerning lipid composition.[50] Moreover, cell membranes contain an abundance of membrane proteins that also influence microdomain formation. For these reasons, microdomains must be also studied on cells. Early work along these lines was done by immunogold labeling and electron microscopy.[136,137] Later, the super-resolution light microscopy techniques PALM[138] and STED[139-141] revealed much more detail about nanometric microdomains in cellular membranes. Due to the very low fluorophore concentration needed by both techniques, delivery efficiency was of no concern. Using LAURDAN as fluorescent sensor, transient laterally ordered micrometer-sized membrane regions were also directly observed in living cells.[142,143] Micrometer-sized domains were also visualized by following the co-localized fluorescence signals of Bodipy-D-erythro-lactoceramide and cholera toxin B subunit, which acted as a microdomain marker.[144]

11.5   Summary

With this short review, we hope to have demonstrated the power of fluorescence-based techniques for studying living cells. In our personal opinion, the state of this specific research field shows a surprising discrepancy. On one hand, we have the highly developed art of fluorescence-based research with specific molecular reporters for almost any parameter of interest and highly sophisticated light microscopic and fluorescence spectroscopic techniques. On the other hand, however, there are surprisingly few efficient techniques to deliver labeled molecules to cells. We are optimistic that fusogenic liposomes will improve this weakness and that they will prove to be a powerful tool for future fluorescence investigations of living cells.

Acknowledgments

The authors acknowledge Tobias Braun, Nils Hersch, Bernd Hoffmann, Anton Hördt, Christian Kleusch, and Elena Naumovska for fruitful scientific discussions in the field of fluorescent membrane sensors and fusogenic liposomes. We also thank Tobias Braun, Christian Kleusch, Christina Tenten, and Marcel Dillenburger for providing micrographs and schemata published in the manuscript. We also acknowledge Tobias Braun, Nils Hersch, and Christian Schuch for critically reading the manuscript and for their valuable suggestions.

Appendix A   Abbreviations

Bodipy	4,4-difluoro-4-bora-3a,4a-diaza-*s*-indacene
Bodipy-FL	4,4-difluoro-5,7-dimethyl-4-bora-3a,4a-diaza-*s*-indacene-3-propionyl
Bodipy-TR	6-(((4-(4,4-difluoro-5-(2-thienyl)-4-bora-3a,4a-diaza-s-indacene-3-yl)phenoxy)acetyl)amino)hexanoic acid
Bodipy-TMR	6-((4,4-difluoro-1,3-dimethyl-5-(4-methoxyphenyl)-4-bora-3a,4a-diaza-*s*-indacene-2-propionyl)amino)hexanoic acid
BSA	bovine serum albumin
CHO	Chinese hamster ovary cell line
DCVJ	9-(2,2-dicyanovinyl)julolidine
di-4-ANEPPS	4-(2-(6-(dibutylamino)-2-naphthalenyl)ethenyl)-1-(3-sulfopropyl)-, hydroxide
$DiOC_2(3)$	3,3'-diethyloxacarbocyanine perchlorate

DiOC$_3$(3)	3,3'-dipropyloxacarbocyanine perchlorate
DiOC$_4$(3)	3,3'-dibuthyloxacarbocyanine perchlorate
DiOC$_6$(3)	3,3'-dihexyloxacarbocyanine perchlorate
DiO (DiOC$_{18}$(3))	3,3'-dioctadecyloxacarbocyanine perchlorate
DiI	1,1'-dioctadecyl-3,3,3',3'-tetramethylindocarbocyanine perchlorate
DiD	1,1'-dioctadecyl-3,3,3',3'-tetramethylindodicarbocyanine 4-chlorobenzenesulfonate salt
DiR	1,1'-dioctadecyl-3,3,3',3'-tetramethylindo-tricarbocyanine iodide
DMSO	dimethyl sulfoxide
DPH	1,2-diphenyl-1,3,5-hexatriene
ER	endoplasmic reticulum
GFP	green fluorescent protein
GUV	giant unilamellar vesicle
FCS	fluorescence correlation spectroscopy
FITC (FL)	fluorescein: 3',6'-dihydroxyspiro [2-benzofuran-3,9'-xanthene]-1-one
FL	fusogenic liposomes
FLIM	fluorescence lifetime microscopy
FRAP	fluorescence recovery after photobleaching
FRET	fluorescence resonance energy transfer
LAURDAN	6-dodecanoyl-2-dimethylaminonaphthalene
L_d	liquid-disordered phase
L_o	liquid-ordered phase
MAM	mitochondria-associated ER membrane
NBD	nitrobenz-2-oxa-1,3-diazol-4-yl

PALM	photoactivated localization microscopy
PC	phosphocholine
PE	phophoethanolamine
PM	plasma membrane
PRODAN	6-propionyl-2-dimethylaminonaphthalene
PS	phosphoserin
SIM	structured illumination microscopy
SM	sphingomyelin
STED	stimulated emission depletion
STORM	stochastic optical reconstruction microscopy
Texas Red	5-(chlorosulfonyl)-2-(1H,2H,3H,5H,6H,7H,11H,-12H,13H, 15H,16H,17H-pyrido[3,2,1-ij] quinolizino[1′,9′:6,7,8]-chromeno [2,3-f]quinolin-4-ium-9-yl) benzenesulfonate
TMR	tetramethylrhodamine

References

1. Lipowsky R, Sackmann E. *Structure and Dynamics of Membranes.* Amsterdam: Elsevier Science & Technology; 1995.

2. Zernike F. Phase contrast, a new method for the microscopic observation of transparent objects. *Physica.* 1942; 9: 686–698.

3. Nomarski G, Inventor. Disositif interférentiel à polarisation pour l'étude des Objects transparents ou opaques appartenant à la classe des objects de phase. US patent 1.059.124 1953.

4. Allen RD, Allen NS, Travis JL. Video-enhanced contrast, differential interference contrast (AVEC-DIC) microscopy: A new method capable of analyzing microtubule-related motility in the reticulopodial network of allogromia laticollaris. *Cell Motility.* 1981; 1: 291–302.

5. Abercrombie M, Dunn GA. Adhesions of fibroblasts to substratum during contact inhibition observed by interference reflection microscopy. *Exp Cell Res.* 1975; 92(1): 57–62.

6. Coons RH, Kaplan MH. Localization of antigen in tissue cells. *J Exp Med.* 1950; 91: 1–13.

7. Chalfie M, Tu Y, Euskirchen G, Ward WW, Prasher DC. Green fluorescent protein as a marker for gene expression. *Science.* 1994; 263(5148): 802–805.

8. Jung G. *Fluorescent Proteins.* Heidelberg: Springer-Verlag Berlin Heidelberg; 2012.

9. Struck DK, Pagano RE. Insertion of fluorescent phospholipids into the plasma membrane of a mammalian cell. *J Biol Chem.* 1980; 255(11): 5404–5410.

10. Klar TA, Engel E, Hell SW. Breaking Abbe's diffraction resolution limit in fluorescence microscopy with stimulated emission depletion beams of various shapes. *Phys Rev E Stat Nonlin Soft Matter Phys.* 2001; 64(6 Pt 2): 066613.

11. Hell SW, Wichmann J. Breaking the diffraction resolution limit by stimulated emission: Stimulated-emission-depletion fluorescence microscopy. *Opt Lett.* 1994; 19(11): 780–782.

12. Betzig E, Patterson GH, Sougrat R, et al. Imaging intracellular fluorescent proteins at nanometer resolution. *Science.* 2006; 313(5793): 1642–1645.

13. Rust MJ, Bates M, Zhuang X. Sub-diffraction-limit imaging by stochastic optical reconstruction microscopy (STORM). *Nat Methods.* 2006; 3(10): 793–795.

14. Heintzmann R, Cramer C. Laterally modulated excitation microscopy: Improvement of resolution by using a diffraction grating. *SPIE.* 1999; 3568: 185–196.

15. Gustafsson MG. Surpassing the lateral resolution limit by a factor of two using structured illumination microscopy. *J Microscopy.* 2000; 198: 82–87.

16. Ishikawa-Ankerhold HC, Ankerhold R, Drummen GPC. Advanced fluorescence microscopy techniques—FRAP, FLIP, FLAP, FRET and FLIM. *Molecules.* 2012; 17: 4047–4132.

17. Reits EAJ, Neefjes JJ. From fixed to FRAP: Measuring protein mobility and activity in living cells. *Nat Cell Biol.* 2001: E145–147.

18. Sprague BL, McNally JG. FRAP analysis of binding: Proper and fitting. *Trends Cell Biol.* 2005; 15: 84–91.

19. Magde D, Elson EL, Webb WW. Thermodynamic fluctuations in a reacting system: Measurement by fluorescence correlation spectroscopy. *Phys Rev Letters.* 1972; 29: 705–708.

20. Schwille P. Fluorescence correlation spectroscopy and its potential for intracellular applications. *Cell Biochem Biophys.* 2001; 34: 383–408.

21. Becker W. Fluorescence lifetime imaging: Techniques and applications. *J Microscopy.* 2012; 247: 119–136.

22. Berezin MY, Achilefu S. Fluorescence lifetime measurements and biological imaging. *Chem Rev.* 2010; 110: 2641–2684.

23. Lavis LD, Raines RT. Bright ideas for chemical biology. *ACS Chem Biol.* 2008; 3(3): 142–155.

24. Ulrich G, Ziessel R, Harriman A. The chemistry of fluorescent Bodipy dyes: Versatility unsurpassed. *Angew Chem Int Ed Engl.* 2008; 47(7): 1184–1201.

25. Beija M, Afonso CAM, Martinho JMG. Synthesis and applications of rhodamine derivatives as fluorescent probes. *Chem Soc Rev.* 2009; 38: 2410–2433.

26. Prescher JA, Bertozzi CR. Chemistry in living systems. *Nat Chem Biol.* 2005; 1(1): 13–21.

27. Jing C, Cornish VW. Chemical tags for labeling proteins inside living cells. *Acc Chem Res.* 2011; 44(9): 784–792.

28. Simons K, Gerl MJ. Revitalizing membrane rafts: New tools and insights. *Nat Rev Mol Cell Biol.* 2010; 11(10): 688–699.

29. Singer SJ, Nicolson GL. The fluid mosaic model of the structure of cell membranes. *Science.* 1972; 175(4023): 720–731.

30. Marsch D. Protein modulation of lipids, and vice-versa, in membranes. *BBA.* 2008; 1778(7–8): 1545–1575.

31. Kusumi A, Fujiwara TK, Morone N, et al. Membrane mechanisms for signal transduction: The coupling of the meso-scale raft domains to membrane-skeleton-induced compartments and dynamic protein complexes. *Semin Cell Dev Biol.* 2012; 23(2): 126–144.

32. Rheinstädter MC, Mouritsen OG. Small-scale structure in fluid cholesterol-lipid bilayers. *COCIS.* 2013; 18: 440–447.

33. Honerkamp-Smith AR, Veatch SL, Keller SL. An introduction to critical points for biophysicists: Observations of compositional heterogeneity in lipid membranes. *Biochim Biophys Acta.* 2009; 1788(1): 53–63.

34. Gregoriadis G. *Liposome Technology.* Vol 2. 3rd ed. New York: Informa Healthcare; 2007.

35. Khalil IA, Kogure K, Akita H, Harashima H. Uptake pathways and subsequent intracellular trafficking in nonviral gene delivery. *Pharmacol Rev.* 2006; 58: 32–45.

36. Cevc G. *Phospholipids Handbook.* 1st ed. New Yourk, Basel: Marcel Dekker, Inc.; 1993.

37. Birks JB. *Photophysics of Aromatic Molceules.* London: Wiley-Interscience; 1970.

38. Valeur B. *Molecular Fluorescence.* Weinheim: Wiley-VCH; 2002.

39. Turro JN, Scaiano JC, Ramamurthy V. *Modern Molecular Photochemistry of Organic Molecules.* Sausalito, CA: University Science Books; 2010.

40. Klan PJ, Wirz J. *Photochemistry of Organic Compounds.* Chichester, UK: John Wiley and Sons; 2009.

41. Robinson RW, Frosch RP. Electronic excitation transfer and relaxation. *J Chem Phys.* 1963; 38: 1187–1203.

42. Nifosi R, Tozzini V. One photon and two-photon excitation of fluorescent proteins. In: Jung G, ed., *Fluorescent Proteins I:* Springer 2012: 1–37.

43. Lakowicz JR. *Principles of Fluorescence Spectroscopy.* 3rd ed. New York: Springer Science+Business Media, LLC; 2006.

44. Swairjo MA, Concha NO, Kaetzel MA, Dedman JR, Seaton BA. Ca(2+)-bridging mechanism and phospholipid head group recognition in the membrane-binding protein annexin V. *Nat Struct Biol.* 1995; 2(11): 968–974.

45. Ioannou PV, Golding BT. Cardiolipins: Their chemistry and biochemistry. *Prog Lipid Res.* 1979; 17(3): 279–318.

46. Chudakov DM, Matz MV, Lukyanov S, Lukyanov KA. Fluorescent proteins and their applications in imaging living cells and tissues. *Physiol Rev.* 2010; 90(3): 1103–1163.

47. Ptaszek M. Rational design of fluorophores for in vivo applications. *Prog Mol Biol Transl Sci.* 2013; 113: 59–108.

48. Johnson I. Fluorescent probes for living cells. *Histochem J.* 1998; 30(3): 123–140.

49. Bai J, Pagano RE. Measurement of spontaneous transfer and transbilayer movement of Bodipy-labeled lipids in lipid vesicles. *Biochemistry.* 1997; 36(29): 8840–8848.

50. Marks DL, Bittman R, Pagano RE. Use of Bodipy-labeled sphingolipid and cholesterol analogs to examine membrane microdomains in cells. *Histochem Cell Biol.* 2008; 130(5): 819–832.

51. Pagano RE, Chen CS. Use of Bodipy-labeled sphingolipids to study membrane traffic along the endocytic pathway. *Ann N Y Acad Sci.* 1998; 845: 152–160.

52. Pagano RE, Watanabe R, Wheatley C, Dominguez M. Applications of Bodipy-sphingolipid analogs to study lipid traffic and metabolism in cells. *Methods Enzymol.* 2000; 312: 523–534.

53. Loudet A, Burgess K. Bodipy dyes and their derivatives: Syntheses and spectroscopic properties. *Chem Rev.* 2007; 107(11): 4891–4932.

54. Zachowski A, Favre E, Cribier S, Herve P, Devaux PF. Outside-inside translocation of aminophospholipids in the human erythrocyte membrane is mediated by a specific enzyme. *Biochemistry.* 1986; 25(9): 2585–2590.

55. Skehel JJ, Wiley DC. Receptor binding and membrane fusion in virus entry: The influenza hemagglutinin. *Annu Rev Biochem.* 2000; 69: 531–569.

56. Maier O, Oberle V, Hoekstra D. Fluorescent lipid probes: Some properties and applications (a review). *Chem Phys Lipids.* 2002; 116 (1–2): 3–18.

57. Kleusch C, Hersch N, Hoffmann B, Merkel R, Csiszár A. Fluorescent lipids: Functional parts of fusogenic liposomes and tools for cell membrane labeling and visualization. *Molecules.* 2012; 17(1): 1055–1073.

58. Coban O, Burger M, Laliberte M, Ianoul A, Johnston LJ. Ganglioside partitioning and aggregation in phase-separated monolayers characterized by Bodipy GM1 monomer/dimer emission. *Langmuir.* 2007; 23(12): 6704–6711.

59. Mikhalyov I, Gretskaya N, Johansson LB. Fluorescent Bodipy-labelled GM1 gangliosides designed for exploring lipid membrane properties and specific membrane-target interactions. *Chem Phys Lipids.* 2009; 159(1): 38–44.

60. Golebiewska U, Nyako M, Woturski W, Zaitseva I, McLaughlin S. Diffusion coefficient of fluorescent phosphatidylinositol 4,5-bisphosphate in the plasma membrane of cells. *Mol Biol Cell.* 2008; 19(4): 1663–1669.

61. Mwongela SM, Lee K, Sims CE, Allbritton NL. Separation of fluorescent phosphatidyl inositol phosphates by CE. *Electrophoresis.* 2007; 28(8): 1235–1242.

62. Mouritsen OG, Zuckermann MJ. What's so special about cholesterol? *Lipids.* 2004; 39(11): 1101–1113.

63. Shaw JE, Epand RF, Epand RM, Li Z, Bittman R, Yip CM. Correlated fluorescence-atomic force microscopy of membrane domains: Structure of fluorescence probes determines lipid localization. *Biophys J.* 2006; 90(6): 2170–2178.

64. Wüstner D. Fluorescent sterols as tools in membrane biophysics and cell biology. *Chem Phys Lipids.* 2007; 146(1): 1–25.

65. Hölttä-Vuori M, Uronen RL, Repakova J, et al. Bodipy-cholesterol: A new tool to visualize sterol trafficking in living cells and organisms. *Traffic.* 2008; 9(11): 1839–1849.

66. Fu YY, Tang SC. Optical clearing facilitates integrated 3D visualization of mouse ileal microstructure and vascular network with high definition. *Microvasc Res.* 2010; 80(3): 512–521.

67. Heinrich L, Freyria AM, Melin M, et al. Confocal laser scanning microscopy using dialkylcarbocyanine dyes for cell tracing in hard and soft biomaterials. *J Biomed Mater Res B Appl Biomater.* 2007; 81(1): 153–161.

68. Staffend NA, Meisel RL. DiOlistic labeling of neurons in tissue slices: A qualitative and quantitative analysis of methodological variations. *Front Neuronat.* 2011; 5(14).

69. Sims PJ, Waggoner AS, Wang CH, Hoffman JF. Studies on the mechanism by which cyanine dyes measure membrane potential in red blood cells and phosphatidylcholine vesicles. *Biochemistry.* 1974; 13(16): 3315–3330.

70. Cohen LB, Salzberg BM, Davila HV, et al. Changes in axon fluorescence during activity: Molecular probes of membrane potential. *J Membr Biol.* 1974; 19(1): 1–36.

71. Bhowmik BB, Basu S, Sil A, Moulik SP. Photophysics of thionine dye in aqueous and liposome media in presence of different reducing agents. *Chem Phys Lipids.* 2001; 111(1): 19–27.

72. Terasaki M, Jaffe LA. Imaging endoplasmic reticulum in living sea urchin eggs. *Methods Cell Biol.* 1993; 38: 211–220.

73. Terasaki M, Reese TS. Characterization of endoplasmic reticulum by co-localization of BiP and dicarbocyanine dyes. *J Cell Sci.* 1992; 101 (Pt 2): 315–322.

74. Terasaki M. Fluorescent labeling of endoplasmic reticulum. *Meth Cell Biol.* 1989; 29: 125–135.

75. Demchenko AP, Mely Y, Duportail G, Klymchenko AS. Monitoring biophysical properties of lipid membranes by environment-sensitive fluorescent probes. *Biophys J.* 2009; 96(9): 3461–3470.

76. Klymchenko AS, Demchenko AP. Multiparametric probing of microenvironment with solvatochromic fluorescent dyes. *Methods Enzymol.* 2008; 450: 37–58.

77. Weber G, Farris FJ. Synthesis and spectral properties of a hydrophobic fluorescent probe: 6-propionyl-2-(dimethylamino)naphthalene. *Biochemistry.* 1979; 18(14): 3075–3078.

78. Parasassi T, Krasnowska EK, Bagatolli L, Gratton E. Laurdan and Prodan as polarity-sensitive fluorescent membrane probes. *J Fluoresc.* 1998; 8(4): 365–373.

79. Dietrich C, Bagatolli LA, Volovyk ZN, et al. Lipid rafts reconstituted in model membranes. *Biophys J.* 2001; 80(3): 1417–1428.

80. Bagatolli LA. To see or not to see: Lateral organization of biological membranes and fluorescence microscopy. *BBA.* 2006; 1758(10): 1541–1556.

81. Bloksgaard M, Brewer JR, Pashkovski E, Ananthapadmanabhan KP, Sorensen JA, Bagatolli LA. Effect of detergents on the physicochemical properties of skin stratum corneum: A two-photon excitation fluorescence microscopy study. *Int J Cosmet Sci.* 2013.

82. Bloksgaard M, Brewer J, Bagatolli LA. Structural and dynamical aspects of skin studied by multiphoton excitation fluorescence microscopy-based methods. *Eur J Pharm Sci.* 2013; 50(5): 586–594.

83. Jin L, Millard AC, Wuskell JP, et al. Characterization and application of a new optical probe for membrane lipid domains. *Biophys J.* 2006; 90(7): 2563–2575.

84. M'Baye G, Mely Y, Duportail G, Klymchenko AS. Liquid ordered and gel phases of lipid bilayers: Fluorescent probes reveal close fluidity but different hydration. *Biophys J.* 2008; 95(3): 1217–1225.

85. Martin OC, Pagano RE. Transbilayer movement of fluorescent analogs of phosphatidylserine and phosphatidylethanolamine at the plasma membrane of cultured cells. Evidence for a protein-mediated and ATP-dependent process(es). *J Biol Chem.* 1987; 262(12): 5890–5898.

86. Devaux PF, Zachowski A, Favre E, et al. Energy-dependent translocation of amino-phospholipids in the erythrocyte membrane. *Biochimie.* 1986; 68(3): 383–393.

87. Smeets EF, Comfurius P, Bevers EM, Zwaal RF. Calcium-induced transbilayer scrambling of fluorescent phospholipid analogs in platelets and erythrocytes. *BBA.* 1994; 1195(2): 281–286.

88. Bevers EM, Smeets EF, Comfurius P, Zwaal RF. Physiology of membrane lipid asymmetry. *LUPUS.* 1994; 3(4): 235–240.

89. Lipsky NG, Pagano RE. A vital stain for the Golgi apparatus. *Science.* 1985; 228(4700): 745–747.

90. Bevers EM, Comfurius P, Dekkers DW, Zwaal RF. Lipid translocation across the plasma membrane of mammalian cells. *BBA.* 1999; 1439(3): 317–330.

91. Sleight RG, Pagano RE. Transport of a fluorescent phosphatidylcholine analog from the plasma memrane to the Golgi apparatus. *J Cell Biol.* 1984; 99: 742–751.

92. Pleyer U, Grammer J, Kosmidis P, Ruckert DG. Analysis of interactions between the corneal epithelium and liposomes: Qualitative and quantitative fluorescence studies of a corneal epithelial cell line. *Surv Ophthalmol.* 1995; 39 Suppl 1: S3–16.

93. Hoffmann PM, Pagano RE. Retrograde movement of membrane lipids from the Golgi apparatus to the endoplasmic reticulum of perforated cells: Evidence for lipid recycling. *Eur J Cell Biol.* 1993; 60(2): 371–375.

94. Pagano RE. Lipid traffic in eukaryotic cells: Mechanisms for intracellular transport and organelle-specific enrichment of lipids. *Curr Opin Cell Biol.* 1990; 2(4): 652–663.

95. Pagano RE, Sepanski MA, Martin OC. Molecular trapping of a fluorescent ceramide analogue at the Golgi apparatus of fixed cells: Interaction with endogenous lipids provides a trans-Golgi marker for both light and electron microscopy. *J Cell Biol.* 1989; 109(5): 2067–2079.

96. Rothman JE. Mechanisms of intracellular protein transport. *Nature.* 1994; 372: 55–63.

97. Bonifacino JS, Glick BS. The mechanisms of vesicle budding and fusion. *Cell.* 2004; 116: 153–166.

98. Jahn R, Scheller, RH. SNAREs: Engines for membrane fusion. *Nat Rev Mol Cell Biol.* 2006; 7: 631–643.

99. Youle RJ, van der Bliek AM. Mitochondrial fission, fusion, and stress. *Science.* 2012; 337(6098): 1062–1065.

100. Levchenko TS, Rammohan R, Volodina N, Torchilin VP. Tat peptide-mediated intracellular delivery of liposomes. *Methods Enzymol.* 2003; 372: 339–349.

101. Torchilin VP, Levchenko TS. TAT-liposomes: A novel intracellular drug carrier. *Curr Protein Pept Sci.* 2003; 4(2): 133–140.

102. Nagai Y, Tadokoro S, Sakiyama H, Hirashima N. Effects of synaptotagmin 2 on membrane fusion between liposomes that contain SNAREs involved in exocytosis in mast cells. *BBA.* 2011; 1808(10): 2435–2439.

103. van Lengerich B, Rawle RJ, Bendix PM, Boxer SG. Individual vesicle fusion events mediated by lipid-anchored DNA. *Biophys J.* 2013; 105(2): 409–419.

104. Csiszár A, Hersch N, Dieluweit S, Biehl R, Merkel R, Hoffmann B. Novel fusogenic liposomes for fluorescent cell labeling and membrane modification. *Bioconj Chem.* 2010; 21(3): 537–543.

105. Rao M, Mayor S. Use of Förster's resonance energy transfer microscopy to study lipid rafts. *BBA.* 2005; 1746(3): 221–233.

106. Struck DK, Hoekstra D, Pagano RE. Use of resonance energy transfer to monitor membrane fusion. *Biochemistry.* 1981; 20(14): 4093–4099.

107. Malinin VS, Haque ME, Lentz BR. The rate of lipid transfer during fusion depends on the structure of fluorescent lipid probes: A new chain-labeled lipid transfer probe pair. *Biochemistry.* 2001; 40(28): 8292–8299.

108. Dutta D, Pulsipher A, Luo W, Mak H, Yousaf MN. Engineering cell surfaces via liposome fusion. *Bioconjug Chem.* 2011; 22(12): 2423–2433.

109. Holthuis JC, Levine TP. Lipid traffic: Floppy drives and a superhighway. *Nat Rev Mol Cell Biol.* 2005; 6: 209–220.

110. Pagano RE, Sleight RG. Defining lipid transport pathways in animal cells. *Science.* 1985; 229(4718): 1051–1057.

111. Alberts B, Johnson A, Lewis J, Raff M, Roberts K, Walter P. *Molecular Biology of the Cell,* 5th ed., New York: Garland Science; 2008.

112. Lynes EM, Simmen T. Urban planning of the endoplasmic reticulum (ER): How diverse mechanisms segregate the many functions of the ER. *Biochim Biophys Acta.* 2011; 1813: 1893–1905.

113. Terasaki M, Loew L, Lippincott-Schwartz J, Zaal K. Fluorescent staining of subcellular organelles: ER, Golgi complex, and mitochondria. *Curr Protoc Cell Biol.* 2001; Chapter 4: Unit 4 4.

114. Terasaki M. Fluorescent labeling of endoplasmic reticulum. *Methods Cell Biol.* 1989; 29: 125–135.

115. Terasaki M, Chen LB, Fujiwara K. Microtubules and the endoplasmic reticulum are highly interdependent structures. *J Cell Biol.* 1986; 103(4): 1557–1568.

116. Terasaki M, Song J, Wong JR, Weiss MJ, Chen LB. Localization of endoplasmic reticulum in living and glutaraldehyde-fixed cells with fluorescent dyes. *Cell.* 1984; 38(1): 101–108.

117. van Meer G, Voelker DR, Feigenson GW. Membrane lipids: Where they are and how they behave. *Nat Rev Mol Cell Biol.* 2008; 9(2): 112–124.

118. Martin OC, Pagano RE. Internalization and sorting of a fluorescent analogue of glucosylceramide to the Golgi apparatus of human skin fibroblasts: Utilization of endocytic and nonendocytic transport mechanisms. *J Cell Biol.* 1994; 125(4): 769–781.

119. Pagano RE, Martin OC, Kang HC, Haugland RP. A novel fluorescent ceramide analogue for studying membrane traffic in animal cells: Accumulation at the Golgi apparatus results in altered spectral properties of the sphingolipid precursor. *J Cell Biol.* 1991; 113(6): 1267–1279.

120. Johnson LV, Walsh ML, Bockus BJ, Chen LB. Monitoring of relative mitochondrial membrane potential in living cells by fluorescence microscopy. *J Cell Biol.* 1981; 88(3): 526–535.

121. Prime TA, Forkink M, Logana A, et al. A ratiometric fluorescent probe for assessing mitochondrial phospholipid peroxidation within living cells. *Free Radical Bio Med.* 2012; 53(3): 544–553.

122. Simons K, Ikonen E. Functional rafts in cell membranes. *Nature.* 1997; 387(6633): 569–572.

123. Bagatolli LA, Ipsen JH, Simonsen AC, Mouritsen OG. An outlook on organization of lipids in membranes: Searching for a realistic connection with the organization of biological membranes. *Prog Lipid Res.* 2010; 49(4): 378–389.

124. Baumgart T, Hunt G, Farkas ER, Webb WW, Feigenson GW. Fluorescence probe partitioning between Lo/Ld phases in lipid membranes. *BBA.* 2007; 1768(9): 2182–2194.

125. Samsonov AV, Mihalyov I, Cohen FS. Characterization of cholesterol-sphingomyelin domains and their dynamics in bilayer membranes. *Biophys J.* 2001; 81(3): 1486–1500.

126. Cicuta P, Keller SL, Veatch SL. Diffusion of liquid domains in lipid bilayer membranes. *J Phys Chem B.* 2007; 111(13): 3328–3331.

127. Veatch SL, Gawrisch K, Keller SL. Closed-loop miscibility gap and quantitative tie-lines in ternary membranes containing diphytanoyl PC. *Biophys J.* 2006; 90(12): 4428–4436.

128. Veatch SL, Keller SL. Seeing spots: Complex phase behavior in simple membranes. *BBA.* 2005; 1746(3): 172–185.

129. Veatch SL, Keller SL. Miscibility phase diagrams of giant vesicles containing sphingomyelin. *Phys Rev Lett.* 2005; 94(14): 148101.

130. Veatch SL, Keller SL. Separation of liquid phases in giant vesicles of ternary mixtures of phospholipids and cholesterol. *Biophys J.* 2003; 85(5): 3074–3083.

131. Veatch SL, Keller SL. A closer look at the canonical "Raft Mixture" in model membrane studies. *Biophys J.* 2003; 84(1): 725–726.

132. Veatch SL, Keller SL. Organization in lipid membranes containing cholesterol. *Phys Rev Lett.* 2002; 89(26): 268101.

133. Baumgart T, Hammond AT, Sengupta P, et al. Large-scale fluid/fluid phase separation of proteins and lipids in giant plasma membrane vesicles. *Proc Natl Acad Sci U S A.* 2007; 104(9): 3165–3170.

134. Sezgin E, Kaiser HJ, Baumgart T, Schwille P, Simons K, Levental I. Elucidating membrane structure and protein behavior using giant plasma membrane vesicles. *Nat Protoc.* 2012; 7(6): 1042–1051.

135. de Almeida RF, Fedorov A, Prieto M. Sphingomyelin/phosphatidylcholine/cholesterol phase diagram: Boundaries and composition of lipid rafts. *Biophys J.* 2003; 85(4): 2406–2416.

136. Prior IA, Muncke C, Parton RG, Hancock JF. Direct visualization of Ras proteins in spatially distinct cell surface microdomains. *J Cell Biol.* 2003; 160(2): 165–170.

137. Wilson BS, Steinberg SL, Liederman K, et al. Markers for detergent-resistant lipid rafts occupy distinct and dynamic domains in native membranes. *Mol Biol Cell.* 2004; 15(6): 2580–2592.

138. Hess ST, Gould TJ, Gudheti MV, Maas SA, Mills KD, Zimmerberg J. Dynamic clustered distribution of hemagglutinin resolved at 40 nm in living cell membranes discriminates between raft theories. *Proc Natl Acad Sci U S A.* 2007; 104(44): 17370–17375.

139. Mueller V, Ringemann C, Honigmann A, et al. STED nanoscopy reveals molecular details of cholesterol- and cytoskeleton-modulated lipid interactions in living cells. *Biophys J.* 2011; 101(7): 1651–1660.

140. Testa I, Wurm CA, Medda R, et al. Multicolor fluorescence nanoscopy in fixed and living cells by exciting conventional fluorophores with a single wavelength. *Biophys J.* 2010; 99(8): 2686–2694.

141. Eggeling C, Ringemann C, Medda R, et al. Direct observation of the nanoscale dynamics of membrane lipids in a living cell. *Nature.* 2009; 457(7233): 1159–1162.

142. Gaus K, Gratton E, Kable EP, et al. Visualizing lipid structure and raft domains in living cells with two-photon microscopy. *Proc Natl Acad Sci U S A.* 2003; 100(26): 15554–15559.

143. Gousset K, Wolkers WF, Tsvetkova NM, et al. Evidence for a physiological role for membrane rafts in human platelets. *J Cell Physiol.* 2002; 190(1): 117–128.

144. Sharma DK, Brown JC, Cheng Z, Holicky EL, Marks DL, Pagano RE. The glycosphingolipid, lactosylceramide, regulates beta1-integrin clustering and endocytosis. *Cancer Res.* 2005; 65(18): 8233–8241.

Index

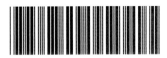